Monograph on
Tropical Fever

Monograph on
Tropical Fever

Editors

Jyotirmoy Pal
MBBS MD (General Medicine) FRCP
FICP FACP WHO Fellow
Professor (General Medicine)
Department of Medicine
Barasat Government Medical College and Hospital
Kolkata, West Bengal, India

Nandini Chatterjee
MD FRCP (Glasgow) FICP
Professor
Department of Medicine
The Institute of Postgraduate Medical Education
and Research (IPGMER) and SSKM Hospital
Kolkata, West Bengal, India

Kamlesh Tewary
MD FICP FRCP (Glasgow) FRCP (Edinburgh)
Senior Consultant and Director
Deo Narayan Hospital and Maternity Center
Former Professor and Head
Sri Krishna Medical College
Muzaffarpur, Bihar, India
Past President
Association of Physicians of India (API)

Forewords
Sahajanand Prasad Singh, Jayesh M Lele
Alaka Deshpande, Shyam Sundar

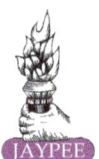

JAYPEE BROTHERS MEDICAL PUBLISHERS
The Health Sciences Publisher
New Delhi | London

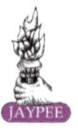 **Jaypee Brothers Medical Publishers (P) Ltd**

Headquarters

Jaypee Brothers Medical Publishers (P) Ltd
EMCA House, 23/23-B
Ansari Road, Daryaganj
New Delhi 110 002, India
Landline: +91-11-23272143, +91-11-23272703
+91-11-23282021, +91-11-23245672
Email: jaypee@jaypeebrothers.com

Corporate Office

Jaypee Brothers Medical Publishers (P) Ltd
4838/24, Ansari Road, Daryaganj
New Delhi 110 002, India
Phone: +91-11-43574357
Fax: +91-11-43574314
Email: jaypee@jaypeebrothers.com

Overseas Office

JP Medical Ltd
83 Victoria Street, London
SW1H 0HW (UK)
Phone: +44 20 3170 8910
Fax: +44 (0)20 3008 6180
Email: info@jpmedpub.com

Website: www.jaypeebrothers.com
Website: www.jaypeedigital.com

© 2023, Jaypee Brothers Medical Publishers

The views and opinions expressed in this book are solely those of the original contributor(s)/author(s) and do not necessarily represent those of editor(s) or publisher of the book.

All rights reserved. No part of this publication may be reproduced, stored or transmitted in any form or by any means, electronic, mechanical, photocopying, recording or otherwise, without the prior permission in writing of the publishers.

All brand names and product names used in this book are trade names, service marks, trademarks or registered trademarks of their respective owners. The publisher is not associated with any product or vendor mentioned in this book.

Medical knowledge and practice change constantly. This book is designed to provide accurate, authoritative information about the subject matter in question. However, readers are advised to check the most current information available on procedures included and check information from the manufacturer of each product to be administered, to verify the recommended dose, formula, method and duration of administration, adverse effects and contraindications. It is the responsibility of the practitioner to take all appropriate safety precautions. Neither the publisher nor the author(s)/editor(s) assume any liability for any injury and/or damage to persons or property arising from or related to use of material in this book.

This book is sold on the understanding that the publisher is not engaged in providing professional medical services. If such advice or services are required, the services of a competent medical professional should be sought.

Every effort has been made where necessary to contact holders of copyright to obtain permission to reproduce copyright material. If any have been inadvertently overlooked, the publisher will be pleased to make the necessary arrangements at the first opportunity.

Inquiries for bulk sales may be solicited at: jaypee@jaypeebrothers.com

Monograph on Tropical Fever

First Edition: **2023**

ISBN: 978-93-5465-506-7

Contributors

Abhishek Kochar
Medical Officer
Department of Neurology
Sardar Patel Medical College and
AG of Hospitals
Bikaner, Rajasthan, India

Adnanul Alam
Senior Resident
Department of Internal Medicine
Bangabandhu Shekh Mujib Medical
University
Dhaka, Bangladesh

Agnibho Mondal
Senior Resident
Department of Tropical Medicine
School of Tropical Medicine
Kolkata, West Bengal, India

Alladi Mohan
Dean and Professor (Senior Grade)
Department of Medicine
Sri Venkateswara Institute of Medical
Sciences
Tirupati, Andhra Pradesh, India

Animesh Ray
Associate Professor
Department of Medicine
All India Institute of Medical Sciences
New Delhi, India

Anivita Agarwal
Senior Resident (Infectious Diseases)
Department of Medicine
All India Institute of Medical Sciences
New Delhi, India

Anupam Prakash
Director Professor of Medicine
and Head
Department of Accident and
Emergency
Lady Hardinge Medical College
and Associated Hospitals
New Delhi, India

Aritra Kumar Ray
Senior Resident (General Medicine)
Department of Medicine
RG Kar Medical College and Hospital
Kolkata, West Bengal, India

Arkaprava Hati
Student
RG Kar Medical College and Hospital
Kolkata, West Bengal, India

Arpana Chatterjee
Junior Consultant
Department of Pulmonology
Apollo Multispecialty Hospital
Kolkata, West Bengal, India

Arunaloke Chakrabarti
Former Head and Professor
Department of Medical Microbiology
Postgraduate Institute of Medical
Education and Research
Chandigarh, India

Atanu Chandra
Assistant Professor
Department of Internal Medicine
Bankura Sammilani Medical College
Bankura, West Bengal, India

Contributors

Atul K Patel
Director
Department of Infectious Diseases
Vedanta Institute of Medical Sciences
and Sterling Hospital
Ahmedabad, Gujarat, India

Bibhuti Saha
Professor and Head
Department of Infectious Diseases
and Advanced Microbiology
School of Tropical Medicine
Kolkata, West Bengal, India

Biswajit Mandal
Associate Professor
Department of Economics and Politics
Visva-Bharati University
Birbhum, West Bengal, India

Biva Bhakat
MBBS MD (General Medicine)
Senior Resident
Department of General Medicine
Nil Ratan Sircar Medical College
and Hospital
Kolkata, West Bengal, India

Chandrasekhar Valupadas MD FICP
Professor
Department of General Medicine
Kakatiya Medical College
Kaloji Narayana Rao University
of Health Sciences
Warangal, Telangana, India
Former Medical Superintendent
MGM Hospital, Warangal
Chairman
API, Telangana State Chapter

D Suresh Kumar
Senior Consultant (Infectious Diseases)
Apollo Hospitals
Chennai, Tamil Nadu, India

Debraj Jash
Consultant Pulmonologist
Apollo Multispecialty Hospitals
Kolkata, West Bengal, India

Dhanpat Kumar Kochar
Former Senior Professor and Head
Department of Medicine
Sardar Patel Medical College
and AG of Hospitals
Bikaner, Rajasthan, India
Chairman
Research Advisory Committee
Multidisciplinary Research Unit
In-charge, Cerebral Malaria
Research Lab

Dhruva Chaudhry
Senior Professor and Head
Department of Pulmonary and
Critical Care Medicine
Postgraduate Institute of Medical
Sciences
Rohtak, Haryana, India

G Bindhu Madhavi
Junior Resident
Department of Medicine
Sri Venkateswara Institute of Medical
Sciences
Tirupati, Andhra Pradesh, India

J Rajkumar DNB (Ped) Fell Ped Inf Dis
Consultant
Infectious Diseases
Gleneagles Global Health City
Chennai, Tamil Nadu, India

Jaya Chakravarty
Professor
Department of Medicine
Institute of Medical Sciences
Banaras Hindu University
Varanasi, Uttar Pradesh, India

Jyotirmoy Pal
MBBS MD (General Medicine) FRCP
FICP FACP WHO Fellow
Professor (General Medicine)
Department of Medicine
Barasat Government Medical College
and Hospital
Kolkata, West Bengal, India

Contributors

Kamlesh Tewary
MD FICP FRCP (Glasgow) FRCP (Edinburgh)
Senior Consultant and Director
Deo Narayan Hospital and
Maternity Center
Former Professor and Head
Sri Krishna Medical College
Muzaffarpur, Bihar, India
Past President
Association of Physicians of India

Ketan K Patel MD
Infectious Diseases Consultant
Vedanta Institute of Medical Sciences
and Sterling Hospital
Ahmedabad, Gujarat, India

Manali Chandra MD
Senior Resident (Medicine)
Department of General Medicine
Kolkata Medical College and Hospital
Kolkata, West Bengal, India

Md Karimulla
Senior Resident
Department of Medicine
The Institute of Postgraduate Medical
Education and Research (IPGMER)
and SSKM Hospital
Kolkata, West Bengal, India

Mehruba Alam Ananna
Associate Professor
Department of Nephrology
and Dialysis
BIRDEM and Ibrahim Medical College
Dhaka, Bangladesh

Mugundhan K
Professor and Head
Department of Neurology
Stanley Medical College
Chennai, Tamil Nadu, India

Muralidharan K
Resident
Department of Neurology
Stanley Medical College
Chennai, Tamil Nadu, India

N Naveen Kumar
Postgraduate in Medicine
Madras Medical College
Chennai, Tamil Nadu, India

Nandini Chatterjee
MD FRCP (Glasgow) FICP
Professor
Department of Medicine
The Institute of Postgraduate Medical
Education and Research (IPGMER)
and SSKM Hospital
Kolkata, West Bengal, India

Pranabananda Pal
General Physician
Department of Medicine
Kolkata Medical College and Hospital
Kolkata, West Bengal, India

Prantiki Halder
Assistant Professor
Department of Tropical Medicine
School of Tropical Medicine
Kolkata, West Bengal, India

Prasanta Kumar Bhattacharya
Professor and Head
Department of General Medicine
North Eastern Indira Gandhi Regional
Institute of Health and Medical
Sciences (NEIGRIHMS)
Shillong, Meghalaya, India

Prasun Chatterjee
Additional Professor
Department of Geriatric Medicine
All India Institute of Medical Sciences
New Delhi, India

Pritam Roy
MBBS MD FRSPH (London, UK)
Physician and Public Health Expert
on Neglected Tropical Diseases
WHO, India

Purbasha Biswas
Junior Resident
Department of Medicine
RG Kar Medical College and Hospital
Kolkata, West Bengal, India

Contributors

V Ramasubramanian
MD FRCP (Glas) DTM & H (Lon) DGUM (Lon) FESCMID
Director
The Capstone Clinic
Consultant
Infectious Diseases and Tropical Medicine
Apollo Hospitals
Adjunct Professor (Infectious Diseases)
Sri Ramachandra Institute of Higher Education and Research;
The Tamil Nadu Dr MGR Medical University;
Saveetha Medical College; and Apollo Hospitals Educational and Research Foundation
President
Clinical Infectious Diseases Society of India

Saikat Datta MBBS MD (Medicine) FICP FIACM
Professor and Head
Department of Medicine
MJN Medical College
Cooch Behar, West Bengal, India

Santanu K Tripathi
MBBS MD DM (Clinical Pharmacology)
Former Head
Department of Clinical Pharmacology
School of Tropical Medicine
Kolkata, West Bengal, India
Professor and Founder President
Association of Clinical Pharmacologists of India (ACPI)

Saswati Chaudhuri PhD
Assistant Professor (Economics)
Department of Commerce and Business Administration
St Xavier's College (Autonomous)
Kolkata, West Bengal, India

Shambo S Samajdar
Clinical Pharmacologist
School of Tropical Medicine
Consultant at Diabetes and Allergy-Asthma Therapeutics Specialty Clinic
Kolkata, West Bengal, India

Shantanu Kumar Kar
MD FAMS FICP Diploma in Clinical Epidemiology
Former Director
ICMR RMRIMS, Patna
Former Director
ICMR RMRC, Bhubaneswar
Director (Research)
Medical and Life Sciences
Directorate of Medical Research
IMS and SUM Hospital
S 'O' A University, BBSR (Retd)
Bhubaneswar, Odisha, India

Sharmistha Bhattacherjee
Associate Professor
Department of Community Medicine
North Bengal Medical College
Darjeeling, West Bengal, India

Shaurya Mehta
DNB Nephrology Trainee
Jaslok Hospital and Research Centre
Mumbai, Maharashtra, India

Shohael Mahmud Arafat
Professor and Chairman
Department of Internal Medicine
Bangabandhu Sheikh Mujib Medical University
Dhaka, Bangladesh

Shreya Singh
Research Associate
Department of Medical Microbiology
Postgraduate Institute of Medical Education and Research
Chandigarh, India

Soumyadip Chatterjee
Consultant
Department of Infectious Diseases
Tata Medical Centre
Kolkata, West Bengal, India

Sowmini PR
Assistant Professor
Department of Neurology
Stanley Medical College
Chennai, Tamil Nadu, India

Contributors

Suba Guruprasad MD
Clinical Registrar
Department of Infectious Diseases
Apollo Hospitals
Chennai, Tamil Nadu, India

Subhra Sankar Sen
MBBS MD (Medicine) MRCP UK
Senior Resident
Department of Internal Medicine
Midnapore Medical College and Hospital
Midnapore, West Bengal, India

Subramanian Swaminathan
MD DNB MNAMS AB (Int Med)
AB (Inf Dis) FIDSA
Director
Infectious Diseases and Infection Control
Gleneagles Global Health City
Chennai, Tamil Nadu, India

Sudhir Mehta
Senior Professor
Department of Medicine
SMS Medical College and Attached Group of Hospitals
Jaipur, Rajasthan, India

Sunanda Ghosh
Post-doctoral Trainee
The Institute of Postgraduate Medical Education and Research (IPGMER) and SSKM Hospital
Kolkata, West Bengal, India

Swati Pal
Assistant Professor (Economics)
Department of Economics
Kidderpore College
Kolkata, West Bengal, India

Tanuka Mandal
Consultant
Department of Medicine
RG Kar Medical College and Hospital
Kolkata, West Bengal, India

Foreword

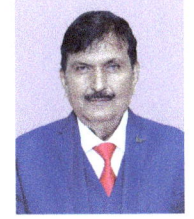

Greetings from Indian Medical Association!

I am delighted to know that you are publishing a book on *Tropical Fever* which covers different types of tropical fever.

India is a tropical country and therefore harbors different tropical diseases depending upon the local weather conditions. Whereas we have succeeded in eradicating some the tropical diseases such as Yaws and Pinta, and controlling diseases such as Kala-azar, the continuous outbreaks of other tropical diseases is a matter of concern.

Differential diagnosis of some of the tropical diseases is not easy especially in endemic areas.

I am confident that this book has been found to be in line with the current scenario as well as ready-reckoner for the practitioners. The more readable it becomes the more popular it would be.

I congratulate Dr Jyotirmoy Pal and his team for the efforts put for the success of the publication.

Best wishes as always.

Long live IMA!!

https://www.youtube.com/channel/UCgLOj1rXZ2G0M23XYsjO7Eg
https://www.ima-india.org/ima/index.php
https://www.facebook.com/indianmedicalassociationofficial
https://twitter.com/IMAIndiaOrg
https://www.linkedin.com/company/indian-medical-association/?originalSubdomain=in

Sahajanand Prasad Singh
National President
Indian Medical Association (IMA)

Foreword

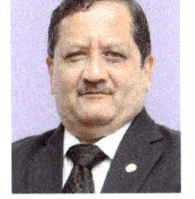

I am immensely happy to note that a *Monograph on Tropical Fever* will be released during the ensuing Meeting of Central Working Committee of Indian Medical Association (IMA).

I am delighted to write a foreword for this book which is the need of hour because sometimes different types of tropical fevers become the challenge for the medical fraternity and a book always proved itself a great guide during any challenge or epidemic.

I am not only sure but confident that this book will also prove itself a very informative and useful for the medical field. This type of book can become a great gift for the medical fraternity which can be used as and when required at large.

However, I wish the authors and book a grand success.

Jayesh M Lele
Honorary Secretary General
Indian Medical Association (IMA)

Foreword

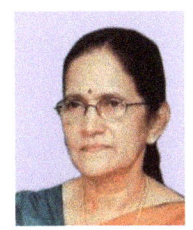

I feel privileged and proud that *Monograph on Tropical Fever* edited by Professor Jyotirmoy Pal, Professor Nandini Chatterjee and Dr Kamlesh Tewary is going to be published very soon. Fevers are a burning problem faced by every physician in their day-to-day practice and it is of immense importance to be aware of the latest information on atypical presentations, newly emerging complications, and latest guidelines for management.

The chapters contributed by various experts give comprehensive information and sharing of clinical experience. This book is a reference guide for all the clinicians.

My congratulations to the entire team of authors for an excellent piece of work which I hope will enrich the readers and be useful in their daily practice.

Alaka Deshpande
MD FIMSA FICP FRCP (London)
Recipient of Padmashree
Dean, Indian College of Physicians
Former Professor and Head (Medicine)
Grant Medical College and
Sir JJ Group of Government Hospitals
Mumbai, Maharashtra, India

Foreword

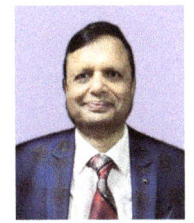

I am delighted to know that *Monograph on Tropical Fever* is being published and will be released at 78th annual meeting of the Association of Physicians of India (APICON), Ahmedabad, Gujarat, India. Fevers in tropical countries are common occurrences and at times, it becomes difficult to pinpoint its etiology. Tropical diseases, unfortunately, do not get attention of the world of medical science, and it is true for our country as well. On the other hand, these tropical illnesses form a major chunk in a tropical country like India. I am very happy to note that this book describes these subjects in great detail. Though enteric fever, kala-azar and malaria attract due attention, but diseases such as dengue, lymphatic filariasis, kala-azar (classified by WHO as Neglected Tropical Disease) need more consideration. Japanese B encephalitis, leptospirosis, scrub typhus and fungal infections are not given enough stress either in undergraduate or postgraduate training.

I have gone through the content of this book, and it is heartening to note that each of the above-mentioned topics has separate chapters and have been written by respective experts on these subjects.

I am certain that this book will be very useful for practicing physicians and under-/postgraduate trainees. Professor Jyotirmoy Pal, Professor Nandini Chatterjee and Professor Kamlesh Tewary have chosen the authors very meticulously and I congratulate them on this endeavor. I am sure that this book will be very popular and my best wishes for the success of this monograph.

Shyam Sundar
MD FRCP (London) FAMS FNASc FASc FNA FTWAS FASTMH
Distinguished Professor of Medicine
President
Association of Physicians of India (API)

Preface

The tropics are regions of the Earth surrounding the Equator. They are defined in latitude by the Tropic of Cancer in the Northern Hemisphere and the Tropic of Capricorn in the Southern Hemisphere. The tropics constitute 40% of Earth's surface area and contain 36% of Earth's landmass. As of 2014, the region was home also to 40% of the world's population. Tropical diseases are diseases that are prevalent in or unique to tropical and subtropical regions. The diseases are less prevalent in temperate climates, as lower temperatures control the insect population. Insects such as mosquitoes and flies are by far the most common disease carrier, or vector. These insects may be a vector for a parasite, bacterium or virus infectious to humans and animals. Current history suggests that tropical areas of the world are more harshly affected by infectious diseases in contrast to the temperate world. Environmental and biological factors are responsible for biodiversity of pathogens, vectors and hosts, but social factors also play a role in the spread of these diseases, common among them being, protozoal diseases, such as malaria, Leishmaniasis, Chagas' disease and sleeping sickness, others being schistosomiasis, onchocerciasis and lymphatic filariasis. Viral diseases such as dengue fever are rampant in these tropical areas.

Human exploration of tropical rainforests, deforestation, rising immigration and increased international air travel and other tourism to tropical regions have led to an increased incidence of such diseases to nontropical countries. Cholera outbreak happened in Jessore district of undivided Bengal in 1818, but the British army spread it to England. During extensive voyages in the 19th century by Europeans, tropical infectious diseases from one part of the continent spread to other continents. In 20th century in the First and Second World War, there was massive troop movements across the world. Diseases spread like wild fire among the soldiers and also globally. Necessity is the mother of invention. There was rapid discovery of drugs for different tropical infections. School of Tropical Disease in London and Kolkata was established in 1889 and 1914 respectively. Post-World War, society moved toward industrialization and urbanization. This led to environmental changes, changes in sewerage system—that favored growth of vectors and spread of disease. Toward the end of 20th century, there was an exponential increase of international travel. That further aggravated the threat of spread of tropical diseases to non-tropical countries also. Poverty and pollution are other challenges to tropical countries. Most of the tropical countries are overcrowded and economically inferior. Poor hygiene, crowded habitation, and slums are rampant in this part of the globe leading to expanding the vector population and human-to-human transmission and repeated epidemics. At the same time due to poor health infrastructure, many of the diseases were not properly diagnosed, which resulted in significant mortality and morbidity, and loss of economy at micro and macro levels. WHO termed it as "neglected tropical diseases". So, "neglected tropical disease" is a vast entity and a subject in itself. And it needs a long way to go in terms of research, infrastructure, investment, training and drug development. The major obstacle is finance of tropical countries and nonprofitability from a commercial point of view. So, initially what was thought to be tropical disease, now has become a global challenge.

With course of time "tropical" diseases emerged as specialty due to diversity in presentation, challenges in management and high mortality. So, "tropical" infectious disease needs to be addressed in a comprehensive way, easily understandable and useful for practitioners and students. This book deals with the subject individual disease-wise and also syndromically. We hope doctors practicing in "tropics" will be benefited from approaches to "tropical fever" described here.

We are thankful to Dr Sahajanand Prasad Singh, President, Indian Medical Association (IMA); Dr Jayesh M Lele, Secretary General, IMA; Professor Alaka Deshpande, Dean, ICP; Professor Shyam Sundar, President, API; Professor Bibhuti Saha, Head, Department of Tropical Medicine, School of Tropical Medicine; Dr YP Munjal, Past President, API; and Professor BB Thakur, Past President, API, for constant encouragement to write this book.

Jyotirmoy Pal
Nandini Chatterjee
Kamlesh Tewary

Contents

SECTION 1: INTRODUCTION TO TROPICAL FEVER

1. **Tropical Fever: A Global Challenge** 3
   Shambo S Samajdar, Santanu K Tripathi, Jyotirmoy Pal, Kamlesh Tewary
   - Dynamic Changes in Etiology of Tropical Fevers   4
   - Physiography of the Tropics   4
   - Climate and Environmental factors in the Tropics   5
   - Population Census   6
   - Addressing Low Resource Setting   6
   - Drug Discovery for Tropical Fever   7
   - Resistance to Antimicrobials   8
   - Neglected Tropical Disease   10
   - The Way Forward—Bridging the Knowledge Gap   11

2. **Pathophysiology of Fever** 14
   Nandini Chatterjee
   - Pathogenesis   14
   - Pyrogens and their Effect   15
   - Cytokines in the Central Nervous System   16
   - Other Consequences of Fever   17
   - Hyperthermia—How is it Different from Fever?   17
   - How do Antipyretics Act?   18

3. **Approach to Tropical Fever** 19
   Jyotirmoy Pal
   - Incubation Period   21
   - Ingestion   21
   - Associated Symptoms   22
   - Day of Appearance of Rash   24
   - Investigations   28
   - Treatment   30

SECTION 2: COMMON TROPICAL FEVER

4. **Dengue** 35
   Shohael Mahmud Arafat, Mehruba Alam Ananna, Adnanul Alam
   - Pathophysiology   35
   - Pathogenesis of Severe Dengue   36

- Transmission 38
- Clinical Features 38
- Diagnosis 40
- Treatment 42
- Pregnancy 45
- Children 46
- Convalescence and Discharge 46
- Adjunctive Therapies 47
- Disease Notification 47
- Prognosis 48
- Long-term Sequelae 48
- Monitoring and Follow-up 48
- Recurrence or Reinfection 48
- Instructions for the Patients 48
- Vector Control 48

5. **Malaria** 52

   Abhishek Kochar, Dhanpat Kumar Kochar, Aritra Kumar Ray
   - Pathogenesis 53
   - Clinical Presentation 55
   - Laboratory Diagnosis 57
   - Treatment 58
   - Vaccine 61
   - Malaria in India 61

6. **Kala-azar** 64

   Jaya Chakravarty, Sunanda Ghosh
   - Organism 64
   - Transmission 64
   - Burden of Disease 64
   - Life Cycle and Pathophysiology 65
   - Clinical Features 66
   - Post-Kala-Azar Dermal Leishmaniasis 66
   - Human Immunodeficiency Virus-Visceral Leishmaniasis Coinfection 66
   - Diagnosis 66
   - Molecular Diagnosis 67
   - Differential Diagnosis 68
   - Treatment 68

7. **Scrub Typhus and Other Rickettsial Diseases** 71

   Prasanta Kumar Bhattacharya, Nandini Chatterjee, Aritra Kumar Ray
   - Epidemiology 71
   - Pathophysiology 71
   - Clinical Features 73
   - Complications 74
   - Diagnosis 74

- Treatment 74
- Indian Perspective 77
- Ricketsial Diseases 78
- Diagnosis 80
- Treatment 80

8. **Leptospirosis** 82

   Subhra Sankar Sen, Biva Bhakat, Manali Chandra, Purbasha Biswas
   - Clinical Features 82
   - Pathogenesis 83
   - Differential Diagnosis 84
   - Diagnostic Tools 86
   - Treatment 86

9. **Zika and Chikungunya** 90

   Anivita Agarwal, Animesh Ray, Tanuka Mandal
   - Zika Virus 90
   - Chikungunya Virus 94

10. **Viral Respiratory Illness** 97

    J Rajkumar, Subramanian Swaminathan, Arkaprava Hati
    - Etiology 97
    - Clinical Manifestations 98
    - Diagnosis 101
    - Prevention 102
    - Treatment 103
    - Indian Perspective 103

11. **Enteric Fever** 105

    Pritam Roy
    - Pathophysiology 105
    - Clinical Definition 106
    - Clinical Features 106
    - Laboratory Evaluation 109
    - Treatment 110
    - Chronic Carrier State 112
    - Immunization 112

12. **Japanese B Encephalitis** 115

    Muralidharan K, Sowmini PR, Mugundhan K, Pranabananda Pal
    - Causative Agent 115
    - Pathophysiology 117
    - Clinical Features 117
    - Diagnosis 119
    - Investigations 119
    - Treatment 120
    - Control Measures 122
    - Prevention 122

13. Filariasis 125
Shantanu Kumar Kar, Md Karimulla
- Pathophysiology *126*
- Clinical Features *128*
- Diagnosis *128*
- Treatment *128*
- Antiparasitic Treatment *129*
- Management of Chronic Filarial Infection *129*

14. Fungal Infections in the Tropics 131
Shreya Singh, Arunaloke Chakrabarti, Md Karimulla
- Pathophysiology *131*
- Clinical Features *131*
- Diagnosis *136*
- Treatment *140*

SECTION 3: SYNDROMIC APPROACH TO FEVER

15. Acute Undifferentiated Fever 147
Saikat Datta, Sharmistha Bhattacherjee, Atanu Chandra
- Etiology and Pathophysiology *147*
- Pathogenesis of Acute Undifferentiated Febrile Illness *148*

16. Fever with Rash: Approach 156
Prantiki Halder, Agnibho Mondal, Bibhuti Saha, Soumyadip Chatterjee
- History *156*
- Investigations *171*

17. Hemorrhagic Fever 173
Ketan K Patel, Atul K Patel
- Etiology and Epidemiology *173*
- Clinical Features *177*
- Diagnosis of Hemorrhagic Fever *177*
- Treatment *178*
- Prevention and Infection Control *178*

18. Fever with Hepatorenal Dysfunction 180
D Suresh Kumar, N Naveen Kumar
- Epidemiology *180*
- Etiology *180*
- Pathophysiology *180*
- Clinical Features *182*
- Investigations *183*
- Treatment *183*
- Diagnostic and Treatment Approach *186*
- Prevention *187*

Contents

19. Fever with Central Nervous System Dysfunction 188
Suba Guruprasad, V Ramasubramanian, Prasun Chatterjee
- Viruses and Central Nervous System Dysfunction *188*
- Bacterial Infections Associated with Central Nervous System Dysfunction *190*
- Protozoal and Helminthic Infections and Central Nervous System Dysfunction *193*
- Approach to a Patient with Fever and Central Nervous System Dysfunction *195*

20. Fever with Acute Respiratory Distress Syndrome 199
Chandrasekhar Valupadas
- Acute Respiratory Distress Syndrome *199*
- Clinical Features *200*
- Etiology *200*
- Pathophysiology *201*
- Course of Acute Respiratory Distress Syndrome *201*
- Diagnosis *203*
- Management of Acute Respiratory Distress Syndrome *203*
- Complications of Acute Respiratory Distress Syndrome *203*
- Management of Undiagnosed Fever with Respiratory Distress *205*

21. Fever with Hepatosplenomegaly/Lymphadenopathy 207
Alladi Mohan, G Bindhu Madhavi
- Clinical Examination: Imaging Correlates *207*
- Evaluation of a Patient with Fever with Hepatosplenomegaly/Lymphadenopathy *209*
- Laboratory Evaluation *210*
- Imaging Studies *211*
- Treatment *211*

22. Fever in Intensive Care Unit..213
Dhruva Chaudhry, Arpana Chatterjee, Debraj Jash
- Definition *213*
- Etiology *213*
- History and Examination *214*
- Different Conditions *215*
- Approach to the Patient *219*

23. Approach to an Adult with Pyrexia of Unknown Origin.................225
Sudhir Mehta, Shaurya Mehta
- Definition *225*
- Causes *225*
- Epidemiology *226*
- Clinical Approach *226*
- Investigations *227*
- Concept of "Therapeutic Trial" in Pyrexia of Unknown Origin *229*
- Outcome of Pyrexia of Unknown Origin *230*

24. **Emerging Tropical Infections in India** 232
   Anupam Prakash
   - Definition *232*
   - About Emerging Infectious Diseases *233*
   - Prevention *234*

25. **Neglected Tropical Diseases** 236
   Aritra Kumar Ray
   - List of Diseases *236*
   - Effects For Patients *242*
   - Social and Economic Impact of Neglected Tropical Diseases *242*
   - Prevention, Treatment, and Eradication *242*
   - Control of Neglected Tropical Diseases *243*

26. **Health Policies and Economic Impact of Fever on Indian Society** 245
   Saswati Chaudhuri, Biswajit Mandal, Swati Pal
   - Economic Repercussions *246*
   - COVID and the Indian Economy *248*
   - Movement of People and the Spread of Infection *249*
   - Effect on Employment *250*
   - Human Capital and Productivity in Days to Come *250*

Index 255

Section

Introduction to Tropical Fever

- **Tropical Fever: A Global Challenge**
  Shambo S Samajdar, Santanu K Tripathi, Jyotirmoy Pal, Kamlesh Tewary

- **Pathophysiology of Fever**
  Nandini Chatterjee

- **Approach to Tropical Fever**
  Jyotirmoy Pal

Chapter 1

Tropical Fever: A Global Challenge

Shambo S Samajdar, Santanu K Tripathi, Jyotirmoy Pal, Kamlesh Tewary

■ INTRODUCTION

Tropical fever refers to the febrile illness of infectious origin, prevalent in, or specific to tropical and subtropical regions. The infection could be of parasitic or viral in nature. Irrespective of their etiologies, tropical fevers are mostly contributed by an insect bite, which leads to transmission of the microbe. Predominantly seasonal in nature, tropical fevers are uncommon in temperate climates. The Indian subcontinent arguably harbors the largest tropical and subtropical regions and thereby carries a huge burden of tropical diseases and tropical fevers. Depending on the nature of vectors and infectious agents, there are various season- and geography-specific (especially monsoon season) and season- and geography-nonspecific (throughout the year) tropical fevers.[1] Regarding burden of tropical fevers, there is a relative paucity of reliable data. According to a World Health Organization (WHO) publication which aggregated different available evidences, it was found that in rural tropical areas the incidence of fever episodes was 10 per person-year in <5 years' pediatric age group and 4 per person-year in rest of age combined age group (>5 years). In urban areas incidence was quite low, estimated as 2.5 and 0.5 per person-year for these two age groups, respectively.[2]

Geography-restricted etiologies, season-specific exacerbations, nonspecific early symptomatology, and lack of diagnostic facility to diagnose offending pathogen or predict severity have always puzzled healthcare providers. The fast-changing ecological balance due to civil wars, population migration, deforestation, global warming, and the ease of international travel, makes the management of tropical fevers more challenging. Infection control is largely influenced by different public health measures including sanitary education, hand washing, vaccination, and appropriate antimicrobial use. Besides infection control, early identification and monitoring deserve equal attention and emphasis. Nonavailability of reliable and low-cost, point-of-care diagnostic tools for human immunodeficiency virus (HIV), malaria, drug-resistant tuberculosis, MRSA (methicillin-resistant *Staphylococcus aureus*) infection, and other endemic tropical diseases make the management more challenging. Monitoring of disease with biomarkers and related effective surveillance tools and techniques is crucial. Application of global informatics skill could be beneficial.

Geopolitical influences on socioeconomic status of people in the tropics impact on the prevalence and outcome of tropical fevers. The living conditions of a vast majority of the population in these regions, their compromised access to healthcare, the over-reliance of traditional medicine practices, often amalgamating with modern medicine, often pose a huge challenge in the control and management of tropical fevers.

■ DYNAMIC CHANGES IN ETIOLOGY OF TROPICAL FEVERS

Due to various factors including weather changes, migration of population, public health measures, and economic dynamicity etiologies of tropical fevers are changing from time to time. Wide differences in etiologies of tropical fevers are noted while we move from tropical Asia to Africa and then to America. Japanese encephalitis or melioidosis were previously not recognized much but have in recent times appeared to contribute noticeably to the tropical fever burden in South and Southeast Asia. Brucellosis and Q fever became the concerning zoonotic bacterial infections in sub-Saharan Africa. In Latin America, arboviruses were raising threats and warranting urgent attention on diagnostic and management workup. Increase in the incidence of leptospirosis or rickettsial diseases in tropical countries have been noted in the last few decades. Across the globe in tropical and subtropical regions there has been a consistent increase in the number of children attending primary healthcare facility with fever due to viral pathogens. Incidence of malaria is however on a declining mode.[3] And the world has witnessed the devastating COVID-19 pandemic in the last two years that has tended to affect the overall infectious disease dynamics. Thus, studies in Southeast Asia and Latin America have shown a decline (44.1% decrease compared to 2019 incidences) in dengue incidences in 2020.[4] Underreporting of dengue cases due to reduced health care seeking behavior of patients, and the reduced availability of laboratory facilities, may have contributed to this low number of dengue cases. Large-scale epidemiological studies of tropical fevers are an urgent need in order to bridge the knowledge and understanding gaps. And this assumes even greater relevance in this post COVID-19 pandemic era.

■ PHYSIOGRAPHY OF THE TROPICS[5]

The tropics are those regions which lie at the center of the globe, on the either side of the equator between the tropic of Cancer and tropic of Capricorn. Tropical region includes parts of Central and South America, parts of Africa, Middle East, India, Oceania, and Australia. The average climate of the tropics is warm throughout the year and the temperature ranges from 25 to 28°C. The reason behind this is that the tropical region lies close to the equator and

CHAPTER 1: Tropical Fever: A Global Challenge

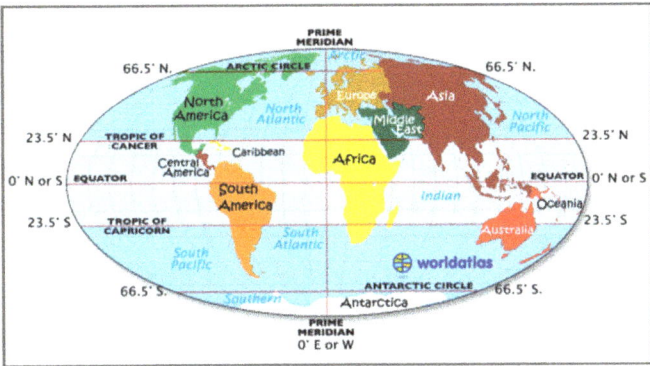

Fig. 1: The tropical and subtropical regions.
(*Courtesy*: WorldAtlas.com)

receives direct sunlight throughout the year. However, there is a variation in the rainfall also with the Amazon Basin recording the highest rainfall and Northern part of Africa receiving scanty to no rainfall most of the year. These climatic conditions help in the development of flora, fauna, insect, and wildlife in the areas. In **Figure 1**, map of the tropical and subtropical regions is depicted.

CLIMATE AND ENVIRONMENTAL FACTORS IN THE TROPICS[5]

The general mean temperature of the tropical region is >18°C. The flora and fauna of the arid tropical regions are greatly affected due to scanty rainfall. The tropical region holds 80% of the world's biodiversity. There are several environmental factors that can be considered, e.g., climate, air pollution, land degradation and deforestation, water scarcity, and pollution, etc.

The climate change can have a wide range of impact on the habitat, species distribution, human health, agriculture, sea level, and frequency and intensity of extreme weather events. Vector-borne diseases such as dengue and malaria are more prevalent in the tropics due to the increase in temperature, changes in rainfall pattern, increased vector distribution, and decreased vector and parasite incubation time period. Air pollution with high carbon dioxide emission is another important environmental factor contributing to causation of tropical fevers. South-East Asia has recorded the highest carbon dioxide emission followed by South Asia and South America. Land degradation is caused by poor agricultural techniques and deforestation which leads to an adversely altered ecosystem promoting incidence of tropical fevers. Although the tropics have 54% of the world's renewable water sources, more than half of them are considered vulnerable water stress because of the inequality of water distribution with South-East Asia having the highest water pollution discharge.[5]

POPULATION CENSUS

About 40% of the world's population and 55% of children younger than age five years resides in the tropical regions. By 2050, it is expected to rise to 50% and 60%, respectively. The life expectancy in the tropics has been increased from 22.8 years to 64.4 years and the infant mortality is reduced by 36% between the years 1950 to 2010. Despite these humungous steps in improving the mortality of the infants, almost 6.9 million infants younger than age five years have died in 2011 out which 99% of the deceased were from low to middle- and low-income families.[5]

ADDRESSING LOW RESOURCE SETTING

As per the State of Tropics Report 2014, it was found that extreme poverty worldwide was decreased by almost 50% since the 1980s. Unfortunately almost two-thirds of the poorest people globally are living in the tropical and subtropical regions. Southeast Asia and Central America have witnessed reduction in poverty along with rapid increase in urbanization. However, rapid urbanization has been responsible for huge increase in the slum dweller populations. This suboptimal and compromised hygiene and sanitation conditions in the urban slums are crucial contributor to the tropical disease burden.[5]

Early diagnosis and prompt initiation of treatment are extremely important steps for successful management of tropical fever. Recognizing etiology early is very difficult due to financial constraints and difficulty in access to sophisticated microbiological investigations. Comprehensive evidence-based clinical algorithm could be useful tool to help in early diagnosis and initiating treatment. It is also important to give emphasize on detection of early warning signs which would guide primary care providers to refer patients timely in higher centers. Importance of malaria-specific rapid diagnostic test is well understood and this test is well utilized in different parts of tropical region. Problems arise in cases of nonmalarial febrile illnesses. Diseases such as human African trypanosomiasis, dengue fever, brucellosis, leptospirosis, leishmaniosis, and enteric fever face challenges in getting early diagnosis. More researches are required to find solutions where cost-effectiveness analysis shows favor to the rapid diagnostic kit. Point-of-care laboratory services with rapid diagnostic kits integrated with algorithm-based syndromic approach need to be developed and validated for providing better care.[6]

Morbidity and mortality are in a huge extent associated with infectious diseases in tropical countries, mostly belonging to low- and middle-income groups. And this is responsible for heavy economic burden to them. In low- and middle-income group, it has been observed that an expenditure of billions of dollars every year is spent due to infectious diseases in tropics.

Estimated annual global cost of dengue was US $8.9 billion in 2013,[7] and another study from Philippines had depicted that schistosomiasis costs loss of an average of 45.4 work days per infected person per year.[8] According to WHO, infectious tropical diseases had resulted in 4 million deaths and the loss of >250 million disability-adjusted life years (DALYs) in 2015.[9] These data clearly emphasize the need of holistic approach to address economic challenges in tropical disease management.

■ DRUG DISCOVERY FOR TROPICAL FEVER[10]

The drug discovery trajectory is a pretty long path involving huge amount of resources of all kinds. This involves discovery of hit and hit expansion with target-based or cell-based screening, finding the lead molecules, lead optimization with different in vivo, proof-of-concept studies, the candidate selection process, and finally target product profiling (TPP). The TPP refers to the desired characteristics needed for the final medicinal product, like duration of treatment, route of drug administration, dosage forms and strengths, contraindications, warnings and precautions, adverse reactions, drug interactions, and use in specific populations. Product pricing, net product valuation, patent and exclusivities are important aspects of TPPs commercial perspective and are given due importance. The TPP guides the drug discovery pathway. A few diseases such as malaria, cryptosporidiosis, Chagas disease, leishmaniosis, and dengue have disease-specific TPPs which could help drug discovery for these diseases, whereas most of other infectious diseases prevalent in tropical region do not have their specific TPPs. Defining TPPs and compound progression criteria need to be developed in this sector which would guide the drug-developing industry to decide on "early go or no go" decision-making.

Developing new small-molecule drugs to treat infectious diseases is challenging. There is insufficient knowledge of pathogen biology. Relevant cellular in vitro model or predictive animal in vivo models of the human infectious disease preparations are obstacles against developing new drugs in this field. To identify a suitable druggable target, fulfilling the assay ability, essentiality, and selectivity criteria is always challenging. Use of newer technologies such as CRISPR–Cas9 could help in this regard providing validated target development.

Use of animal model is another challenge in reference to drug development for infectious diseases. The causative microorganism for river blindness, *Onchocerca volvulus* can infect primates only; so related different species are utilized in cattle or rodent models during drug development. *Plasmodium falciparum*, responsible to develop severe form of human malaria, could not infect mice or rats. A genetic autosomal recessive mutation designated Prkdc^{scid} mice model having severe combined immunodeficiency affecting both B and T lymphocytes could be infected by *P. falciparum*. The

SCID model is important to help in therapeutics development program for falciparum malaria. Researches are ongoing to develop suitable rodent model for *Plasmodium vivax*. Mostly rodent models are not useful for tuberculosis research, because formed granulomas are not matching with human tuberculosis. Development of the right animal model can be revolutionary in developing the right drug. CYP51 inhibiting drugs such as azoles were not established as successful therapeutics in different clinical trials of Chagas disease, unless a rodent model was developed which helped to identify benznidazole as a successful therapeutic option for Chagas disease.

Quiescence and dormancy are also important factors for some tropical diseases. *Plasmodium ovale* and *P. vivax* could reside in human hepatocytes for weeks to years as hypnozoites, which cause relapse. Patient may remain asymptomatic for a long duration with a potential to develop clinical symptoms of tuberculosis. There is an estimation of one-third global population could be suffering from latent tuberculosis. *Trypanosoma cruzi* had a potential to be in dormant state for prolonged duration. Pathogens in quiescent and dormant stages have reduced metabolic state, which make difficult environment for drugs to act. This is an important area to be addressed by future research to get more drugs which would be effective in quiescent and dormant stages of microorganisms.

Physicochemical properties of drugs such as molecular weight, number of hydrogen bond donors and acceptors, solubility, electrostatic charge, and lipophilicity are crucial factors governing drugs' penetration into the microorganisms. Hydrophilic nature of drugs helps them to enter into microorganisms through channels such as porins. When drugs need to enter into microorganisms via diffusion, their lipophilicity could help out. After entrance into cytoplasm drugs need to be polar to stay within and execute their action. In presence of efflux pump, there is a high probability of being eliminated from the cytoplasm. Drug accessibility to microorganisms such as Trypanosoma cruzi, *Chlamydia trachomatis*, *Mycobacterium tuberculosis*, and different viruses becomes more compromised when they live maximum time of their life cycle in host cells. *Leishmania* and *Salmonella* could stay in intracellular acidic environment and *M. tuberculosis* could localize themselves in necrotic granulomas. Presence of microorganisms in extremes of host environment is a challenge to develop drug in this regard and need design modifications during drug development which help to penetrate via nonvascularized lipid-rich caseum to access the pathogen.

■ RESISTANCE TO ANTIMICROBIALS[11]

Improper management of infective diseases would lead to develop of antimicrobial resistance (AMR). Around 700,000 deaths per year happen due to AMR. Low- and middle-income countries in tropical area are facing huge economic loss due to AMR. Statistical models are predicting AMR would be going to surpass cancer as the leading cause of death within next 30 years. There are multiple factors which have a complex interplay between them. Poor clinical decision-making, antimicrobial over consumption, surveillance gap, weak diagnostics, antimicrobial agent use in agricultural and fishery field, veterinary antibiotic usage, and improper disposal policy of unused antimicrobials are key factors to generate AMR gene. Overcrowding and poor sanitation, hospitalization, and travel or migrations are detrimental factors in spreading AMR.

There are a few resistance genes found on plasmids which are clinically relevant like extended spectrum β-lactamase enzymes (ESBL-E) or for carbapenemases in *Enterobacteriaceae* (CPE). They are responsible for producing resistance to most β-lactam antibiotics. In gastrointestinal tract or environmental or direct contact between human to human, resistance genes can be rapidly spread. In European hospitals, ESBL-E were first time reported in 1980s. Though in Europe and America, fecal carriage rates were less but in low- and medium-income tropical countries, the rate is very high due to contaminated water and poor sanitary condition. Unfortunately, it was estimated that >1.1 billion in South-East Asia, 110 million in Africa, and 280 million in Western Pacific habitants were carrying ESBL-E.

Hospitalization of foreign travelers in tropical countries such as Asia, sub-Saharan Africa, and Latin America seems to carry additional risks to have ESBL-E, CPE, or MRSA. Presence of carbapenem-resistant *Acinetobacter* in war zones and conflict areas followed by transmission of AMR via soldiers to different parts of world is also a concern. At the beginning of Operation Iraqi Freedom, carbapenem-resistant *Acinetobacter baumannii* (CRAB) infections due to production of oxacillinases among injured soldiers were 12% which increased to 97.4% subsequently. There are a good number of studies suggesting that multidrug-resistant (MDR) *Enterobacteriaceae* can be transmitted to travelers without hospitalization too. Evidence-based applied travel medicine and focused decision-making in designing strategies to combat against AMR should be implemented to combat against such adversities. The One Health Approach for mitigation and control of AMR, involving interdisciplinary coordination and shared decision-making, is a potential solution, albeit too demanding, to the problem of AMR.

An important step taken by WHO in 2017 could be immensely helpful for mitigation of AMR is "AWaRe" (Access–Watch–Reserve) classification[12] of antibiotic to increase awareness on rational prescription of antibiotic. Access (amoxicillin, amoxicillin plus clavulanic acid, metronidazole, doxycycline, clindamycin, nitrofurantoin, sulfamethoxazole plus trimethoprim, gentamycin, and amikacin), watch (macrolides, fluoroquinolone, piperacillin plus tazobactam, and third-generation cephalosporin), and reserve (linezolid, aztreonam, third- and fourth-generation cephalosporin, fosfomycin, tigecycline, and polymyxin B) group of antibiotics would ensure use of "The Right Antibiotic at the Right Time".

■ NEGLECTED TROPICAL DISEASE[13]

More than one billion people worldwide is suffering from neglected tropical diseases (NTDs). Buruli ulcer, foodborne trematodes, mycetoma, chromoblastomycosis and other deep mycoses, soil-transmitted helminthiases, Chagas disease (American trypanosomiasis), human African trypanosomiasis (sleeping sickness), onchocerciasis (river blindness), snakebite envenoming, dengue, leishmaniasis, rabies, taeniasis and cysticercosis, dracunculiasis (Guinea worm), leprosy, scabies and other ectoparasitoses, trachoma, echinococcosis, lymphatic filariasis, schistosomiasis, and Yaws (endemic treponematoses) are different NTDs which are prevalent in 149 tropical and subtropical countries. The poor and the marginalized people are the ones suffering from these diseases predominantly as they live in dismal sanitary conditions, and often are in close contact with domestic livestock. Since these diseases mostly affect those with little paying capacity, NTDs are often referred to as orphan diseases; obviously the pharma industries by and large are reluctant to invest in development of therapeutics for them.

World Health Organization in January 2021 launched a new roadmap for NTDs for 2021–2030—"Ending the neglect to attain the Sustainable Development Goals: a road map for NTDs 2021–2030"—which carries a ray of hope for this special group of diseases **(Box 1)**.

Annual World NTD Day is observed on 30th January since 2020, with a purpose to increase awareness and engagement of the common man to combat against NTDs. In 2022, the third World NTD Day was celebrated with the theme of "Achieving health equity to end the neglect of poverty-related diseases". Poverty and inequity are two important intrinsic factors acting as barriers for managing NTDs. NTD-related stigmatization and disability promote poverty and suffering of the family as a whole. Apart from physical well-being, it is also important to promote social, mental, and spiritual well-being of the patients. Leaving no one behind should be the aim of NTD control programs.

Innovative scientific approaches are required in this field. Adequate resources for translational research need to be pooled; this can strengthen

---

BOX 1: Neglected tropical diseases (NTDs)—goals for 2021–2030 decade.

- To reduce the number of people requiring treatment for NTDs by 90%
- To eliminate at least one NTD in 100 tropical countries
- To eradicate two diseases (dracunculiasis and yaws)
- To reduce by 75% the disability-adjusted life years (DALYs) related to NTDs

existing strategies for NTDs. For example, the novel vector control tools such as introducing Wolbachia infected *Aedes aegypti* reduced dengue incidence by 77% as seen in a community trial conducted in Indonesia. Developing "Tiny Targets" to control Gambian human African trypanosomiasis was a cost-effective trapping system for tsetse fly vector.

▪ THE WAY FORWARD—BRIDGING THE KNOWLEDGE GAP

The vast areas of tropical fevers remain unexplored. Extensive dearth of etiological knowledge in most parts of the continents, such as Western and Central Africa, the Middle East, Central Asia and Latin America, has been embarrassing since long. Only recently many national and international research groups have focused their attention on this matter. Planning and execution of well-designed studies in these underexplored geographical locations can prove very useful to the ailing population. Special attention should be given to the vulnerable groups such as neonates, pregnant females, immunocompromised persons (e.g., Diabetes, HIV, on immunosuppressant drugs), and the aged. Multicentered, multicountry studies are currently underway aiming at ready investigation and diagnosis of tropical fevers and hopefully the existing knowledge gaps would soon be bridged. The challenges to conduct such studies in these low resource settings are enormous which can only be tackled by large industry-academia collaboration. Epidemiological studies of tropical fevers shall prove useful in gathering information and data particularly in those tropical regions where paucity of data has been rather a norm. With an increasing emphasis on global health security in all socioeconomic levels of the society, more meaningful research is the need of the hour. Integrated surveillance should be reinforced with emphasis on single case studies. Improvement in the diagnostic infrastructure would be helpful in the long run. Digital data integration should be implemented at country and regional levels. Distinct diagnostic tools such as multi-analyte detection platforms, biomarker-based tools, and rapid phenotypic diagnostics for antimicrobial resistance detection, both at the point of care and at the laboratory levels, should be made available. Special evidence-based clinical algorithms and electronic device should be designed which will be useful in providing geographically relevant disease-specific rapid diagnosis.

The fundamental goal of the diagnostic research in tropical fevers has evolved over the past decades. Relevant clinical and cost-effective end points have been developed in the targeted population in tropical regions. Access to management aids and improvement in diagnostic infrastructure and facilities that are much needed in the low resource settings can only be made feasible through suitable investment in the general qualification of the frontline health workforce on one hand, and the availability of simple point-of-care diagnostics and treatment algorithms, on the other.

Lastly, it may be reasonably hoped that the availability of quality point-of-care diagnostics for tropical fevers shall be poised to change the overall disease and healthcare dynamics of tropical fevers in the coming years.

> **TAKE HOME MESSAGE**
> - Geography-restricted etiologies, season-specific exacerbations, non-specific early symptomatology, and lack ofdiagnostic facility to diagnose offending pathogen or predict outcome are different challenges in tropical fevermanagement.
> - Geopolitical influences on socioeconomic status of people in the tropics impact on the prevalence and outcomeof tropical fevers.
> - Physiography of tropics is unique compared to other parts of the world and need considerations in details whiletargeting disease.
> - Dynamic changes in aetiology of tropical fever need special attention from researchers, treatment providers andregulatory authorities.
> - Drug discovery is another challenge in tropical fever sector.
> - Resistance to anti microbial agents require dedicated implementation of "One Health Approach".
> - There should be scientific rational way to address neglected tropical diseases where poor and marginalisedpeoples are at the suffering end.

REFERENCES

1. From: The Indian Society of Critical Care Medicine Tropicalfever Group, Singhi S, Chaudhary D, Varghese GM, Bhalla A, Karthi N, et al. Tropical fevers: management guidelines. Indian J Crit Care Med. 2014;18(2):62-9.
2. D'Acremont V, Bosman A. Global Malaria Programme W. WHO Informal Consultation on fever management in peripheral health care settings: a global review of evidence and practice. In: Malar policy adviscomm meet 13–15 March 2013. Geneva: World Health Organization HQ; 2013. pp. 1-10.
3. Bottieau E, Yansouni CP. Fever in the tropics: the ultimate clinical challenge? Clin Microbiol Infect. 2018;24(8):806-7.
4. Chen Y, Li N, Lourenço J, Wang L, Cazelles B, Dong L, et al. Measuring the effects of COVID-19-related disruption on dengue transmission in Southeast Asia and Latin America: a statistical modelling study. Lancet Infect Dis. 2022;22(5):P657-67.
5. Rupali P. Introduction to tropical medicine. Infect Dis Clin North Am. 2019;33(1):1-15.
6. Chappuis F, Alirol E, d'Acremont V, Bottieau E, Yansouni CP. Rapid diagnostic tests for non-malarial febrile illness in the tropics. ClinMicrobiol Infect. 2013;19(5):422-31.
7. Shepard DS, Undurraga EA, Halasa YA, Stanaway JD. The global economic burden of dengue: a systematic analysis. Lancet Infect Dis. 2016;16(8):935-41.
8. Conteh L, Engels T, Molyneux DH. Socioeconomic aspects of neglected tropical diseases. Lancet. 2010;375(9710):239-47.
9. World Health Organization. Global Health Estimates 2015: Deaths by Cause, Age, Sex, by Country and by Region, 2000–2015. Geneva: World Health Organization; 2016.

10. De Rycker M, Baragaña B, Duce SL, Gilbert IH. Challenges and recent progress in drug discovery for tropical diseases. Nature. 2018;559(7715):498-506.
11. Semret M, Haraoui LP. Antimicrobial resistance in the tropics. Infect Dis Clin North Am. 2019;33(1):231-45.
12. Sharland M, Pulcini C, Harbarth S, Zeng M, Gandra S, Mathur S, et al. Classifying antibiotics in the WHO essential medicines list for optimal use—be AWaRe. Lancet Infect Dis. 2018;18(1):18-20.
13. Taylor MJ. Specialty grand challenge: embracing the need for research and innovation as fundamental enablers for programmatic progress for all neglected tropical diseases. Front Trop Dis. 2021;2:669726.

Pathophysiology of Fever

Nandini Chatterjee

■ INTRODUCTION

Fever is defined to be the elevation of an individual's core body temperature in conjunction to a raised hypothalamic "set-point" that is normally regulated by the body's thermoregulatory center in the hypothalamus.

A morning temperature (around 6 AM) >37.2°C (98.9°F) and an afternoon temperature (around 4 PM) >37.7°C (99.9°F) are designated as fever.

The pathogenesis of fever is the culmination of various exogenous and endogenous variables that ultimately lead to the elevation of thermoregulatory set point and lead to many metabolic, behavioral, and circulatory changes.

■ PATHOGENESIS

The normal core body temperature varies in the range of 36.5–37.5°C (97.7–99.5°F) through the course of the day. This variability of the core temperature is the result of the circadian rhythm of the body and its related effects on sleep/wake cycles, metabolic changes, and hormonal alterations.

During fever, this variation is maintained albeit at a higher level.

Core temperature is primarily controlled by hypothalamus whose thermoregulatory center balances excess heat production with heat dissipation.

Thermoregulation is achieved by peripheral mechanisms, which balance heat production and loss, and a hypothalamic thermoregulatory center controlling these mechanisms. This center receives signals through thermoreceptors sensing the temperature of the blood as it passes through the brain (the core temperature) and signals from thermoreceptors in the skin via the dorsal horn of the spinal cord. Thermoreceptors have cold and warm receptor types. The aim of thermoregulation is to maintain a relatively constant body temperature at 37°C.

> At rest, the brain, muscles, liver, heart, thyroid, pancreas, and adrenal glands contribute to heat production at the cellular level involving adenosine triphosphate (ATP). Nonshivering thermogenesis may also occur in brown adipose tissue (BAT), localized mainly in the neck and scapular area, which is highly vascularized and contains a large

quantity of mitochondria. Fatty acid oxidation in these mitochondria can increase heat production to twofold in response to cold.

Cold exposure normally leads to shivering due to skeletal muscle contraction that increases heat production.

With a rise in body temperature above 37°C (or ambient temperature above 30–31°C), heat is lost from the body by four physical means such as evaporation, radiation, convection, and conduction. The following are the mechanisms by which heat loss occurs at rest:
- *Evaporation:* About one-fourth is lost by evaporation from the skin and lungs
- *Radiation:* 60% of the total heat is lost by radiation (transfer of heat from the skin surface to the atmosphere)
- *Convection:* (12% of the heat loss) by increasing blood flow to body surfaces
- *Conduction:* (3% of the heat loss) is the heat transfer from the core to the surface.

These normal phenomena are accentuated during fever.

■ PYROGENS AND THEIR EFFECT (FLOWCHART 1)

The term Pyrogen comes from the Greek word "pyro" meaning fire. Exogenous pyrogens are microorganisms, their breakdown products or toxins, for example lipopolysaccharide (LPS) from Gram-negative bacteria, or enterotoxins from *Staphylococcus aureus*.

Fever is produced when such exogenous stimuli activate bone-marrow-derived phagocytes. Mononuclear cells are mainly responsible for the

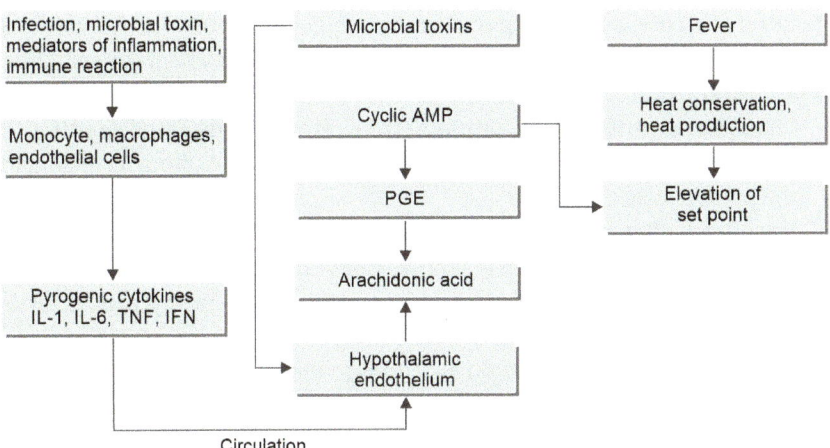

Flowchart 1: Pathogenesis of fever.

(AMP: adenosine monophosphate; IL: interleukin; TNF: tumor necrosis factor; PGE: prostaglandin E)

production of interleukin 1 (IL-1) and fever induction. These cells play a key role in host defense, including engulfing and destroying the microbe (phagocytosis), recognition of antigen and presenting it to attached lymphocytes, and activation of T lymphocytes. The mononuclear cells release fever-inducing cytokines (endogenous pyrogens now called pyrogenic cytokines).

Interleukin 1, IL-6, tumor necrosis factor (TNF) alpha, and interferon (IFN) are the pyrogenic cytokines which influence the thermoregulatory center of the hypothalamus to cause an elevation in the "set-point" for core temperature. Prostaglandin E2 (PGE2) is the central molecule for this process which is produced from the hypothalamic endothelium that leads to increase in cyclic adenosine monophosphate (cAMP) release from glial cells and directly or indirectly alter the set point. The concentration of PGE2 is highest near the circumventricular vascular organs rich in enlarged capillaries surrounding the hypothalamic regulatory centers. Interaction of the cytokines with the endothelium of these capillaries is the preliminary step in altering the set point.[1]

Sometimes noninfective inflammatory processes such as pericarditis, stroke, trauma, and immunization also release these cytokines and cause fever.

■ CYTOKINES IN THE CENTRAL NERVOUS SYSTEM

Cerebral hemorrhage, trauma, and viral infections of the brain may lead to microglial and neuronal production of IL-1, TNF alpha, and IL-6. They bypass the circumventricular organs. Much lower concentrations may account for hyperpyrexia of cerebral hemorrhage trauma or central nervous system (CNS) infection.

The change in the set point in the hypothalamic thermostat causes an elevation in core body temperature by triggering several physiological reactions. Temperature-increasing mechanisms may be by heat conservation or heat production.

- Posterior hypothalamic sympathetic center is stimulated leading to vasoconstriction in the peripheries decreasing heat loss from the skin and the person feels cold.
- Heat production is achieved through shivering, sympathetic stimulation, and thyroxine release. The shivering is stimulated through signals from the skin rather than the core temperature. The energy produced is released as heat.
- Nonshivering heat production also adds to the core temperature.
- Behavioral modifications such as curling up, putting on warm blankets, or clothes also help in raising body temperature.

These processes continue till temperature of blood bathing hypothalamic neurons matches the new thermostat setting.

When fever lyses, heat loss through evaporation (causing sweating) becomes the primary mechanism of heat loss. This is the result of cutaneous vasodilatation, the mechanism being cholinergic relaxation of the vascular smooth muscles.[2]

OTHER CONSEQUENCES OF FEVER

- Increased need for oxygen that leads to increases in heart rate and respiratory rate.
- Increased use of body proteins as an energy source. During fever, body switches from using glucose (an excellent medium for bacterial growth) to metabolism based on protein and fat breakdown.
- Enhanced immune function with increased migration of polymorphonuclear leukocytes, and mononuclear cell activation. Also there is interferon gamma production and subsequent activation of T cells.
- Inhibition of growth of certain microbial agents as microbial agents that cause infection often grow at normal body temperatures.
- Acute-phase response follows (within hours or days) the onset of fever in response to infections or local damage to a tissue. These changes (IL-6 being the primary inducer) are beneficial to the host. It is found that various proteins, namely C-reactive protein (CRP) and serum amyloid A, are produced in abundance and released in circulation. CRP influences complement cascade, opsonization, and platelet function. Although acute-phase response is closely associated with fever, CRP levels can be normal in viral infections and high in diseases without fever (e.g., tumors).
- Synthesis of albumin, transferrin, and concentration of iron and zinc diminishes, while copper levels and ferritin increases. The decreased iron is due to reduced absorption and increased liver storage. These changes are beneficial to host defense as microorganisms are deprived of essential nutrients. The process is designated as nutritional immunity.[3,4]

HYPERTHERMIA—HOW IS IT DIFFERENT FROM FEVER?

In this context, another entity, i.e., hyperthermia should be discussed. It is characterized by uncontrolled rise of body temperature in presence of an unaltered hypothalamic set point. The body's ability to lose heat is overwhelmed either by exogenous heat exposure or endogenous heat production.

There is no role of pyrogens here and antipyretics are ineffective. Exercise at high environmental temperature or drugs that interfere with thermoregulation may cause it.

This condition may lead to damage to liver, muscle, and neural tissue and become rapidly fatal if not intervened.

HOW DO ANTIPYRETICS ACT?

The synthesis of PGE2 depends on the enzyme cyclooxygenase. The reduction of fever is achieved by decreasing the concentration of PGE2 in the thermoregulatory center. Antipyretics are cyclooxygenase inhibitors in the brain that prevent the rate limiting step of action on arachidonic acid by cyclooxygenase that leads to PGE2 synthesis.[5]

> **TAKE HOME MESSAGE**
> - Fever is defined to be the elevation of an individual's core body temperature in conjunction to a raised hypothalamic "set point".
> - IL-1, IL-6, and TNF alpha are the pyrogenic cytokines which influence the thermoregulatory center of the hypothalamus.
> - Peripheral vasoconstriction, shivering, and behavioral changes raise body temperature to match the altered set point.
> - Hyperthermia is characterized by uncontrolled rise of body temperature in presence of an unaltered hypothalamic set point.

REFERENCES

1. Menkin V. Chemical basis of fever. Science. 1944;100(2598):337-8.
2. Mackowiak PA. Pathophysiology and management of fever—we know less than we should. J Support Oncol. 2006;4(1):21-2
3. Dinarello CA, Bunn PA Jr. Fever. Semin Oncol. 1997;24(3):288-98.
4. Dalal S, Zhukovsky DS. Pathophysiology and management of fever. Support Oncol. 2006;4(1):9-16.
5. Gery I, Waksman BH. Potentiation of the lymphocyte response to mitogens: cellular source pf potentiating mediators. J Exp Med. 1972;136(1):143-54.

Chapter 3

Approach to Tropical Fever

Jyotirmoy Pal

■ INTRODUCTION

The world is divided into two zones—the tropics and the temperate. The tropics are characterized by hot humid climate, excessive rainfall, population explosion, poverty, and pollution. These factors favor growth of specific organisms and vectors producing an enormous biodiversity. Thus, the tropics are a unique world and a paradise for different diseases.[1]

The tropical infectious diseases have varied clinical presentations and atypical manifestation which are different from the temperate areas of the world. Also, as a result of poverty and overcrowding, diseases spread rapidly and larger populations are easily affected. Many of the diseases are not properly diagnosed because of lack of health infrastructure and empirical therapy is instituted. So, a syndromic approach to diagnosis is often appropriate in poor, resource-constrained countries of the tropics.

Tropical fevers are usual manifestations of different tropical infections. It can be due to viruses, bacteria, fungus, parasites, and rickettsia.[2]

But fever in tropics can also happen due to some infections which are not restricted to the tropics—such as tuberculosis, human immunodeficiency virus (HIV), and influenza or it can be due to noninfectious etiology **(Table 1)**.

Tropical diseases are defined as diseases that are more prevalent or unique in tropical or subtropical zones.

Typical characteristics are:
- Most of the diseases are transmitted by insects. Rodents and mammals are natural hosts.

TABLE 1: Etiology of tropical fever.	
Virus	Dengue, chikungunya, rotavirus, Ebola, Nipah, measles, EB virus, CMV, and varicella zoster
Bacteria	*Salmonella, Leptospira, Clostridia, Bartonella, Brucella, Burkholderia,* and *Rickettsia*
Protozoa	*Plasmodium, Leishmania, Trypanosoma,* and *Schistosoma*
Fungus	*Cryptococcus, Coccidioidomycosis, Histoplasma, Mucor,* and *Aspergillus*
(CMV: cytomegalovirus; EB: Epstein–Barr; HIV: human immunodeficiency virus)	

- Some occur throughout the year, some have seasonal predilection.
- Often patients have atypical or overlapping signs and symptoms.
- Concomitant infections are possible.
- Serology is often cross-reactive.

Many a times patients become critical within few days of onset of fever resulting in high mortality. Physicians have to rely on clinical judgment and empiric therapy. In sick patients, the idea is to avert the crisis until definite diagnosis is achieved.

So syndromic approach to tropical is often appropriate.

To start with physicians have to take a detailed history of fever and associated conditions:
- Onset of fever and pattern of fever and duration (acute or chronic)
- Any prodrome
- Associated symptoms such as yellowish discoloration of urine and eyes, abdominal pain, headache, body ache, rash, nausea, vomiting, confusion, seizure, photophobia, and conjunctivitis
- Associated signs—hepatosplenomegaly, lymphadenopathy, and crepitation at chest
- Geographic location of patient
- Knowledge of areas with recent outbreak
- Onset of illness in relation to incubation period and time of possible exposure can help in assessing causative etiology.
- Travel history within and outside the country to any specific endemic zone
- Occupational history, animal contact, insect bite, and sexual exposure
- Immunization and drug history
- Important past illness and associated noncommunicable disease.

Atypical or overlapping feature is often present and may confuse physicians. Use of antipyretics can change pattern of disease. Absence of classical pattern should not rule out a typical infection.

Common tropical infections are malaria, dengue, rickettsial disease, leptospiral disease, typhoid, chikungunya, different bacterial, and fungal and viral diseases.

On the basis of clinical signs and symptoms, syndromic approach of tropical fever is formulated as follows:[3]
- *Acute undifferentiated fever:* Patients with acute onset fever within 2 weeks but usually with no localizing signs and symptoms. For examples, malaria, dengue, leptospirosis, scrub typhus, typhoid, and other common viral infections.
- *Fever with rash:* Acute onset fever along with a transient or persistent skin rash or exanthems (popular, macular, vesicular, and purpuric) with or without thrombocytopenia: Dengue, leptospirosis, measles, rubella,

rickettsial infections, meningococcal infections, malaria, and other viral exanthems.
- *Fever with acute respiratory distress syndrome (ARDS):* Acute onset fever with respiratory distress such as SpO_2 <90% at room air or frank ARDS with PaO_2/FiO_2 ratio <200: Scrub typhus, *falciparum* malaria, influenza (including H_1N_1), Hantavirus infection, melioidosis, and community-acquired pneumonia.
- *Acute febrile encephalopathy/acute encephalitic syndrome:* Fever with confusion with or without convulsion within 7 days of onset of fever
- *Fever with multiorgan dysfunction:* Particularly fever with hepatorenal syndrome, e.g., *falciparum* malaria, leptospirosis, bacterial sepsis, dengue, etc.
- Fever with arthralgia.

Knowledge of incubation period can help in categorizing tropical infections in different four categories. Time of possible exposure or travel to endemic zone and onset of symptoms may be helpful in suspecting possible etiology.

INCUBATION PERIOD
- *Short (<10 days):* Arboviral infection. Dengue, chikungunya, and plague
- *Intermediate (10–14 days):* Malaria, enteric fever, leptospirosis, and toxoplasmosis
- *Long (>1 month):* Brucellosis, Kala-azar, and viral hepatitis
- *Variable:* Filariasis, brucellosis, and melioidosis.

Type of Exposure or Contact with Vectors
Identifying vectors which can transmit the organism or suspecting habitat of vectors where the patient had traveled can be often helpful. Transmission may be via bite of a vector, ingestion of contaminated water or food, skin contact with mud, sand, and water, or by sexual contact.

Bites
- *Mosquito:* Malaria, dengue, filariasis, Japanese encephalitis (JE), and yellow fever
- *Flies:* Kala-azar
- *Ticks:* Lyme disease, Q fever, and tularemia
- *Mites:* Scrub typhus
- *Rodents:* Leptospirosis, Monkeypox, and Hantavirus infection.

INGESTION
Water
- Hepatitis A and E, salmonellosis, shigellosis, giardiasis, poliomyelitis, cryptosporidiosis, and dracunculiasis

- *Daily (unpasteurized):* Brucellosis, enteric fever, tuberculosis, and Q fever
- *Raw food (meat, vegetables, fish):* Toxoplasmosis and amoebiasis.

Skin Contact
- *Freshwater skin contact:* Schistosomiasis and *Mycobacterium marinum*
- *Sand and mud skin contact:* Strongyloidiasis, cutaneous larva migrans, melioidosis, and fungal infections (mucormycosis)
- Body piercing and transfusion
- Hepatitis B and C, malaria, *Mycobacterium fortuitum* and *chelonae*.

Sexual Contact
- Hepatitis B and C, syphilis, herpes, and gonococcal infection
- Clinical manifestation
- So, type of contact and onset of symptom and duration between the two may be the first step in suspecting possible etiology.

The most common manifestation of infection is fever. Usually with each degree of temperature rise, there will be rise of pulse of 10/min. If the rise in pulserate is less than 10/min it is called temperature pulse dissociation. This happens in enteric fever, brucellosis, dengue fever, and leptospirosis.

In immunocompromised patient, patient with chronic kidney disease, chronic liver disease, on steroid therapy may not have manifestation of typical fever. Even hypothermia may be present in septic shock.

Periodicity is another characteristic of some tropical infections. For example, in *Plasmodium vivax*, fever appears every third day and in *Plasmodium malariae* every fourth day. In *Borrelia* infection, there is a febrile period, followed by 1 week of afebrile period, then again relapse of fever.

■ ASSOCIATED SYMPTOMS

Fever with Rash
Fever with rash particularly in acutely ill patient is a challenge to physician. Still pattern of rash helps in prompt clinical diagnosis and empiric therapy in critically ill patients **(Table 2)**.

Following patterns in rash should be noted:
- Distribution of rash
- Appearance of rash according to day of onset of illness
- Characteristics of rash.

Centrally Distributed Maculopapular Rash
- *Rubeola (measles):* Initially to start erythematous macule at back of ear, neck, hairline, discrete lesion, and spread downward (sparing palm and sole). Gradually becomes confluent and fades in reverse order.

TABLE 2: Febrile syndromes.

Syndrome	Pathogens
Altered mental status and psychiatric illness	Malaria, enteric fever, typhus, and brucellosis
Acute meningoencephalitis	Dengue, West Nile virus, JE virus, and leptospirosis
Encephalitis	Nipah virus, Zika, dengue, and chikungunya
Focal lesion (stroke and abscess)	Dengue, melioidosis, and tuberculosis
Movement disorder	JE virus
Cranial or peripheral neuropathy	Lyme disease, chikungunya, and tuberculosis

(JE: Japanese encephalitis)

- *Rubella (German measles):* Maculopapular rash usually presents for 3 days. Spread downward with clearing previous rash. Difficult to detect in dark skin persons.
- *Endemic typhus:* Maculopapular eruption starts from axilla, spreading to trunk and extremities (sparing palm, sole, and face). Eventually confluent and petechial rash may appear.
- *Scrub typhus:* Diffuse macular rash starting on trunk, eschar at the site of mite bite
- *Rickettsial spotted fever:* Eschar at the site of bite. Maculopapular rash in extremity, trunk, and face
- *Leptospirosis:* Maculopapular eruption and conjunctival hemorrhage
- *Lyme disease:* Classical erythema migrans lesion. Papule converted to erythematous annular lesion with central clearing
- *Typhoid fever:* Transient, blanchable, and erythematous rash on trunk.
- *Dengue fever:* Diffuse, flushing rash predominantly on trunk, maculopapular, pruritic, eventually spread to periphery. Later on petechial rash
- *Relapsing fever:* Central rash at end of febrile episode may be petechial.
- *Rheumatic fever:* Erythematous annular papules and plaques occurring as polycyclic lesions in waves in trunk, proximal extremities, and fades within hours.
- *West Nile fever:* Maculopapular eruptions involving trunk, trunk, extremity, head, and neck
- *Zika virus:* Pruritic maculopapular rash spread from trunk to extremity. Conjunctival injection and petechial rash may appear.

Peripheral Lesion

- *Rocky Mountain spotted fever:* Rash appears first on wrist and ankle, spreading centripetally, palm, and sole at later stage. Blanchable to petechial spot

- *Chikungunya fever:* Maculopapular rash on periphery and trunk. Children often develop bullous lesion. Appear on third day of disease. Gradually desquamate.

Vesiculobullous Lesion
- *Varicella:* Macules, then papules, then vesicles, erythematous base. Appear in crops in face, trunk, limbs, and pruritic. Gradually lesions become pustular, then crusting. Different stages of development at any point of time. Smallpox or variola more prominent at face, whereas varicella at trunk
- *Rickettsialpox:* Eschar found at the site of bite mark (differentiate from varicella). Generalized rash involving face, trunk, and extremities. Some may be converted to vesicle and pustules.

Nodular Lesion
- *Disseminated fungal infections:* Subcutaneous nodules, fluctuating, necrotic. Fever, myalgia, and eruptive nodules found in disseminated candidiasis. Disseminated cryptococcosis resembles molluscum contagiosum. Necrosis of nodule raises suspicion of *Aspergillosis* or *Mucor*.
- Urticaria-like eruption
- Common in different parasitic disease
- Eruption with eschar.

■ DAY OF APPEARANCE OF RASH

Fever with Rash
- *Rash appearing on first day of fever:* Varicella and vesicular type
- *Rash appearing on second day of fever:* Scarlet fever and maculopapular rash
- *Rash appearing on third day of fever:* Smallpox, vesicular, and pustular rash
- *Rash appearing on fourth day of fever:* Measles and maculopapular rash
- *Rash appearing on fifth day of fever:* Scrub typhus eschar, also macular rashes spreading to arms and legs
- *Rash appearing on sixth day of fever:* Dengue, confluent macular rash, generalized erythema with islands of skin sparing, more in trunk and face
- *Rash appearing on seventh day of fever:* Enteric fever—rose spots often not recognized in dark complexion.

Fever with Purpura
Dengue, leptospirosis, malaria, and leukemias.

Fever with Palpable Purpura
Systemic vasculitis, thrombotic thrombocytopenic purpura, and Henoch–Schönlein purpura.

Fever with Confusion
Fever with altered sensorium can occur due to different viral, bacterial, and parasitic infections. Presentation may be from encephalopathy to demyelination. History of contact, exposure, travel, bite from insect or animal, endemicity, and other associated signs and symptoms will help in appropriate diagnosis.

Viral
- *Dengue:* Encephalitis, meningitis, meningoencephalitis, myelitis, seizure, coma, and rarely intracerebral hemorrhage
- *Nipah virus:* Myoclonus, seizure, cerebellar ataxia, brainstem involvement, and coma
- *Chikungunya:* Encephalitis, meningoencephalitis, neuropathy, and myelopathy can occur in 25% cases.
- *Zika virus:* Guillain–Barré (GB) syndrome, acute demyelination, encephalitis, and stroke
- *JE virus:* Seizure, extrapyramidal symptoms, opsoclonus-myoclonus, and altered sensorium.

Bacterial
- *Melioidosis:* Intracerebral abscess, epidural abscess, brainstem encephalitis, and transverse myelitis
- *Lyme disease:* Meningitis, cranial nerve palsy, radiculopathy, mononeuritis multiplex, and cerebellar ataxia
- *Enteric fever:* Altered sensorium, delirium, and psychotic symptoms.

Protozoal and Helminthic Disease
- *Malaria:* Altered sensorium, delirium, and encephalopathy. Neck rigidity and focal sign are rare.
- *Neurocysticercosis:* Headache, seizure, and psychiatric symptoms.

Fever with Jaundice

Common tropical infections that can involve liver include hepatitis A and E, dengue, scrub typhus, malaria, leptospirosis, amoebic liver abscess, hydatid disease of liver, and many other bacterial, protozoal, or fungal infections. Infections are mostly food or water borne, may be from insect bite. History of travel to endemic zone must be obtained. In some infections such as hepatitis, symptoms start with fever, anorexia, and malaise but fever subsides with appearance of jaundice. But if fever persists in spite of appearance of jaundice, other etiologies should be considered, e.g., malaria, leptospirosis, dengue, and scrub typhus. Most of tropical infections present with either acute liver injury or acute liver failure (ALF) **(Flowchart 1)**.

Malaria is the most common tropical infection precipitating both liver injury to liver failure. Predominantly *falciparum*, nowadays *vivax*, also causes asymptomatic elevation of liver enzymes, clinical jaundice to fulminant hepatic Failure. Jaundice in malaria is due to hemolysis as well as hepatocellular dysfunction. Soft hepatosplenomegaly and anemia are almost invariable. There is elevation of serum bilirubin with borderline disproportionately less elevation of liver enzymes. International normalized

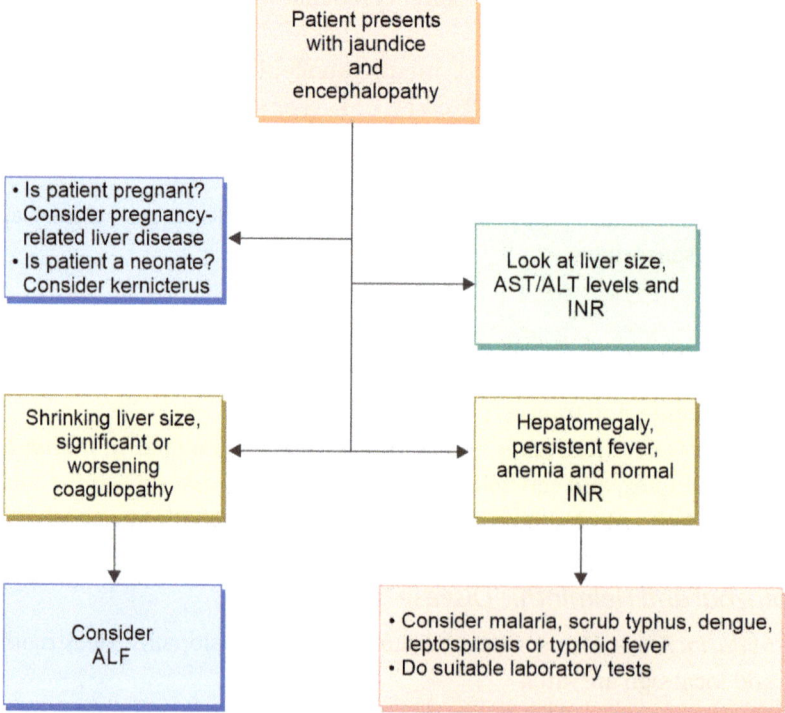

Flowchart 1: Syndromic approach to fever.

(ALF: acute liver failure; ALT: alanine transaminase; AST: aspartate transaminase; INR: international normalized ratio)

ratio (INR) is not elevated as in ALF. This differentiates malarial jaundice with jaundice due to hepatitis. In dengue, enzyme elevation is almost universal and rarely causes hepatic failure. Leptospirosis has biphasic clinical illness. Fever, jaundice, conjunctival hemorrhage, and renal failure hint diagnosis of leptospirosis. Jaundice appears on 4–9 days of illness. Fever, jaundice, and tender hepatomegaly are hallmarks of hepatic involvement. Raised bilirubin is not only due to hepatic involvement, but also due to hemolysis. Bilirubin level is relatively much higher in comparison to enzyme levels. This is in contrast to viral hepatitis. *Yellow fever* is another tropical virus disease characterized by high fever, jaundice, heart and kidney failure, and hemorrhagic diathesis.

In enteric fever, jaundice usually appears in the second week. Jaundice, hepatomegaly, or elevation of enzyme are seen frequently. ALF is rather uncommon. But etiology of ALF or acute-on-chronic liver failure (ACLF) is hepatitis E infection. There will be jaundice, tender hepatomegaly, raised serum bilirubin, enzymes, and elevated INR. Fever will subside with appearance of jaundice. In tropics, tuberculosis is a common infection that can involve the liver. In 50–80% of all patients of pulmonary tuberculosis, hepatic involvement occurs. Granulomatous hepatitis is the most common presentation. Common symptoms include abdominal pain, fever, anorexia, weight loss, hepatosplenomegaly, and jaundice.

Fever with Renal Failure

Tropical infections that cause acute renal failure (ARF) are malaria, salmonellosis, shigellosis, leptospirosis, and cholera. Dengue hemorrhagic fever can be associated with ARF.

In malaria particularly *falciparum*, malaria may be complicated by ARF in 1–5% cases. Oliguric ARF is common. Leptospirosis causes renal failure due to glomerulonephritis. In leptospirosis, renal failure is usually nonoliguric in dengue hemorrhagic fever or dengue shock syndrome, ARF may occur. In salmonellosis abnormal renal function is found in 16% of cases though acute renal failure is uncommon and reversible if it occurs. In shigellosis acute tubular necrosis may occur due to dehydration.

Fever with Lymphadenopathy

Plague, filariasis, brucellosis, tuberculosis, rickettsial disease, and infectious mononucleosis.

Fever with Hepatosplenomegaly

Malaria, Kala-azar, schistosomiasis, enteric fever, amoebic liver abscess, hepatitis, and leptospirosis.

Fever with Acute Respiratory Distress Syndrome[4]

Scrub typhus, leptospirosis, H_1N_1, and complicated malaria.

■ INVESTIGATIONS

Many of these infections have overlapping symptoms, judicious advice of investigations depends on local epidemiology and common infections.

Dengue
- Nonstructural protein 1 antigen detection on day 1[5]
- Sensitivity 76–93% and specificity 98%
- Immunoglobulin M (IgM) and IgG detection after 4th day of symptom onset (IgG >1:1,280 is 90% sensitive and 98% specific).

Malaria—Smear both Thick and Thin Smear[6]
- Thick smear—rapid detection
- Thin smear—identification of species, assess parasitemia and prognostication.

Rapid Antigen Test
- Immunochromatographic tests (**Fig. 1**)
- Capture of the parasite antigens from the peripheral blood using either monoclonal or polyclonal antibodies
  - Histidine-rich protein 2 of *Plasmodium falciparum*
  - Pan-malarial *Plasmodium* aldolase

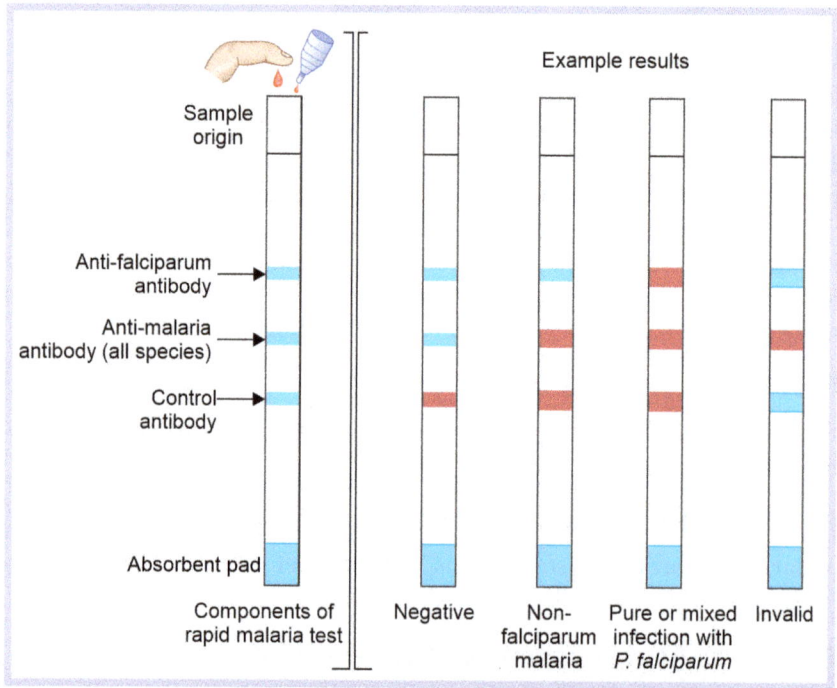

Fig. 1: RDT for malaria.

- Parasite-specific lactate dehydrogenase (LDH)
- Sensitivity and specificity >95%.

Histidine-based Rapid Test
- Inexpensive, rapid diagnosis
- Sensitivity same as thick film
- Can detect only *falciparum* species
- Remain positive after 2–6 weeks after infection
- Diagnostic failure due to polymorphism of *HRP2* gene.

Lactate Dehydrogenase-based Rapid Test
- Rapid and inexpensive:
  - Pan malarial antigen test
  - In case of *vivax* can miss low parasitemia (<100 parasite count/µL)
  - Malaria microscopy is still the best method and gold standard for malaria diagnosis.
  - Rapid detection tests (RDTs) have changed the malaria diagnosis at large, but they have failed to detect when the level is <100 parasites/µL blood.

Enteric Fever
- *Typhidot (RDT):* Sensitivity 95–97%, and specificity >89%
- *Widal test:* Nonspecific
- *Blood cultures:* Gold standard, positive in 40–80% patients
- *Bone marrow cultures:* Sensitivity 80–95% may remain positive even after 5 days of pretreatment.[7]

Leptospirosis
- *IgM enzyme-linked immunoassay (ELISA):* Sensitivity 52–89%, specificity >94%
- Positive serology
- Raised creatine phosphokinase levels, culture.[8]

Scrub Typhus
- *Weil–Felix test:* Poor sensitivity and specificity
- *Indirect fluorescent antibody:* Gold standard
- *ELISA for IgG/IgM:* Sensitivity and specificity >90%.[9]

Japanese Encephalitis
- *IgM capture ELISA:* Sensitivity 85–93% and specificity 96–98%
- *Cerebrospinal fluid (CSF):* Sensitivity 65–80% and specificity 89–100%
- *Magnetic resonance imaging (MRI) of the brain:* Involvement of thalamus, brainstem, and basal ganglia.[10]

Serological tests have a tendency to cross react and this interaction should be kept in mind while doing interpretation of laboratory results. Also to remember tropical infections are often life-threatening and investigation facilities are often not available in developing countries and reports may take time to arrive, so empiric treatment should be started as soon as possible without delay.

■ TREATMENT

Treatment of tropical infection should be based on identification of causative organism. But many a times, it may not be possible to identify etiology at emergency **(Table 3)**. So the emergency duty of medical officer is to stabilize the patient. To ensure airway, circulation, and breathing, circulatory shock, ARDS, and bleeding disorder are the three most common clinical condition of an acutely ill patients. Shock should be managed with isotonic saline. Oxygen device should be chosen according to the flow rate. Invasive procedure should be avoided, as often tropical infections present with thrombocytopenia. If physician cannot identify causative organism at emergency, at least should exclude few infections for whom RDT is available (malaria). Empiric therapy should be started with injection ceftriaxone or doxycycline. These two will cover leptospirosis, scrub typhus, enteric fever, and pyogenic meningitis.

TABLE 3: Syndrome-based treatment guidelines for critical tropical infections.

Fever with thrombocytopenia	• Antipyretics for control of fever IV fluids for fluid balance • Monitor PCV and platelet • Avoid aspirin/anticoagulants • Platelet transfusion if the platelet count <10,000 or bleeding manifestation occur. Steroid should not be used • Antipyretics for control of fever
Fever with jaundice	• Injection ceftriaxone 2 g IV BD doxycycline 100 mg BD (will cover leptospirosis, scrub typhus) • Artemisinin if *falciparum* malaria etiology • Watch for urine output, seizures, encephalopathy, and bleeding • Specific therapy once the diagnosis is established • Antipyretics for control of fever • Injection ceftriaxone 2 g IV BD or doxycycline 100 mg BD IV fluids according to CVP
Fever with renal failure	• Hemodialysis as required • Fluid balance must. Watch for encephalopathy, bleeding, seizures, ARDS renal replacement therapy (intermittent HD/CRRT) • Specific therapy once the diagnosis is established • Antipyretics for control of fever • Control of seizure by phenytoin or levetiracetam or lorazepam • Injection ceftriaxone 2 g IV BD<

Contd...

Contd...	
Fever with encephalopathy	• IV acyclovir 10 mg/kg in adults (up to 20 mg/kg in children) intravenously every 8 hours • IV fluids • IV mannitol for raised ICP • Specific therapy once the diagnosis is established • Antipyretics for control of fever • IV fluids • Oxygen by Venturi mask (level IV) Injection ceftriaxone 2 g IV BD injection azithromycin 500 mg IV OD • Tablet oseltamivir 150 mg BD, if H1N1 is a possibility (Level IA)
Fever with respiratory distress	• Watch for impending respiratory failure, shock, renal failure, and alveolar hemorrhage • Specific therapy once diagnosis is established

(ARDS: acute respiratory distress syndrome; CRRT: continuous renal replacement therapy; CVP: central venous pressure; ICP: intracranial pressure; IV: intravenous)

But empiric therapy with antimalarial drugs should not be given as it will create more resistance. If there is no improvement after 48 hours of empiric therapy, alternative diagnosis should be thought of.[11]

In spite of thorough search, often causative agent is not identified, or due to resource constrained state many a times investigation facilities are not available. So in tropical countries syndromic approach to management is often warranted.

■ CONCLUSION

Tropical infection is often challenging to diagnose and to treat. Symptoms often overlap and may be atypical. Tropical countries are usually poor, overpopulated, with paucity of well-equipped healthcare system. Lack of awareness and poor healthcare facilities often leads to late diagnosis and critical illness at presentation. After initial stabilization, physician should approach in syndromic manner, if specific etiology is not identified. Early recognition of infectious syndromes and prompt management based on clinical clues are often the bread and butter of a physician from tropical countries.

■ REFERENCES

1. John TJ, Dandona L, Sharma VP, Kakkar M. Continuing challenge of infectious diseases in India. Lancet. 2011;377:252-69.
2. Frean J, Blumberg L. Tropical fevers part A. Viral, bacterial and fungal infections. Primer of Tropical Medicine. Ch. 5A. Brisbane: ACTM Publication; 2005. pp. 1-18.

3. Bhalla A, John M. Syndromic approach to tropical infections. Update on Tropical Fever. Association of Physicians of India. [online] Available from https://www.icp-api.org/pdf/monograph_2015_update_on_tropical_fever/002_syndromic_approach.pdf. [Last accessed June 2022].
4. Kothari VM, Karnad DR, Bichile LS. Tropical infections in the ICU. Review Article. JAPI. 2006;54.
5. Singh MP, Majumdar M, Singh G, Goyal K, Preet K, Sarwal A, et al. NS1 antigen as an early diagnostic marker in dengue: report from India. Diagn Microbiol Infect Dis 2010; 68:50-4.
6. World Health Organization. Guidelines for the Treatment of Malaria, 2nd edition. Geneva: World Health Organization; 2010.
7. Ismail TF. Rapid diagnosis of typhoid fever. Indian J Med Res. 2006;123:489-92.
8. Toyokawa T, Ohnishi M, Koizumi N. Diagnosis of acute leptospirosis. Expert Rev Anti Infect Ther 2011;9:111-21.
9. Chaudhry D, Goyal S. Scrub typhus-resurgence of a forgotten killer. Indian J Anaesth. 2013;57:135-6.
10. Sarkari NB, Thacker AK, Barthwal SP, Mishra VK, Prapann S, Srivastava D, et al. Japanese encephalitis (JE). Part I: clinical profile of 1,282 adult acute cases of four epidemics. J Neurol. 2012;259:47-57.
11. Singhi S, Chaudhary D, Varghese GM, Bhalla A, Karthi N, Kalantri S, et al. Tropical fevers: management guidelines. Indian J Crit Care Med. 2014;18(2):62-9.

Section 2

Common Tropical Fever

- **Dengue**
  Shohael Mahmud Arafat, Mehruba Alam Ananna, Adnanul Alam
- **Malaria**
  Abhishek Kochar, Dhanpat Kumar Kochar, Aritra Kumar Ray
- **Kala-azar**
  Jaya Chakravarty, Sunanda Ghosh
- **Scrub Typhus and Other Rickettsial Diseases**
  Prasanta Kumar Bhattacharya, Nandini Chatterjee, Aritra Kumar Ray
- **Leptospirosis**
  Subhra Sankar Sen, Biva Bhakat, Manali Chandra, Purbasha Biswas
- **Zika and Chikungunya**
  Anivita Agarwal, Animesh Ray, Tanuka Mandal
- **Viral Respiratory Illness**
  J Rajkumar, Subramanian Swaminathan, Arkaprava Hati
- **Enteric Fever**
  Pritam Roy
- **Japanese B Encephalitis**
  Muralidharan K, Sowmini PR, Mugundhan K, Pranabananda Pal
- **Filariasis**
  Shantanu Kumar Kar, Md Karimulla
- **Fungal Infections in the Tropics**
  Shreya Singh, Arunaloke Chakrabarti, Md Karimulla

Chapter 4

Dengue

*Shohael Mahmud Arafat,
Mehruba Alam Ananna, Adnanul Alam*

■ INTRODUCTION

Dengue fever is one of the most common arthropod-borne diseases caused by a virus all over the globe. In most temperate countries around the world, it has a considerable economic and health impact.[1] Dengue fever has spread more quickly than any other infectious disease, with an increase of 400% between 2000 and 2013.[2] The illness has now spread to over one hundred countries, primarily in Southeast Asia, the western Pacific, and the Americas.[3] Severe presentations such as dengue hemorrhagic fever (DHF) and dengue shock syndrome (DSS), as well as other atypical manifestations, are increasingly being recorded in previously unaffected areas.[4]

Dengue infections were estimated to be over 400 million per year, with around 25% of those being clinically evident.[5] Dengue causes over 10% of all febrile episodes in highly endemic countries. In Asia, 19% of dengue-induced fever episodes necessitated hospitalization.[6]

■ PATHOPHYSIOLOGY

The Virus

Dengue viruses (DENVs) are members of the *Flavivirus* genus in the *Flaviviridae* family. Four different serotypes of the virus have been discovered.[7] DENV contains a single positive-strand RNA genome that is encapsulated by the C (capsid) protein. It is further enveloped by a lipid bilayer membrane containing the E (envelope) and M (membrane) proteins. Apart from these structural proteins, the genome also codes for seven nonstructural proteins (NS1, NS2A, NS2B, NS3, NS4A, NS4B, and NS5). The replication complex, which amplifies the viral genome, is made up of NS1 to NS5. They also serve an important role in interacting with host proteins, which is required for viral replication to be successful.[8]

The Vector

The main vector is *Aedes aegypti*, a day biting peridomiciliary mosquito capable of stinging multiple humans in a short period of time. It can breed in a variety of human-made water containers.

Aedes albopictus is another vector which is gradually expanding its range into tropical and subtropical countries. Climate change allows *Aedes* mosquitos to spread more widely over the globe, perhaps raising the risk of a dengue epidemic in temperate areas.[7] Main factors responsible for the increasing dengue incidence include population growth and increased population density, migration from rural to urban area, deteriorated urban environment, lack of reliable water source, and disorganized vector control programs.[9] As a result of increased human migration with advanced means of transportation, DENVs have spread fast around the world. Dengue fever has surpassed malaria as the primary cause of fever in returning travelers to Southeast Asia.[10]

■ PATHOGENESIS OF SEVERE DENGUE

Antibody-dependent Enhancement

Type-specific antibodies are generated following infection with one DENV. They provide long-term protection against the homologous serotype of the virus, but protection from other heterologous serotypes are temporary. Trial showed that this cross-protection lasted about 3 months.[11]

Infection with one of the DENV variant in fact raises the chance of severe disease in case of subsequent disease with a heterologous virus.[12]

Similarly, DENV infection in infants increase the risk of severe dengue when maternal antibodies reduce to subneutralizing concentrations.[13] This can be explained by antibody-dependent enhancement (ADE). This concept was proposed by Halstead and colleagues that suggests that subneutralizing antibody concentrations may bind heterologous variant of DENV, allowing viral entrance through Fc receptors expressed on target cells. Antibody-dependent enhancement thus induces mismatched proinflammatory and anti-inflammatory responses resulting in capillary endothelial pathology, vascular leak, and hypovolemic shock. According to a study, people who have cross-reactive antibodies that are over certain levels are more likely to develop ADE.

During ADE, the virus interacts with the host to escape antiviral and immunological responses that might otherwise limit infection. As a result, the risk of ADE is not the same for all secondary DENV infections, but it does require the right antibody-to-virus ratios.

Viral Determinants

Viral factors may have a key role in pathogenesis, according to long-term epidemiological findings. Dengue virus is continually evolving due to its RNA-dependent RNA polymerase, which is prone to errors. Dengue viruses that improve their ability to avoid host responses against them achieve enhanced viability by being able to grow to a higher titer in their hosts.

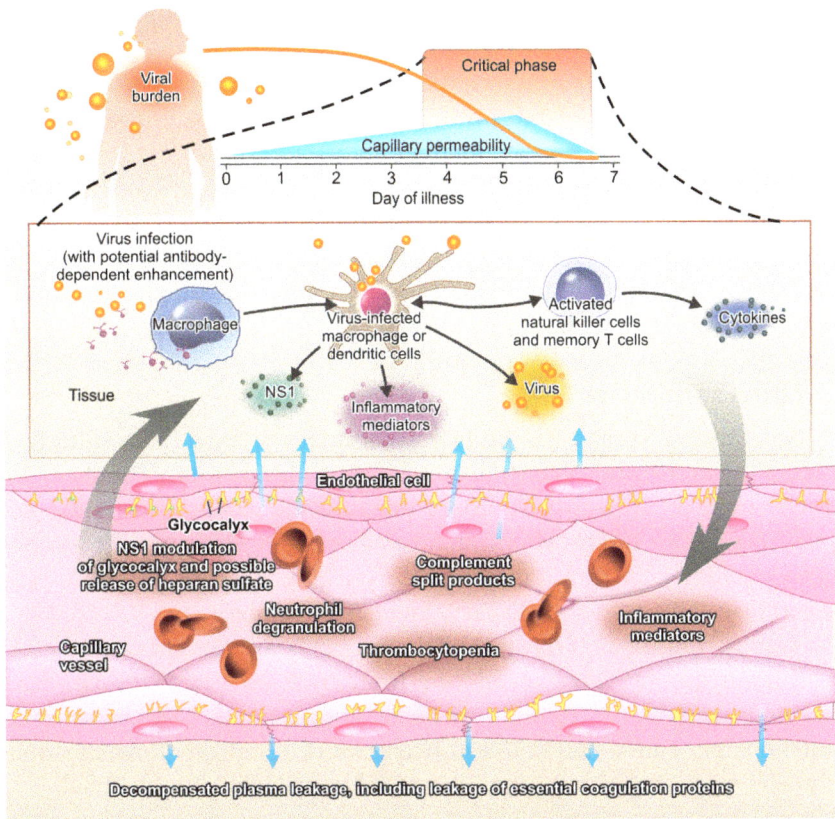

Fig. 1: Pathophysiology of dengue infection.[7]

Dengue virus strains that are less evasive, on the other hand, are clinically weakened. The NS1 protein is a viral component that may play a key role in dengue pathogenesis. NS1 is a component of the DENV genome's replication complex. It binds to a wide range of host proteins. Infected cells release a hexameric version of NS1 that protects the virus from complement and lectin-mediated neutralization. Recent research suggests that NS1 may have toxic qualities that affect the endothelium glycocalyx, causing vascular permeability and contributing to dengue-related vascular leakage. Finally, secreted NS1 may contribute to the enhancement of flaviviral infection in mosquito vectors. As a result, NS1 has been identified as a potential target for antiviral therapy and immunization **(Fig. 1)**.

Host Factors

Dengue virus infection's clinical consequences are also influenced by host variables. Several studies have discovered genetic polymorphisms linked to more serious disease. The polymorphisms include—activation of Fc gamma receptor, cytokines (both proinflammatory and anti-inflammatory), HLA (human leukocyte antigens), and genes in the different metabolic pathways.

Persons of African origin are thought to be less susceptible to severe dengue due to such polymorphisms in the OSBPL10 (oxysterol binding protein-like 10) and RXRA (retinoid X receptor alpha) genes.[8]

Susceptibility loci in the major histocompatibility complex (MHC) class I chain-related protein B (MICB) and phospholipase C epsilon 1 (PLCE1) genes were discovered in a Vietnamese investigation. Another study in Thailand found that lower and higher DSS risks were linked to single-nucleotide polymorphisms in the PLCE1 and MICB genes.[8]

■ TRANSMISSION

Dengue fever is spread via the bite of an infected female mosquito that carries the virus. Nonvector transmissions are also possible. For example, transfusion, organ transplantation, needle stick wounds, and mucosal splashing are the modes of nonvector transmission. Dengue fever has not been recorded to be transmitted sexually yet. However, a recent single-case report revealed persistent DENV shedding in the semen.

Vertical transmission can occur if the mother is viremic during the period of childbirth; however, transmission from illnesses that begin earlier in the pregnancy is not thought to occur. Although no cases have been documented, DENV was found in two-third of 12 infected breastfeeding mothers, suggesting that transmission via breast milk may be possible.[9]

■ CLINICAL FEATURES

History

Suspicion of dengue fever is high in anyone who lives in a country where the dengue infection is endemic or has traveled there during the last two weeks. Symptoms usually appear suddenly following the incubation period. Fever is the principal symptom that appears suddenly, usually with high temperature of 39.4–40.5°C. It can occur in two phases with a remittent pattern or low grade. Fever usually lasts for 5–7 days. Children may develop febrile seizures. Fast defervescence may trigger entering the critical phase of the infection.

Backache, arthralgia, myalgia, and bone pain are all common. Infection-related headaches are also typical, and they are usually continuous and located in the front of the head. Within a few days, it normally improves. It is also frequent to have severe retro-orbital discomfort while moving the eyes or applying a small amount of pressure to the eyeball.

Possible gastrointestinal symptoms are loss of appetite, nausea or vomiting, epigastric pain, or discomfort. Patients frequently complain of a loss of appetite or a change in taste experience. In DHF, gastrointestinal symptoms, weakness, and disorientation may be more prominent. Upper respiratory symptoms (such as cough and soreness of throat) are usually not present, though may appear in mild infections.

Physical Examination

Early infection causes diffuse flushing of skin, especially in the face, neck, and chest. On the third or fourth day of the fever, this develops into a maculopapular or rubelliform rash that covers the entire body. When the skin is squeezed, blanching might occur. The rash fades with time and appears as pale regions throughout the convalescent phase **(Fig. 2)**.

Petechiae, purpura, and a positive tourniquet test are all indicators of hemorrhage. Tourniquet test is considered to be positive if 10 or more petechiae per square inch occur on the forearm when blood pressure cuff is kept inflated to a point between systolic and diastolic pressures for at least 5 minutes. Nose bleeds (epistaxis), gum bleeding, hematemesis, bleeding per rectum or vagina, or bleeding from a venepuncture site are all features of more serious hemorrhage. Dengue fever or DHF might cause these symptoms. Hepatomegaly can be also found **(Fig. 3)**.

Plasma leakage, evidenced by ascites, postural dizziness, and pleural effusion, is a symptom of DHF.

Dengue shock syndrome is suspected when circulatory collapse is evident by cold, clammy skin, rapid and week pulse, narrow pulse pressure, postural drop, delayed capillary refill time (>3 seconds), and decreased urine output.

Phases of Infection

The three stages of dengue fever are febrile, critical, and convalescent.

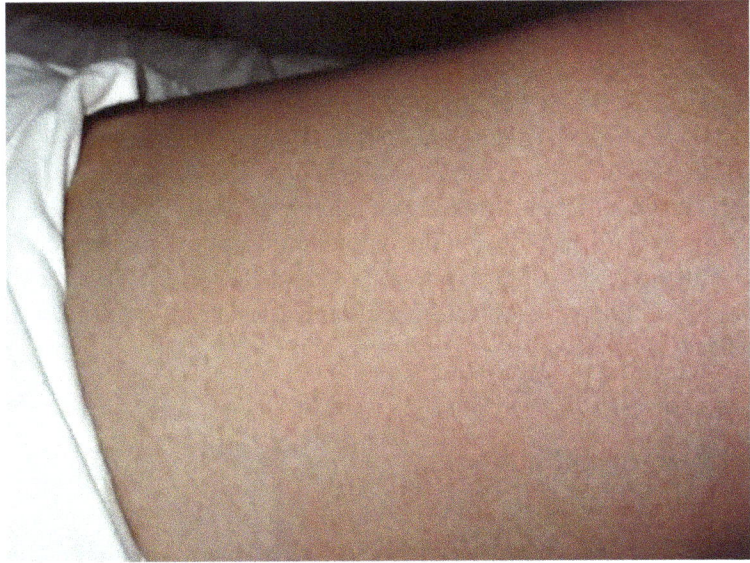

Fig. 2: Convalescent rash.[14]

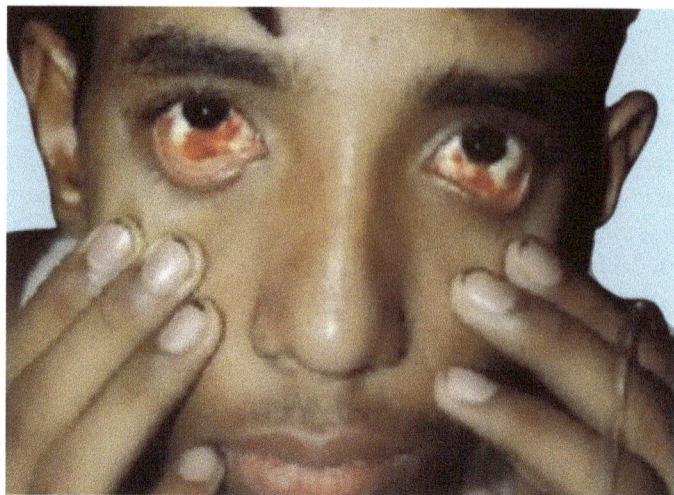

Fig. 3: Conjunctival hemorrhage.[14]

A rapid high-grade fever and dehydration characterize the febrile phase, which can last 2–7 days. Plasma leakage, hemorrhage, shock, and organ dysfunction characterize the critical phase. This phase usually lasts for about 24–48 hours.

It normally begins during the time of defervescence most of the time, usually between days 3 and 7.

All three stages are experienced by patients with DHF as well as DSS. In patients with dengue fever, the critical phase is skipped.[15]

Expanded Dengue Syndrome

Expanded dengue syndrome (EDS) is a name coined by the World Health Organization (WHO) in 2011 to describe the rare manifestations of dengue fever that cause serious damage to the liver, kidneys, bone marrow, heart, or brain. They could be the result of underlying co-morbidities, co-infections, or shock. Pregnant mothers, newborns, the elderly, and people with coronary artery disease, hemoglobinopathies, and immunocompromised individuals are all at greater risk of developing EDS. Clinicians must be aware of these uncommon symptoms in order to detect dengue fever early, especially during epidemics **(Table 1)**.[16]

■ DIAGNOSIS

Laboratory Investigations

Initial Laboratory Investigations

In all patients with symptoms, a complete blood count should be ordered first. Leukopenia and thrombocytopenia usually appear on the second day

TABLE 1: Unusual presentations of dengue infection.[14]

Expanded dengue syndrome

Neurological involvement	• Encephalopathy • Encephalitis • Intracranial hemorrhages • Mononeuropathies • polyneuropathies • Guillain–Barré syndrome • Transverse myelitis
Cardiac involvement	• Conduction abnormalities • Myocarditis • Pericarditis
Pulmonary involvement	• Pleural effusion • Acute respiratory distress syndrome • Pulmonary hemorrhage • Pneumonitis
Liver and gut involvement	• Hepatitis • Fulminant hepatic failure • Acalculous cholecystitis • Acute pancreatitis • Acute parotitis
Renal involvement	• Acute renal failure • Proteinuria • Immunoglobulin a nephropathy • Glomerulonephritis • Hemolytic uremic syndrome
Blood and bone involvement	• Hemophagocytic lymphohistiocytosis • Idiopathic thrombocytopenic purpura • Disseminated intravascular coagulopathy • Hepatomegaly • Splenomegaly • Cytopenia • Lymphadenopathy

of a fever. In a dengue-endemic area, leukopenia combined with a positive tourniquet test has a positive predictive value of 70–80%. Throughout the febrile episode, leukopenia (together with neutropenia) persists. Thrombocytopenia is usually modest in basic dengue fever, but it can occasionally be severe. Dehydration can cause the hematocrit to rise by roughly 10% in patients with dengue fever. The findings of liver function tests, notably for alanine and aspartate aminotransferases, are frequently elevated. Clotting investigations are not required for diagnosis, although they can help with infection management when hemorrhagic symptoms are present.

Confirmatory Laboratory Investigations

Confirmatory testing should be performed if possible. This is critical since dengue fever can be mistaken for a variety of other conditions. Dengue virus infection can be confirmed using one of four diagnostic tests. Numerous factors influence test selection, including geographic availability, cost, time to collect sample, facilities available, and knowledge. Direct approaches (viral nucleic acid or antigen detection) are more specific than indirect approaches (such as serology). But they are more expensive and needs more time while indirect approaches are more accessible, faster, and less expensive. Combined serology for the detection of viral nucleic acid or antigen as well as antibody response, is better than either of the technique alone.

Virus nucleic acid or antigen detection is mostly done in the first five days of sickness. Serological tests can be done after this period. Some assays distinguish between virus serotypes, however this is irrelevant in clinical practice. Virus isolation is possible during the early stages of a viremic outbreak. This test is only available in a few areas and is not widely advised because findings are rarely available in a clinically useful time frame.[14]

Imaging

Imaging scans are required only if the clinicians suspect DHF or DSS. Lateral decubitus chest X-ray can be done to reveal clinically minimal pleural effusion in the early stages of plasma leakage. Ultrasonography of the abdomen can identify ascites, plasma leaks, and other changes in abdominal organs such as the liver, gallbladder, and kidneys.

■ TREATMENT

Treatment Approach

There is no specific antiviral medicine for dengue illness. Treatment is supportive and based on the recommendations of WHO and other regional authorities.

Maintaining appropriate hydration is the mainstay of treatment for dengue fever, and fluid replacement therapy is used to treat DHF and DSS.

Clinically suspected dengue should preferably be triaged in a specific location of the health facility in dengue-endemic areas.

Severity of Infection

World Health Organization developed the most commonly used and adoptable treatment approach depending on the severity of infection.

Depending on the clinical presentation, patients are classified into one of three groups.[14]

Group A

These patients can be taken care of at home:
- Absence of warning signs.
- Can take an appropriate amount of fluids orally and can pass urine at the rate of once every 6 hours.
- Normal or near normal hematocrit or packed cell volume and other blood counts.

Group B

Group B patients have the following characteristics and need to be admitted to the hospital:
- Having warning signs
- Co-existing risk factors that may lead to serious infection (e.g., pregnancy, very young or old age, obesity, diabetes mellitus, renal function impairment, hemolytic diseases)
- Lack of family or social support (e.g., patients living by themselves or away from medical centers)
- Rising hematocrit or packed cell volume or a rapidly decreasing platelet count.

Group C

These patients have the following key features and needs immediate attention:
- Confirmed warning features.
- In the critical phase of infection defines by either severe plasma leakage, severe blood loss, or severe organ dysfunction (e.g., liver or kidney function impairment, cardiomyopathy, and encephalopathy).

Management of Group A Patients

Group A patients can be taken care of at home. Rest and drinking plenty of fluids orally should be encouraged. Daily fluid intake is usually about 2,500 mL for adults.

Alternative fluids such as ORS (oral rehydration solutions), juices, and soups can be taken instead of water. Colored fluid fluids should be avoided. Fever can be treated with tepid sponging and paracetamol in standard doses. Nonsteroidal anti-inflammatory medicines (NSAIDs) should not be taken because they may increase the likelihood of bleeding episodes. Patients should be counseled regarding the warning signals and told to go to the health facility as soon as possible if any appear. Blood counts should be done on a daily basis.

Management of Group B Patients

These patients will need to be admitted to the hospital. It is necessary to determine the severity of the infection.

Patients should be encouraged to take fluids orally if they are not in the early stages of acute illness (i.e., no plasma leakage). Daily fluid requirement is about 2,500 mL for adults.

If patient cannot take oral fluid or is in the critical phase, intravenous (IV) fluid replacement therapy with 0.9% saline (or Ringer's lactate) should be commenced. Elevated hematocrit, reduced albumin, progressive leukopenia, thrombocytopenia, fluid loss in the third space, and narrowing of pulse pressure with postural drop are all signs of the critical phase.

The formula for fluid replacement is maintenance (M) + 5% fluid deficit.

Following clinical parameters should be monitored closely: Vital signs, urine output. temperature, and peripheral perfusion. Biochemical parameters that need close monitoring are hematocrit, platelet count, blood glucose, hepatic function tests, renal function test, and coagulation profile.

Management of Group C Patients

Immediate medical assistance is needed for these patients. Patients may be in shock at the time of presentation.

Blood transfusions and intensive care facilities should be available **(Table 2)**. According to WHO guidelines, intravenous crystalloids and colloids delivered quickly are advised. Attempts to determine the length of time in the critical phase as well as their prior fluid balance should be taken. The next 48 hours total fluid requirement should be calculated. Following formula can be used:

$$\text{Maintenance (M) fluid} + 5\% \text{ fluid deficit}$$

where Maintenance fluid = 100 mL per kg for the first 10 kg of body weight, 50 mL per kg for the second 10 kg of body weight, and 20 mL per kg for over

TABLE 2: Indications of blood and platelet transfusion.[14]

When to give whole blood	1. Low hemoglobin (≤5 g%) 2. Bleeding causing loss of >10% of total blood volume (80 mL/kg) 3. Hidden bleeding manifested by fall of hematocrit and unstable vital signs despite appropriate fluid replacement. Dose: 10 mL/kg/dose at a time
When to give platelet concentrate: Role is very limited except in some special conditions. Whole blood may be given as an alternative in case of unavailability	1. When surgery is needed in patients with very low platelet count 2. Judgment of the clinician

20 kg of body weight up to 50 kg. 5% fluid deficit is calculated as 50 mL per kg of body weight up to 50 kg.

According to this formula, 4,600 mL fluid is required for a 50 kg adult in 48 hours.

This formula can be used for patients of any age group including children. Following local protocols should be preferred as rate of administering treatment differs between patient groups. For children, the formula should be based on their ideal body weight. The infusion rate should be adjusted according to the usual monitoring variables, and therapy is usually required for only 24–48 hours, with a gradual reduction once the rate of plasma leakage decreases toward the end of the critical phase.

Colloids (e.g., dextran 70% or 6% starch) are not superior to crystalloids and has no added clinical benefit.

Colloids should be used when clearly indicated by WHO guidelines (e.g., intractable shock, resistance to crystalloid resuscitation).

Clinical and biochemical parameters should be closely monitored throughout. Organ function tests should be carried out as indicated.

Within a few hours of starting fluid therapy, the patient's condition should stabilize.

Other contributing factors should be explored and addressed accordingly if patients remain unstable. Such conditions are metabolic acidosis, electrolyte imbalance, low serum calcium, low blood glucose, myocarditis, and liver necrosis.

Internal bleeding should be under consideration if the patient's condition does not get better and the hematocrit drops. Blood transfusion should be commenced as soon as possible in this case **(Table 2)**; however, caution should be exercised due to the risk of fluid overload.

In refractory unstable patients, there is now widespread agreement on the use of colloids and blood transfusions early on.

Fluid overload can result from overzealous therapy and quick hydration. Features of fluid overload are pulmonary edema, congested face, elevated jugular venous pressure, pleural effusion, and ascites.

Until patients are stable, these problems should be addressed with intravenous fluid restriction and bolus doses of intravenous furosemide (frusemide).

The disease may follow a different course as a result of the complications even if they are less common.

■ PREGNANCY

Pregnancy is linked to an increased risk of maternal death and poor prenatal outcomes. Maternal risks are increased chance of caesarean sections, pre-eclamptic toxemia, and delivery before term. Low birth weight of infant and vertical transmission of disease are also common. In this patient group, close observation and precise management are essential. Fluid intake should be the same as for normal adult, and the calculation must be based on prepregnancy body weight. As clinical (rapid pulse rate, low blood pressure, broader pulse pressure) and biochemical parameters (lower hemoglobin and hematocrit and decreased platelet count) are disrupted during pregnancy, baseline observations should be documented on the first day. Subsequent observations should be compared with prior ones cautiously.

Pre-eclamptic toxemia and HELLP (hemolysis, elevated liver enzymes, low platelet count) syndrome are illnesses related to pregnancy that might affect test results as well. In pregnant women, detecting plasma leakage (for example, ascites, pleural effusion) is challenging, hence early ultrasonography is recommended.

■ CHILDREN

Laboratory indicators should be evaluated on a frequent basis as children are more prone to develop severe dengue in the form of DHF or DSS.[14] When compared to older children and adults, determining the severity of symptoms in newborns under the age of one year is challenging. Infants have a lower respiratory reserve, making them more vulnerable to electrolyte imbalance and liver failure. Children's plasma leakage may be short-lived and respond to fluid resuscitation more quickly.

■ CONVALESCENCE AND DISCHARGE

The betterment in clinical indicators, patient's appetite, and general well-being, are all signs of convalescence. Patients may experience diuresis, which can lead to hypokalemia. IV fluids should be replaced with fluid rich in potassium if hypokalemia arises. Rash or generalized itching may appear while recovery. Patients can be discharged after achieving wellness with no fever for 48 hours with an increasing platelet count and persistently normal hematocrit **(Box 1)**.

BOX 1: Discharge criteria.[14]

When to discharge
- Afebrile for at least 24 hours without antipyretic medication
- Two days passed after the patient recovered from shock
- General well-being and good appetite
- Hematocrit gone back to baseline value or around 38–40%
- Absence of respiratory distress due to pleural effusions
- Absence of ascites
- Platelet count above 50,000/mm^3
- Absence of any other complications

■ ADJUNCTIVE THERAPIES

Prophylactic platelet transfusions are needed very rarely and not advised unless active bleeding is present. Fresh frozen plasma, corticosteroids, intravenous immunoglobulin, and antibiotics are all problematic in clinical practice, and more data is needed before they can be prescribed.

Vaccines

CYD-TDV or Dengvaxia is the world's first licensed dengue vaccine. It is manufactured by Sanofi Pasteur that got its licensed in 2015. It is a live-attenuated vaccine, based on the yellow fever 17D backbone. It is indicated for persons aged 9–45 years. In 2018, it was revealed that there is an excess risk of severe dengue in seronegative recipients of this vaccine. It does, however, give protection in case of the patients who are seropositive. This can be explained by the most plausible hypothesis for the increased risk in seronegative individuals is that in fact CYD-TDV triggers a first immune response to dengue in seronegative individuals. This makes them vulnerable to a risk of severe disease when they get their first wild infection. In April 2018, WHO suggested that this vaccine should be given to only dengue-seropositive individuals and screening prior to vaccination should be done.

Rapid diagnostic techniques to detect for dengue seropositivity are currently being developed and evaluated. Cross-reactivity with certain other *Flaviviruses*, however, will continue to be a problem.

There is also a need for research to test vaccine regimens with lesser number of doses. Determining which populations will get the most benefit from this vaccine should also be addressed.

Two chimeric second-generation dengue vaccines are now being tested in phase 3 trials. It is unclear whether these vaccines will have the same safety issues in seronegative patients like its predecessor.

Antiviral Drugs

A safe and equally effective antiviral drug for dengue is still on search. In spite of continuous attempts, no fruitful results have been found. A pro-drug called, balapiravir, which is an inhibitor of hepatitis C replication, was a candidate drug in a trial of adults with dengue fever. But it was found to be ineffective.

■ DISEASE NOTIFICATION

Notification of dengue cases should be done routinely in dengue endemic areas. Both suspected and confirmed cases of dengue infection should be notified to the health authorities. This may help to take necessary steps to stop transmission.

■ PROGNOSIS

The mortality rate for severe dengue fever is 0.8–2.5%. Children are at an increased risk of severe infection and death, although severe infection in adults is increasingly being reported. The risk of children aged 1–5 years dying from dengue fever is fourfold higher than in children aged 11–15 years. Even though DHF and DSS are uncommon in adults, a higher morbidity and mortality rate has been reported, especially in older people, which is related to an increased risk of organ impairment.

■ LONG-TERM SEQUELAE

Dengue fever has minimal long-term consequences once patients have recovered; nevertheless, some patients may have postviral fatigue syndrome. During convalescence, the platelet count gradually rises, albeit some patients may experience transient thrombocytosis. It may take up to four weeks for liver function test values to return to normal.

■ MONITORING AND FOLLOW-UP

Beyond the acute infectious period, patients do not require monitoring or regular follow-up. Blood counts and liver function should be monitored for up to four weeks after discharge.

■ RECURRENCE OR REINFECTION

A different DENV serotype might cause recurrence, resulting in secondary dengue infection. Recurrences of clinical infection on the third and fourth occasions are possible, although their clinical significance is unknown. Development of immunity to all four serotypes gives protection for life.

■ INSTRUCTIONS FOR THE PATIENTS

Patients should be reassured that dengue fever has no long-term consequences and that they can resume normal activities once they are physically capable. Patients should be counseled to avoid alcohol and heavy exercise during convalescence, based on empirical research, because liver function can take up to three weeks to recover to normal.

■ VECTOR CONTROL

World Health Organization is promoting an integrated vector control strategy to countries in order to minimize dengue mortality and morbidity.

Biological methods are aimed at control of larval stages of mosquito. Use of larvicidal bacteria such as *Bacillus thuringiensis israelensis*, raising larvivorous fish (e.g., *Poecilia reticulata*), and crustaceans such as copepods are the example of these methods. Chemical methods are namely insecticide spray for indoors, use of materials (mosquito nets) treated with insecticide and use of chemical larvicides for outdoors such as temephos or pyriproxyfen.

Mosquito breeding places can be reduced using environmental measures.

Evidence that shows community mobilization may improve vector control and reduce dengue cases came from a recent multicenter randomized study.

Because of low compliance rates, daytime protective clothing against *Aedes* mosquito bites is difficult.

Insecticide-treated clothing to guard against mosquito bites can be a research priority.

The discharge of mosquitoes infected with *Wolbachia* and the insects expressing dominant lethal genes (RIDL) are two unique techniques to control *A. aegypti* are in the development.

There is growing interest in merging mosquito interventions with vaccination, as no single intervention can successfully reduce the burden of the disease.

■ CONCLUSION

Although death rate is often minimal in nations with adequate clinical infrastructure for the management of acute dengue, consequences in adults are still poorly understood.

Despite significant breakthroughs in our knowledge about the disease etiology and significant funding in antiviral drug research, progress toward the development of successful therapies has been slow.

A regional platform comprised of well-established centers with the requisite infrastructure and clinical competence across dengue-endemic nations could also be beneficial for trials of other therapies, such as antiviral medicines.

Several interesting DENV detection technologies are currently being developed. A test that differentiates between cross-reactive antibodies might speed up the process of developing vaccines.

Finally, all countries affected by dengue fever need a better monitoring program to guide infection prevention and control efforts.

> **TAKE HOME MESSAGE**
> - *A. aegypti* and *A. albopictus* mosquitos are the primary carriers of DENV. Dengue virus can infect a person up to four times in their lifetime.
> - Dengue infections might be asymptomatic in 40–80% of cases. A sudden onset of high fever, headache, and retro-orbital pain, myalgia, arthralgia, maculopapular rash, and mild bleeding are all common clinical signs.
> - Severe dengue, termed as DHF/DSS, is defined by an increase in vascular permeability, which can lead to life-threatening hypovolemic shock.
> - The theory is that following a "primary" infection with one serotype, "secondary" infections with one or more other serotypes might generate "antibody dependent enhancement" (ADE), which is the cause of severe dengue fever.

- When mosquitoes bite on a viremic host, they pick up the virus. When virus-containing saliva is injected into a nonimmune host during successive blood meals, new infections in humans can develop.
- Reverse transcription polymerase chain reaction (RT-PCR) can detect the dengue viral genome in blood samples up to five days of illness. The non-structural-1 (NS1) dengue antigen can also be detected up to four days after the commencement of the disease.
- From days 5–6 of sickness, serological diagnosis can be made by looking for dengue immunoglobulin M (IgM) antibodies in a serum sample.
- The only treatment option is supportive therapy, with aspirin and other anticoagulants strictly avoided.
- A licensed dengue vaccination for persons who have already been exposed to the virus has just been launched.
- Mosquito nets (ideally insecticide-treated), sleeping in screened or air-conditioned rooms, wearing garments that cover the majority of the body and using mosquito repellent are all effective personal mosquito protection strategies.
- Multisectoral collaboration and community participation are required for integrated vector management programs that aim to reduce mosquito vector density in a sustainable way.

REFERENCES

1. Bhatt S, Gething PW, Brady OJ, Messina JP, Farlow AW, Moyes CL, et al. The global distribution and burden of dengue. Nature. 2013;496(7446):504-7.
2. Fitzmaurice C, Allen C, Barber RM, Barregard L, Bhutta ZA, Brenner H, et al. Global, regional, and national cancer incidence, mortality, years of life lost, years lived with disability, and disability-adjusted life-years for 32 cancer groups, 1990 to 2015: a systematic analysis for the global burden of disease study. JAMA oncology. 2017;3(4):524-48.
3. Halstead SB. Dengue. Lancet. 2007;370(9599):1644-52.
4. Teixeira MG, Barreto ML. Diagnosis and management of dengue. BMJ. 2009;339:b4338.
5. Beatty ME, Beutels P, Meltzer MI, Shepard DS, Hombach J, Hutubessy R, et al. Health economics of dengue: a systematic literature review and expert panel's assessment. Am J Tropical Med Hygiene. 2011;84(3):473-88.
6. L'Azou M, Moureau A, Sarti E, Nealon J, Zambrano B, Wartel TA, et al. Symptomatic dengue in children in 10 Asian and Latin American countries. New England Journal of Medicine. 2016;374(12):1155-66.
7. Simmons CP, Farrar JJ, van Vinh Chau N, Wills B. Dengue. N Engl J Med. 2012;366(15):1423-32.
8. Wilder-Smith A, Ooi EE, Horstick O, Wills B. Dengue. Lancet. 2019;393(10169):350-63.
9. Wilder-Smith A, Ooi EE, Vasudevan SG, Gubler DJ. Update on dengue: epidemiology, virus evolution, antiviral drugs, and vaccine development. Curr Infect Dis Rep. 2010;12(3):157-64.
10. Schwartz E, Weld LH, Wilder-Smith A, von Sonnenburg F, Keystone JS, Kain KC, et al. Seasonality, annual trends, and characteristics of dengue among ill returned travelers, 1997–2006. Emerging infectious diseases. 2008;14(7):1081.

11. Snow GE, Haaland B, Ooi EE, Gubler DJ. Research on dengue during World War II revisited. Am J Trop Med Hyg. 2014;91(6):1203-17.
12. Guzman MG, Halstead SB, Artsob H, Buchy P, Farrar J, Gubler DJ, et al. Dengue: a continuing global threat. Nature reviews microbiology. 2010;8(12):S7-16.
13. Chau TN, Hieu NT, Anders KL, Wolbers M, Lien LB, Hieu LT, et al. Dengue virus infections and maternal antibody decay in a prospective birth cohort study of Vietnamese infants. The Journal of infectious diseases. 2009;200(12):1893-900.
14. DGHS. National Guideline for Clinical Management of Dengue Syndrome. [Internet] 4th Ed. Dhaka;2018 Available from: https://old.dghs.gov.bd/index.php/en/publications/guideline
15. Kularatne SA. Dengue fever. BMJ. 2015;351:h4661.
16. Umakanth M, Suganthan N. Unusual Manifestations of dengue fever: a review on expanded dengue syndrome. Cureus. 2020;12(9):e10678.

Chapter 5

Malaria

Abhishek Kochar, Dhanpat Kumar Kochar, Aritra Kumar Ray

■ INTRODUCTION

Malaria is a protozoan disease caused by *Plasmodium falciparum*, *Plasmodium vivax*, *Plasmodium ovale*, *Plasmodium malariae*, and *Plasmodium knowlesi*. It is transmitted by the bite of the female *Anopheles* mosquito and its incidence depends on environmental suitability for local vectors in terms of altitude, climate, vegetation, and implementation of control measures, and is also linked to poverty, natural disasters, and war. *P. falciparum* and *P. vivax* are the predominant species worldwide and the great majority of *falciparum* malaria occurs in sub-Saharan Africa. In Asia and Oceania, the proportions caused by *P. vivax* and *P. falciparum* are similar, whereas in the Americas, *P. vivax* malaria is more common. *P. knowlesi* is seen mainly in Malaysia and other Southeast Asian countries. *P. falciparum* accounts for most deaths globally. However, the *P. vivax* infection, which was traditionally considered to cause uncomplicated disease, also causes severe disease and death. *P. malariae* and *P. ovale* infection usually cause uncomplicated malaria.

The lifecycle of *P. falciparum* is summarized in **Figure 1**. The female *Anopheles* mosquito inoculates the infective form of the parasite (sporozoites) when feeding upon humans. The circulating sporozoites invade hepatocytes and remain there for 7–14 days and replicate. This pre-erythrocytic stage equals to the incubation period because no symptoms occur during this period. In *P. vivax* and *P. ovale* infection, this stage may last for a very long period, as some parasites remain dormant in the liver as hypnozoites, causing relapse at a latter period up to many months. After emerging from liver, merozoite enters the bloodstream and invades circulating red blood cell (RBC) and multiplies into schizont which bursts and releases merozoites to reinvade other RBCs and perpetuate the blood stage of the cycle. During this period, clinical symptoms appear. A small percentage of merozoites develop into the sexual stages or gametocytes. In order to continue transmission into human being, the female and male gametocytes require to be taken by another mosquito to complete the sexual cycle in the vector's mid gut. After a period of 9–14 days, the mosquito cycle ends with the sporozoite migrating to the salivary glands, and able to infect another person by bloodstream inoculation during a subsequent blood meal.[1]

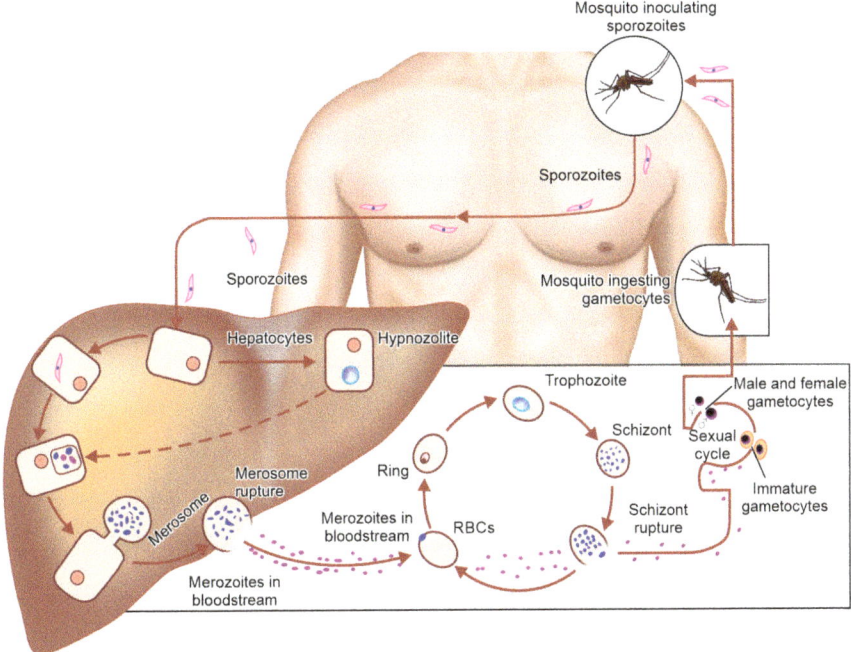

Fig. 1: Life cycle of malarial parasite.
(RBC: red blood cell)

■ PATHOGENESIS

Usually malaria presents clinically with periodic fever paroxysms which coincide with the parasite's intraerythrocytic cycles of each species (24 hours for *P. knowlesi*; 48 hours for *P. falciparum*, *P. vivax*, and *P. ovale*; and 72 hours for *P. malariae* infection). Both parasite and host determinants contribute to the onset and outcome of severe malaria (SM) infection including cerebral malaria (CM). RBC sequestration, inflammation, and endothelial dysfunction are key components, which lead to SM. Sequestration is mediated through the adherence of mature infected RBCs to host receptor expressed on the endothelium lining host capillaries, on uninfected RBCs to form rosettes, and on platelets to form platelet-mediated clumps. Cytoadhesion, a key feature of the pathogenesis of *P. falciparum* infections, is mediated through *P. falciparum* erythrocyte membrane protein 1 (PfEMP1), which binds to numerous host receptors importantly intercellular adhesion molecule (ICAM), vascular cell adhesion molecule (VCAM), chondroitin sulfate, E-selectin, P-selectin, CD-36, integrin alpha beta, thrombospondin-1 (TSP), etc. **(Fig. 2)**. There are a number of bioactive molecules that also influence the pathogenesis of CM due to release of cytokines or secondary messengers, and these include mitogens, polar lipids, and hemozoin. They act on host cells such as macrophages, monocytes, and T cells. Malarial antigens can

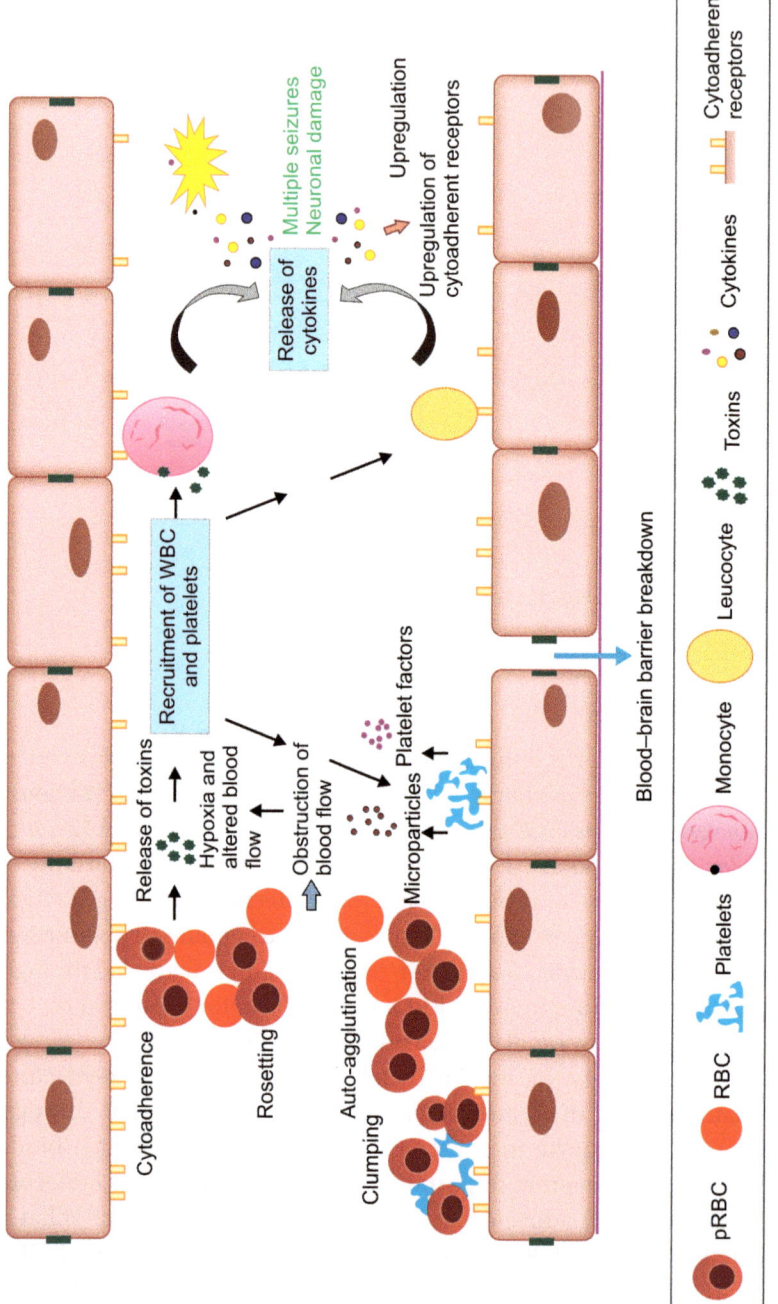

Fig. 2: Pathogenesis of cerebral malaria.
(RBC: red blood cell; WBC: white blood cell)

also stimulate T cells and macrophages to produce various cytokines such as interferon γ (IFN-γ), interleukin 4 (IL-4), IL-2, and IL-3 from T lymphocyte and tumor necrosis factor α (TNF-α), IL-1, and IL-6 from macrophages or monocytes. TNF is produced by macrophages or monocytes that are exposed to malarial toxins, hemozoin, or soluble antigens, especially glycophosphatidylinositol (GPI). These events are thought to lead to blood-brain barrier (BBB) dysfunction. Cells of the BBB are damaged and undergo apoptosis; this allows entry of foreign materials into the brain parenchyma, creating hemorrhagic lesions and edema of the brain. The role of nitric oxide (NO) in CM pathogenesis is still a matter of controversy. Although NO has been primarily associated with protection against CM, studies reveal that it may also contribute to pathogenesis. Second, SM may be due to an excessive host immune response resulting in a deregulated inflammatory state. Third, endothelial dysfunction may be a key component of SM pathogenesis linking sequestration and inflammation. High parasite biomass is also directly related to SM as it enhances the RBC sequestration, inflammation, and endothelial dysfunction **(Fig. 2)**. The clinical effect of sequestration and associated endothelial dysfunction depend on the organ(s) involved. In brain, it causes CM; in the lungs, it predisposes to respiratory failure; and in pregnant women, it causes placental malaria with its consequences causing low birth weight, preterm labor, and increased risk of abortion and stillbirth. Placental cytoadherence is mediated by binding to chondroitin sulfate and the effects are most severe in primigravid women.

Repeated exposure over a long period to malaria leads to premunition, which means protection from symptomatic disease in spite of ongoing blood stage infection. Asymptomatic *falciparum* or *vivax* parasitemia are common in areas of high endemicity and use of polymerase chain reaction (PCR) has revealed that parasites can persist for longer period. This asymptomatic infection in community is a real problem for malaria elimination.[2-4]

■ CLINICAL PRESENTATION

The majority of infections presents as uncomplicated malaria and only about 1% of *P. falciparum* infections present with severe clinical manifestations. An uncomplicated malaria presents with high fever, which may or may not be associated with chills and rigor along with general malaise, fatigue, arthralgia, myalgia, headache, abdominal discomfort, nausea, vomiting, and orthostatic hypotension. In nonendemic areas, malaria needs to be suspected in patients with a travel history to endemic countries. SM is a complex multisystem disease depending on the principal organ affected by disease and clinically present as CM, repeated convulsions, severe malarial anemia (SMA), acute kidney injury, acute respiratory distress syndrome (ARDS), jaundice, pulmonary edema, thrombocytopenia with or without significant

TABLE 1: Features of complicated/severe malaria*.

Impaired consciousness	Glasgow Coma Score <11 in adults or Blantyre Coma Score <3 in children
Prostration	*Generalized weakness:* Unable to sit, stand, or walk without assistance
Multiple convulsions	More than two episodes within 24 hours
Shock	• *Compensated shock:* Capillary refill ≥3s, but no hypotension • *Decompensated shock:* Systolic BP <70 mm Hg in children or <80 mm Hg in adults, with evidence of impaired perfusion
Pulmonary edema	Radiologically confirmed or SpO_2 <92% on room air with a respiratory rate >30/min
Significant bleeding	Recurrent or prolonged bleeding from nose, gums, or venepuncture sites; hematemesis or melena
Severe malarial anemia	• Hb ≤5 g/dL or hematocrit ≤15% in children <12 years of age • Hb ≤7 g/dL or hematocrit ≤20% in adults with parasite count >10,000/μL
Jaundice	Plasma or serum bilirubin >50 μmol/L (3 mg/dL) with parasite count >100,000/μL
Renal impairment	Plasma/serum creatinine >265 μmol/L (3 mg/dL) or blood urea >20 mmol/L
Acidosis	• A base deficit of >8 mEq/L or a plasma bicarbonate level of <15 mmol/L or venous plasma lactate • ≥5 mmol/L, manifesting clinically as rapid, deep, labored breathing
Hypoglycemia	Blood or plasma glucose <2.2 mmol/L (<40 mg/dL)
Hyperparasitemia	*Plasmodium falciparum* parasitemia >10%

*WHO Treatment Guidelines for Malaria, – 2015, 2021.
(BP: blood pressure; Hb: hemoglobin)

bleeding, hemoglobinuria, hyperparasitemia, shock, hypoglycemia, acidosis/hyperlactatemia (clinically manifested as respiratory distress) **(Table 1)**. Clinical manifestations of malaria differ between adults and children, with jaundice, shock, and multiorgan dysfunction being more frequent in the former and CM, anemia, and acidosis in the latter. Irrespective of the age, neurological involvement, ARDS, renal impairment, and multiorgan dysfunction are associated with poor outcomes. CM is characterized by severe impairment of consciousness (deep coma) in which other causes had been ruled out by relevant investigation. It is associated with high case fatality rate and neurological sequelae in the form of cognitive dysfunction and other neurological deficits in the survivors. Neurological complications following an episode of CM range from a reversible postmalaria neurological syndrome to permanent deficits including visual, motor, or language disorders and epilepsy. Brain swelling is a key pathogenetic event as evidenced by magnetic resonance imaging (MRI). Respiratory distress is common in both adults and children and presents with deep (acidotic) and labored breathing, tachypnea, lower chest indrawing, and sustained nasal flaring. Anemia is common and is typically multifactorial in origin importantly filtration in spleen of both infected and damaged uninfected RBCs, intravascular hemolysis, bone marrow suppression, and dyserythropoiesis. In the last decade, the pathogenic potential of *P. vivax* or *P. knowlesi* has also become evident and they are no longer considered to be benign. Severe *vivax* malaria can present with both sequestration and nonsequestration-related complications as seen in *P. falciparum* malaria including multiorgan dysfunction and death. Severe *knowlesi* malaria is associated with high parasite densities, acute kidney injury, shock, and respiratory failure.[1,5,6]

Pregnant women especially primigravida are particularly vulnerable as they have more chances of intrauterine growth restriction (IUGR), pregnancy loss, severe anemia, pulmonary edema, and hypoglycemia. Congenital malaria is rare in endemic countries where mothers have high levels of antibodies which they transmit to their offspring, however, this can also occur in naïve pregnant women with no immunity against malaria travel to endemic areas and get infected there. The diagnosis of congenital malaria is easy to miss, especially if the mother is asymptomatic. The clinical presentation mimics neonatal sepsis. Human immunodeficiency virus (HIV) coinfection increases malaria severity and parasite densities tend to be higher.[1,7]

■ LABORATORY DIAGNOSIS

The gold standard for malaria diagnosis remains light microscopy of stained blood films, thick films providing sensitivity, and thin films allowing speciation and quantification. However, rapid diagnostic tests (RDTs) now predominate as the first-line investigation. The commonly used *Plasmodium falciparum* histidine rich protein (PfHRP2) antigen-based tests remain positive for several weeks even after parasite clearance because of persisting pitted RBCs. With the recent reports of HRP2, gene deletion in certain areas of endemic malaria, its reliability, and usefulness had diminished. Parasite lactic dehydrogenase (pLDH) based RDT may be useful in these situations. Sometimes very high *falciparum* parasitemias can also produce negative results due to the prozone effect. The threshold of detection for these methods is approximately 50 parasites per μL (microscopy) and 200 parasites per μL for RDTs. Nucleic acid amplification-based tests (PCR) provide much greater sensitivity (often below one parasite per μL) but not useful for field study and routine examination.

TREATMENT

The principle aim of malaria treatment is preventing progression to severe disease and death, preventing malaria relapse and recrudescence, interrupting the transmission of malaria and preventing drug resistance. The treatment of uncomplicated *P. falciparum* malaria, and mixed malaria is artemisinin-based combination treatments (ACTs) except in the first trimester of pregnancy. These are combinations of two active drugs with different mechanisms of action and different half-lives. The leading ACTs in use are artemether–lumefantrine, artesunate–amodiaquine, dihydroartemisinin–piperaquine, artesunate–mefloquine, and artesunate plus sulfadoxine–pyrimethamine. Quinine remains efficacious, although it requires a long course of treatment (7 days). It is poorly tolerated, particularly by children, and needs to be combined with a second agent such as doxycycline or clindamycin. Along with this a single dose of 45 mg primaquine is also advocated **(Box 1)**.

Uncomplicated *P. vivax* patients are treated with chloroquine, and chloroquine-resistant *P. vivax* cases are treated with ACT as in *P. falciparum*. This should be followed by primaquine for 14 days to eradicate dormant hypnozoites. Although it is in use globally for nearly seven decades, its toxicity in G6PD-deficient individuals (severe or even life-threatening hemolysis) and compliance issues have made the treatment suboptimal. More recently, tafenoquine, a single-dose treatment with similar antihypnozoitic potential, has been approved by stringent regulatory authorities, but it has also similar toxicity in G6PD-deficient individuals, and thus G6PD screening becomes essential. The decision to admit a patient with uncomplicated malaria to hospital depends on the patient's condition and local guidelines. Early detection of malaria in pregnancy is vital. The patient of uncomplicated *falciparum* malaria in the first trimester is treated with a 7-day course of quinine and clindamycin and in second and third trimesters by ACT. *Vivax* malaria in pregnancy is treated with chloroquine unless resistance is suspected (when quinine should be given), but radical cure with primaquine is contraindicated.

Patients with SM (both *P. falciparum* and *P. vivax*) should be preferably admitted in intensive care ward as malaria complications may develop very fast, and may lead to death within few hours after the first symptoms. Parenteral artesunate is now widely accepted as the standard treatment, both in adults and children because of its definite superiority over quinine in achieving a rapid reduction of the parasite biomass. Intramuscular artemether seems to be inferior to intravenous (IV) artesunate in adults but is more effective that quinine. Parenteral treatment must be shifted to oral when the patient improves and is able to take orally **(Box 1)**.

BOX 1: Principles for the drug treatment of malaria*.

Severe malaria

Treatment of choice:
- Artesunate (IV or IM) 2.4 mg/kg* immediately, then at 12, 24 hours and daily until patient is able to take orally (*For children <20 kg, the parenteral artesunate dose is 3 mg/kg)

Alternatives:
- Artemether (IM) 3.2 mg/kg initial dose followed by 1.6 mg/kg daily he can take orally
- Quinine dihydrochloride (20 mg salt/kg) by slow intravenous infusion over 4 hours or by IM injection split to both anterior thighs, followed by 10 mg salt/kg 8 hours until patient is able to take orally.

Uncomplicated malaria

Plasmodium falciparum malaria:
- Artemether 1.4–4 mg/kg body weight + lumefantrine 10–16 mg/kg body weight, twice daily for 3 days
- Artesunate 4 mg/kg body weight + amodiaquine 10 mg/kg body weight, once daily for 3 days
- Artesunate 4 mg/kg body weight + mefloquine 8.3 mg/kg body weight, once daily for 3 days
- Dihydroartemisinin 4 mg/kg body weight + piperaquine 18 mg/kg body weight, once daily for 3 days (for children <25 kg, the dose of dihydroartemisinin is at least 2.5 mg/kg per day)
- Artesunate 4 mg/kg body weight + sulfadoxine–pyrimethamine 25/1.25 mg/kg body weight, once daily for 3 days
- Artesunate 4 mg/kg body weight + pyronaridine 7.5–15 mg/kg body weight, once daily for 3 days
- Quinine 10 mg/kg three times a day along with doxycycline 3 mg/kg for 7 days (doxycycline is combination in pregnant women and children 8 years instead use clindamycin 10 mg/kg, 12 hourly for 7 days).

Chloroquine sensitive *Plasmodium vivax* malaria:
- Chloroquine dose of 10 mg base/kg body weight at days 1 and 2 followed by 5 mg base/kg body weight at day 3.

*WHO Treatment Guidelines for Malaria – 2015, 2021; NVBDCP Guidelines for Diagnosis and Treatment of Malaria in India – 2014.

The presence of SM and multiorgan dysfunction influences the patient's overall outcome and requires vigorous and meticulous treatment simultaneously. The hyperpyrexia is treated by tepid sponging and paracetamol. Convulsions are treated by IV lorazepam followed by loading dose of phenytoin or fosphenytoin. Convulsive status should be treated with usual protocols. Hypoglycemia is very common in children and pregnant women and should be treated by IV 25–50% glucose. Usually, hypoglycemia responds well to standard therapy, although hyperinsulinemic hypoglycemia in association with quinine therapy responds well to long-acting somatostatin analogs. Blood transfusion is generally recommended if the hemoglobin level is <5 g/100 mL (hematocrit <15%). In acute renal failure or severe metabolic acidosis, hemofiltration or hemodialysis should be started early. The fluid balance is critical in SM because of narrow window between overhydration (pulmonary edema) and underhydration (exacerbation of renal impairment and tissue hypoperfusion). Pulmonary edema is treated by avoiding excessive hydration and use of oxygen, whereas overhydration requires stopping IV fluids and use of a diuretic (furosemide: 40 mg IV) along with withdrawing 3 mL/kg of the blood by venesection into a donor bag. Circulatory collapse, shock, and algid malaria are treated by parenteral antimicrobials and vasopressors, along with correction of hemodynamic disturbances. Bleeding and disseminated intravascular coagulation (DIC) require transfusion of fresh blood or clotting factors, along with vitamin K (10 mg IV). Bleeding associated with marked thrombocytopenia may require platelet transfusion. Hyperparasitemia (>20%) should be treated by exchange transfusion. A close monitoring of pregnant women is essential because of high incidence of pulmonary edema and hypoglycemia. Parenteral treatment (artesunate or quinine) should be given for at least the first dose in congenital *falciparum* malaria, followed by ACT. Congenital *vivax* malaria can be treated with oral chloroquine unless the infant is very unwell, in which case parenteral drugs should be used.[8,9]

Treatment Failure

When malaria treatment is not successful, symptoms may recur with an associated positive parasitemia 2-6 weeks after initial regimen and is not always due to drug resistance but may be due to high parasite densities (particularly in nonimmune individuals), poor drug bioavailability, nonadherence to therapy, and resistance of partner drugs in ACT and substandard antimalarials. Relapse of *vivax* malaria is common in Southeast Asia including India and is not regarded a treatment failure.

Antimalarial Drug Resistance

Emergence of antimalarial drug resistance has a strong impact on providing effective antimalarial drug treatment, malaria control, and elimination. It has been observed with almost all antimalarials including artemisinins. The sporadic case reports of delayed clearance times for artemisinins have been reported in Southeast Asia, including some parts of India. Polymorphisms in the kelch13 (k13) propeller gene of *P. falciparum* have been associated with artemisinin resistance. Triple artemisinin-based combinations (dihydroartemisinin-piperaquine with mefloquine and artemether-lumefantrine with amodiaquine) are being evaluated in an attempt to bridge the gap until newer more effective medicines become available.

Adjunctive Therapies for Severe Malaria

In spite of treatment with highly effective drugs such as artemisinin and quinine, the death or neurological disability is very high in patients of SM. Thus, the adjunctive therapies are used in combination with primary antimalarial treatment, with the aim of improving clinical outcomes, reducing mortality, and preventing neurocognitive sequelae. Several adjunctive therapies such as high-dose steroid therapy, anti-TNF antibodies, iron chelators, pentoxifylline, IV immunoglobulins, cyclosporine A, N-acetylcysteine, heparin, aspirin, ibuprofen, cytoadherence, and/or rosetting inhibitors, immunomodulators (rosiglitazone, pantethine, and statins), antiapoptosis molecules (fasudil), NO modulators (L-arginine, inhaled NO), or neuroprotectors (erythropoietin, citicoline), mannitol, NO, or exchanges transfusions have been evaluated in last three decades but they are either ineffective or have proved to be more harmful. Thus, presently, we have no such drug which can be advocated.[10]

■ VACCINE

Malaria is prevented by chemoprophylaxis, bite-avoidance, vector-control measures, and vaccination. The RTS,S/AS01 malaria vaccine, approved by stringent regulatory authorities (European Medicines Agency) in the year 2015, has shown consistently significant levels of protection, both against clinical malaria and severe malarial disease. A pilot and large-scale implementation program, promoted by the World Health Organization (WHO), was launched in 2019, to evaluate the impact on overall infant mortality and the safety of its routine use. A clear recommendation will expand the program of immunization throughout *falciparum* endemic settings. The use of merozoite stage proteins vaccine and transmission blocking vaccines against sexual-stage antigens has not shown any robust evidence of protection against disease.

■ MALARIA IN INDIA

The World Malaria Report (WMR) 2020, released by WHO, indicates that India has made considerable progress in reducing its malaria burden. India is the only high endemic country which has reported a decline of 17.6% in 2019 as compared to 2018. India has also contributed to the largest drop in cases region-wide, from approximately 20 million to about 6 million. The percentage drop in the malaria cases was 71.8% and deaths was 73.9% between 2000 and 2019. India achieved a reduction of 83.34% in malaria morbidity and 92% in malaria mortality between the year 2000 (2,031,790 cases, 932 deaths) and 2019 (338,494 cases, 77 deaths). The figures and trends between last two decades clearly show the drastic decline in malaria and in this regard, the malaria elimination target of 2030 looks achievable.[7,11]

Plasmodium vivax remains a substantial health problem and economic burden in India with proven difficulties to control it, particularly in urban areas. Although the number of malaria cases has declined in the recent years, the relative proportions of *P. vivax* cases are increasing. *P. vivax* is transmitted by a variety of vectors across diverse ecological habitats and shows polymorphism in the patterns of relapse. It can also be overlooked as a pathogen where a mixed infection with *P. falciparum* is present. During last two decades, there is substantial evidence that *P. vivax* is associated with all sorts of SM including CM and death in India. This may be because of improved diagnostic facilities, reporting, investigation, and/or changes in *P. vivax* pathogenicity, which may be specific to individual parasite populations in different areas. As there is heterogeneity in transmission intensities of the *P. vivax*, there is tremendous scope for research in India for studying the parasite biology; detection and treatment of hypnozoites to ensure radical cure.[1,2]

> **TAKE HOME MESSAGE**
>
> - The presentation of malaria in India is very complex due to uneven distribution of *P. vivax* and *P. falciparum* in different geographical region. Although the total number of malaria cases and deaths is showing decreasing trend, the number of *P. vivax* malaria is increasing. Current data shows that India is harboring the largest number of *P. vivax* cases in the world. There is substantial evidence that *P. vivax* is associated with both sequestration and nonsequestration-related severe presentation including CM and death, which were commonly reported with *P. falciparum* malaria infection only. This may be because of changes in *P. vivax* pathogenicity and human immune system in a given population and location. However, the intricacies of host parasite inter-relationship are not clear.
> - According to the Guidelines for Diagnosis and Treatment of Malaria in India (2014), the uncomplicated *P. vivax* should be treated with standard dosage of chloroquine and 14 days primaquine (after G6PD determination), whereas uncomplicated *P. falciparum* cases should be treated with ACT and single-dose primaquine. The treatment of SM in the first trimester of pregnancy is parenteral quinine and clindamycin. However, if quinine is not available, artemisinin derivatives may be used to save the life of the mother. In the second and third trimesters of pregnancy and all other male and female patients should be treated with parenteral artemisinin.

■ REFERENCES

1. Kochar DK, Das A, Kochar A, Middha S, Acharya J, Tanwar GS, et al. A prospective study on adult patients of severe malaria caused by Plasmodium falciparum, Plasmodium vivax and mixed infection from Bikaner, northwest India. J Vector Borne Dis. 2014;51(3):200-10.
2. Ohiagu FO, Chikezie PC, Aahneku CC, Chikezie CM. Pathophysiology of severe malaria infection. Asian J Health Sci. 2021;7(2):1-16.
3. Schiess N, Villabona-Rueda A, Cottier KE, Huether K, Chipeta J, Stins MF. Pathophysiology and neurologic sequelae of cerebral malaria. Malar J. 2020;19(1):266.

4. Hora R, Kapoor P, Kaur K, Mishra PC. Cerebral malaria—clinical manifestations and pathogenesis. Metab Brain Dis. 2016;31(2):225-37.
5. Siddiqui AJ, Adnan M, Jahan S, Redman W, Saeed M, Patel M. Neurological disorder and psychosocial aspects of cerebral malaria: what is new on its pathogenesis and complications? A minireview. Folia Parasitologica. 2020;67:015.
6. Luzolo AL, Ngoyi DM. Cerebral malaria. Brain Res Bull. 2019;145:53-8.
7. World Health Organization. Severe Malaria. Trop Med Int Health. 2014;19 (Suppl 1):7-131.
8. World Health Organization. Guidelines for the Treatment of Malaria, 3rd edition. Geneva: WHO; 2015.
9. Guidelines for Diagnosis and Treatment of Malaria in India – 2009, Government of India. [online] Available from https://nvbdcp.gov.in/Doc/Guidelines_for_Diagnosis___Treatment.pdf. [Last accessed July 2022].
10. Zou Y, Tuo F, Zhang Z, Guo J, Yuan Y, Zhang H, et al. Safety and efficacy of adjunctive therapy with artesunate in the treatment of severe malaria: a systematic review and meta-analysis. Front Pharmacol. 2020;11:596697.
11. World Health Organization. World Malaria Report 2020. Geneva: World Health Organization; 2020. [online] Available from https://www.who.int/publications/i/item/9789240015791. [Last accessed July 2022].
12. Kochar DK, Kochar A. Malaria in India with special reference to severe vivax malaria. JIMA. 2020;118(7):56-63.

Chapter 6

Kala-azar

Jaya Chakravarty, Sunanda Ghosh

■ INTRODUCTION

Leishmaniasis is caused by an intracellular protozoa of the genus *Leishmania* which mainly affects the reticuloendothelial system. It causes varying clinical syndromes ranging from cutaneous ulcers to fatal visceral disease which may be broadly classified as—visceral leishmaniasis (VL), cutaneous leishmaniasis (CL), and mucosal leishmaniasis (ML).

■ ORGANISM

Visceral leishmaniasis is caused by the *Leishmania donovani* complex. In the Indian subcontinent and Africa, *L. donovani*, is the causative organism of VL, while *Leishmania infantum* (*Leishmania chagasi*) causes VL in the Mediterranean basin, Central and South America.

■ TRANSMISSION

The disease is transmitted by the bite of the female sandfly of genus *Phlebotomus* in the Old World (Asia, Africa, and Europe) and *Lutzomyia* in the New World (America). Transmission is anthroponotic in South Asia and the Horn of Africa, where humans with kala-azar or post-kala-azar dermal leishmaniasis (PKDL) are the main reservoir. In the Mediterranean, the Middle East, and Brazil, the transmission is zoonotic, with the domestic dog being the most important reservoir. Human-to-human transmission of VL through infected needles has been reported among intravenous (IV) drug users in the Mediterranean region.

■ BURDEN OF DISEASE

Annually an estimated 50,000–90,000 new cases of VL occur worldwide. In 2020, >90% of new cases reported to World Health Organization (WHO) occurred in 10 countries: Brazil, China, Ethiopia, Eritrea, India, Kenya, Somalia, South Sudan, Sudan, and Yemen. Out of these most cases occurred in Brazil, East Africa, and in India. In India, a total of 1,276 cases were reported to the National Vector Borne Disease Control Programme in 2021 with most of them coming from the state of Bihar, Jharkhand, West Bengal, and Uttar Pradesh.

Most cases of human immunodeficiency virus (HIV)-VL infection were initially reported from southwestern Europe where 70% cases of VL in adults were associated with HIV infection. Now cases are being reported from sub-Saharan Africa, especially Ethiopia, Brazil, and South Asia. Studies from India showed that 1.8–5.6% of VL patients were HIV-positive. While in Ethiopia, 10.4–40% of VL patients were coinfected with HIV.

■ LIFE CYCLE AND PATHOPHYSIOLOGY

Leishmania occurs in two forms:
1. Extracellular, flagellate promastigotes in the sandfly
2. Intracellular, nonflagellate amastigotes in humans.

Promastigotes enter through the proboscis of the female sandfly into the skin of the human. These are first attacked by the neutrophils of the body at the site of entry. The infected neutrophils are then taken up by the macrophages and dendritic cells—where the organisms multiply in their amastigote form—infecting other healthy macrophages. When an infected individual is bitten by an uninfected sandfly, the amastigote forms are transformed into promastigote form inside the sandfly and stored in their midgut for further transmission.

Most infections are asymptomatic as the parasites are cleared by host immune response. Asymptomatic *Leishmania* infection is nine times more frequent than incident VL disease in India and Nepal. However, coinfection with HIV increases the risk of developing active VL by 100 and 2,320 times.

The reticuloendothelial hyperplasia that follows infection with *L. donovani* or *L. infantum* affects the spleen, the liver, the mucosa of the small intestine, the bone marrow, the lymph nodes, and the other lymphoid tissues. The lifespan of leukocytes and erythrocytes is reduced, causing granulocytopenia and anemia. The liver function may be normal or altered. Altered liver function with decreased prothrombin and thrombocytopenia may lead to severe mucosal hemorrhage. Hypoalbuminemia is associated with edema and other features of malnutrition. Diarrhea may occur as a result of intestinal parasitization and ulceration or secondary enteritis. In the advanced stage, intercurrent infections are frequent.

The immune response in patients developing active VL is complex, in addition to increased production of multiple inflammatory cytokines and chemokines, patients have marked increase in interleukin (IL)-10 levels (which further promotes the survival of the pathogen in the macrophages). While secretion of interferon-gamma (IFN-γ), tumor necrosis factor-alpha (TNF-α), and other proinflammatory cytokines by the T helper 1 (Th1) subset of lymphocytes help to clear the infection.

CLINICAL FEATURES

The most common presentation of VL is subacute onset of fever, splenomegaly, hepatomegaly, pancytopenia, progressive anemia, and weight loss. Lymphadenopathy is only encountered in the patients of East Africa. Secondary infections such as measles, pneumonia, tuberculosis, bacillary or amebic dysentery, and gastroenteritis are common in late stage. Patients with thrombocytopenia and liver dysfunction may present with mucosal bleeding such as epistaxis, retinal hemorrhages, and gastrointestinal bleeding. The patients also have generalized weakness, cachexia, and hyperpigmentation. Untreated, the disease is fatal in most patients.

POST-KALA-AZAR DERMAL LEISHMANIASIS

In the Indian subcontinent, 5–15% patients (highest in Bangladesh) with VL develop hypopigmented macules, papules, and/or indurated nodules; 6 months to 3 years after treatment which is called PKDL. Spontaneous resolution is rare in the Indian subcontinent and they can be the source of infection. On the other hand in East Africa especially Sudan, up to 60% patients may develop PKDL, and is seen concurrently with VL or immediately thereafter within 6 months. In most patients, the skin manifestations resolve spontaneously, and only in a small minority treatment is needed.

HUMAN IMMUNODEFICIENCY VIRUS-VISCERAL LEISHMANIASIS COINFECTION

Human immunodeficiency virus infection not only increases the risk of developing VL, but it also reduces the likelihood of a therapeutic response, and increases the chances of relapse. The clinical features are usually similar to a classic VL patient; however, some may have involvement of uncommon sites, e.g., infiltration of skin, oral mucosa, gastrointestinal tract, lungs, and other organs.

DIAGNOSIS

Hematological and Biochemical Abnormalities

Patients usually present with pancytopenia; leukopenia and anemia occur early followed by thrombocytopenia. There is a marked polyclonal increase in serum immunoglobulins with reversal of albumin globulin ratio. Serum levels of hepatic aminotransferases are raised in a significant proportion of patients, and serum bilirubin levels are elevated occasionally. Renal dysfunction is uncommon.

Parasite Detection

The visualization of the amastigotes from tissue aspirates (sensitivity of splenic, bone marrow, and lymph node aspirates is 93–99, 53–86, and 50%, respectively) is the gold standard for the diagnosis of VL. It is mandatory for the diagnosis of relapse or recurrence of the disease. Culture of tissue samples often increases sensitivity. Splenic aspiration has the risk of developing life-threatening hemorrhage if done by untrained person.

Serological Tests

Several serologic tests are currently used to detect antibodies to *Leishmania*. An enzyme-linked immunosorbent assay (ELISA), DAT (direct antibody test), and indirect immunofluorescent antibody test (IFAT) are used in sophisticated laboratories. In the resource-limited settings, a rapid immunochromatographic test based on the detection of antibodies to a recombinant antigen (rK39) consisting of 39 amino acids conserved in the kinesin region of *L. infantum* is widely used. The test requires only a drop of fingerprick blood or serum, and the result can be read rapidly. Sensitivity of the rK39 rapid diagnostic test (RDT) in immunocompetent individuals is ~98% and its specificity is ~90%. Thus, it has been adopted by the national program for diagnosis of kala-azar in the field.

Tests detecting antibodies have some drawbacks. Since the antibodies remain positive for years after cure, these tests cannot be used for measurement of cure or detection of relapse. Moreover, up to 32% healthy individuals living in endemic areas with no history of VL may be positive for antileishmanial antibodies due to asymptomatic infection. Thus, antibody-based tests must always be used in combination with a standardized clinical case definition. Febrile illness associated with hepatosplenomegaly, pancytopenia along with hypergammaglobulinemia, and rK39 test positive in patients from endemic region suggests the diagnosis of VL.

■ MOLECULAR DIAGNOSIS

Qualitative detection of leishmanial nucleic acid by polymerase chain reaction (PCR) or by loop-mediated isothermal amplification (LAMP) and quantitative detection by real-time PCR is highly sensitive; however, as they can be performed only in specialized laboratories, they have yet to be used for routine diagnosis of VL in endemic areas. Polymerase chain reaction can distinguish among the major species of *Leishmania* infecting humans.

Thus, to conclude, at present, rK39-based rapid tests are mainly used for the diagnosis of VL. However, their persistent positivity long after cure and in a high proportion of individuals staying in endemic areas is a major drawback.

DIFFERENTIAL DIAGNOSIS

The differential diagnosis of VL often mimics other tropical febrile illnesses such as malaria, typhoid fever, tuberculosis, brucellosis, and histoplasmosis. Huge splenomegaly secondary to portal hypertension, chronic myeloid leukemia, or tropical splenomegaly syndrome may also be confused with VL.

TREATMENT

General Management

Anemia in VL should be corrected by red cell transfusion, and other coinfections should be managed.

Antileishmanial Drugs

Pentavalent Antimonial Compounds

Two pentavalent antimonial (SbV) preparations are available: Sodium stibogluconate (SSG) and meglumine antimoniate. The daily dose is 20 mg/kg by IV/intramuscular (IM) route, and duration is 28–30 days. Risks of ventricular arrhythmia, sudden death, and pancreatitis are there. Due to widespread resistance of antimonials in the Indian subcontinent, it is no longer used here.

Amphotericin B

Amphotericin B (AmB) is currently considered as a first-line drug in Bihar, India. In rest of the world, it is used when antimonial treatment fails. Conventional AmB deoxycholate is administered in doses of 0.75–1.0 mg/kg on alternate days for total of 15 infusions. Fever with chills is an almost universal adverse effect to AmB infusions. Nausea, vomiting, and thrombophlebitis are common. Acute toxicities can be minimized by premedications such as antihistamines (chlorpheniramine) and antipyretics (acetaminophen). AmB can cause renal dysfunction, hypokalemia, hypersensitivity reactions, bone marrow suppression, and myocarditis.

Liposomal AmB (L-AmB) has been used extensively to treat VL in all parts of the world. This is the only drug approved by the United States Food and Drug Administration (US FDA) for the treatment of VL. The dose of L-AmB required varies with region. In the Indian subcontinent, a single dose of 10 mg/kg results in a cure rate of >95%, and is currently one of the preferred treatments for VL in this region. In the Mediterranean region, Africa, and South America, a total dose of 18–21 mg/kg has been recommended. Adverse effects of L-AmB are usually mild and include infusion reactions, backache, and occasional reversible nephrotoxicity.

Paromomycin

Paromomycin (PM) (aminosidine) is an aminocyclitol-aminoglycoside antibiotic with antileishmanial activity. It is approved in India for the treatment of VL at an IM dose of 11 mg of base/kg daily for 21 days; this regimen produces a cure rate of 94.6%. The main drawback is the need for IM injections. A few patients may develop hepatotoxicity, reversible ototoxicity, and rarely nephrotoxicity and tetany.

Miltefosine

Miltefosine, an alkylphosphocholine, is the first oral compound approved for the treatment of VL. This drug has a long half-life (150–200 hours) and the recommended dose for patients of Indian subcontinent is a daily dose of 50 mg for 28 days in patients weighing <25 kg, a twice-daily dose of 50 mg for 28 days for patients weighing ≥25 kg. Because miltefosine is teratogenic in rats, its use is contraindicated during pregnancy. Adverse effects such as nausea and vomiting is common. Asymptomatic elevation of liver enzymes and rarely nephrotoxicity may occur. Recently, ocular toxicity has been reported in patients with PKDL.

Multidrug Therapy

Multidrug therapy for leishmaniasis is likely to be preferred in the future. Its potential advantages in VL are: (1) Better compliance, lower costs along with shorter treatment courses, and decreased hospitalization, (2) less toxicity due to lower drug doses, and (3) a reduced chances of developing resistance. In a study from India, one dose of L-AmB (5 mg/kg) followed by miltefosine for 7 days, PM for 10 days, or both miltefosine and PM simultaneously for 10 days (in their usual daily doses) produced a cure rate of >97% (all three combinations).

Treatment Guidelines

Visceral Leishmaniasis

Recent treatment guidelines recommend a single dose of L-AmB or combination therapy (miltefosine with PM) as the preferred treatment options in the Indian subcontinent. The combination of SSG with PM for 17 days is the treatment of choice in East Africa and Yemen, whereas L-AmB up to a total dose of 18–21 mg/kg remains the drug of choice in Mediterranean Basin, Middle East, Central Asia, and America.

Human Immunodeficiency Virus-Visceral Leishmaniasis Coinfection

Liposomal AmB at a total dose of 40 mg/kg in the dose of 3–5 mg/kg/day on days 1–5, 10, 17, 24, 31, and 38 is recommended but relapse is common.

Post-kala-azar Dermal Leishmaniasis

In India, miltefosine for 12 weeks or AmB 60–80 doses over 4 months are the recommended regimens for PKDL. In East Africa, PKDL is not routinely treated, as the majority of cases (85%) heal spontaneously. Patients with severe or disfiguring disease, persistent lesions (>6 months), or concomitant anterior uveitis and young children with oral lesions that interfere with feeding are treated with SSG (20 mg/kg/ day) for up to 2 months or a 20-day course of L-AmB at 2.5 mg/kg/day.

REFERENCES

1. Control of the Leishmaniasis. Report of a meeting of the WHO Expert Committee on the Control of Leishmaniases. Geneva;2010.
2. Chakravarty J, Sundar S. Current and emerging medications for the treatment of leishmaniasis. Expert Opin Pharmacother. 2019;20(10):1251-65.
3. Pan American Health Organization. Leishmaniasis in the Americas: treatment recommendations.Washington, D.C.: PAHO;2018. http://iris.paho.org.
4. Sundar S, Chakravarty J, Agarwal D, Rai M, Murray HW. Single-dose liposomal amphotericin B for visceral leishmaniasis in India. N Engl J Med. 2010;362(6):504-12.
5. National centre for Vector Borne Diseases Control. Ministry of Health & Family Welfare, Government of India. https://nvbdcp.gov.in/index1.php?lang=1&level=1&sublinkid=5774&lid=3692.

Chapter 7

Scrub Typhus and Other Rickettsial Diseases

*Prasanta Kumar Bhattacharya,
Nandini Chatterjee, Aritra Kumar Ray*

■ INTRODUCTION

Scrub typhus is an acute infectious disease presenting with fever. It is caused by a rickettsial organism, *Orientia tsutsugamushi*, and is transmitted to humans through bites of infected larvae (chiggers) of trombiculid mites. It is one of the most common rickettsial diseases found in India. The word "Typhus" meaning "smoke" in Greek has been used to describe the confused state of mind associated with these high fevers, and "Scrub" describes the terrain with scrub vegetation where these mites are commonly found. The disease is also known as tsutsugamushi disease, mite-borne typhus, Japanese-river fever, and tropical typhus.

■ EPIDEMIOLOGY

First described from Japan in 1899, Scrub typhus is endemic in the geographical *"tsutsugamushi triangle"* (**Fig. 1**) extending from northern Japan and far-eastern Russia in the north, to northern Australia in the south, and to Pakistan in the west. However, with its sporadic detection in Africa and South America and the newly discovered *Orientia chuto sp. nov.* in UAE, this territorial extent has extended beyond this "triangle" to have possibly distributed around the tropical/subtropical belt globally, rather than confined to Asia.[1,2] Typhus is under-recognized in Asia; nearly 30% of malaria-negative fevers are attributed to rickettsial infections, scrub typhus being the most common.[3] In Southeast Asia alone, an estimated 1 million cases of scrub typhus occur yearly, which translates into approximately 50,000–80,000 deaths per year. In India, outbreaks have been reported among troops during World War II in Assam and (undivided) Bengal, and in the 1965 Indo-Pak war. Several other outbreaks have been reported from areas located in the sub-Himalayan belt, from Jammu to Nagaland.[4]

■ PATHOPHYSIOLOGY

Transmission

The trombiculid mites act as both vectors and reservoir of *O. tsutsugamushi* due to transovarial transmission. The infected larva of the mites (chiggers) feed on small rodents (field mouse, rats, squirrels, and bandicoot)

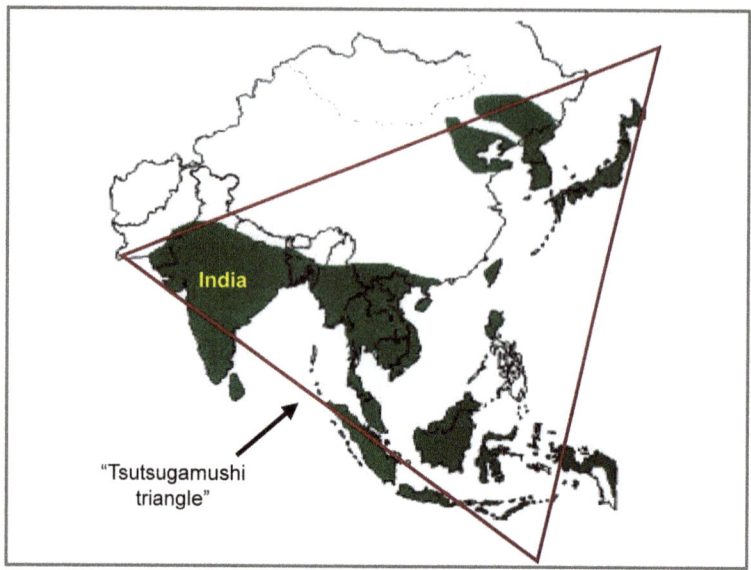

Fig. 1: The "Tsutsugamushi triangle".

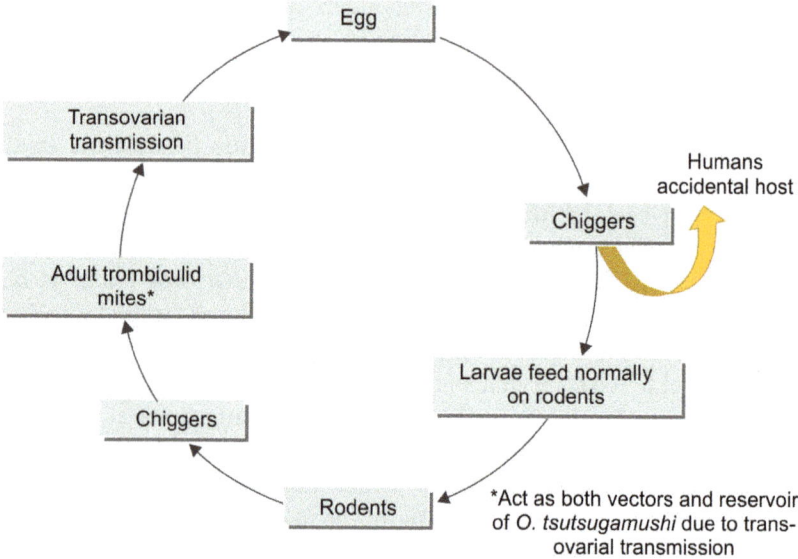

Fig. 2: Transmission of *Orientia tsutsugamushi* from trombiculid mite to humans.

transmitting the disease. Humans are accidental hosts with no person-to-person transmission **(Fig. 2)**.

Pathophysiology

The pathophysiological hallmark of the disease is disseminated vasculitis, followed by vascular injury of the involved tissues and organs. Such injury to the skin leads to macular and maculopapular rash; involvement of the internal organs such as liver, brain, kidney, meninges, and lungs leads to multiorgan dysfunction (MOD).

The organism multiplies at the site of inoculation which leads to ulceration and necrosis, evolving into an "eschar". Within a few days, the patients develop rickettsemia with involvement of the vascular endothelium leading to vascular injury of several organs, which may progress to MOD.

■ CLINICAL FEATURES

The variability and nonspecific presentation often make it difficult to diagnose the disease clinically.[5] Clinically it ranges from a mild, self-limiting disease to a fatal illness (35–50% cases), with MOD, if not promptly diagnosed and appropriately treated. After a variable incubation period ranging from 7 to 21 days, acute fever is the most common presenting symptom, often associated with rigors, chills, breathlessness, regional lymphadenopathy, cough, nausea, vomiting, diarrhea, constipation, conjunctival suffusion, myalgia, and headache. A maculopapular rash may appear at the end of first week, first on the chest, abdomen, and trunk and then on proximal extremities.[5] A painless papule occurs at the bite site, prior to development of other disease symptoms. This later ulcerates, and transforms into a black crust or "eschar" in a variable proportion (10–92%) of patients, depending upon how thoroughly the patient was examined by the clinician, besides other factors such as host immunity and bacterial virulence. Eschars develop usually at sites where the skin surfaces meet, such as axilla, groin, and inguinal areas **(Fig. 3)**, but multiple eschars may also be seen.

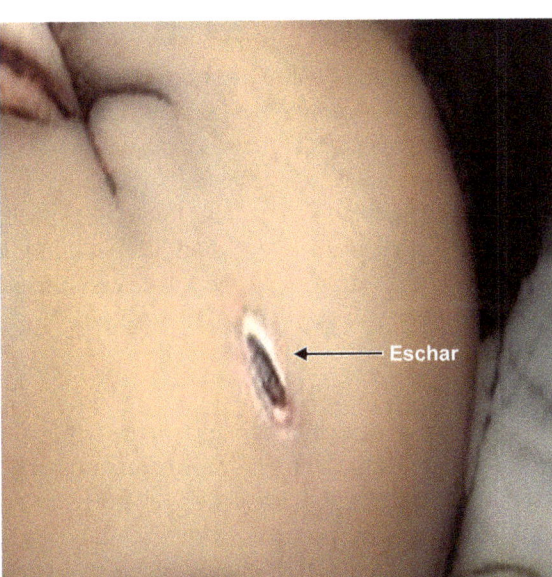

Fig. 3: Eschar.

COMPLICATIONS

Scrub typhus is associated with various systemic complications, commonly involving the respiratory, cardiovascular, renal, hepatic, central nervous systems and often leads to multiple-organ involvement. Severe complications, including acute respiratory distress syndrome, shock, hepatitis, acute kidney injury, meningoencephalitis, and myocarditis, may occur in varying proportions of patients. These complications increase the mortality. Sepsis has also been recognized as a complication in up to 49% of cases, which increases the mortality of the disease.[6]

DIAGNOSIS

Scrub typhus usually presents as undifferentiated fever, without any apparent localization like the respiratory or urinary tract infections. Accordingly the symptoms and signs are nonspecific and several diagnostic possibilities such as malaria, enteric fever, dengue, leptospirosis, spotted fever rickettsioses, and Hantavirus fever have to be considered, especially in the tropics. A detailed clinical history, examination, and relevant laboratory tests are necessary to arrive at an etiological diagnosis. The presence of an eschar makes the diagnosis of scrub typhus highly likely, although its presence is variable and is usually not found in the critically sick patients.[2] Hence, there should be a high index of suspicion for scrub typhus in any undifferentiated fever with a strongly suggestive epidemiological setting.

Accurate and early diagnosis of scrub typhus is very crucial for initiating early treatment with the best prognosis. Unfortunately, this remains as a challenge because the clinical features are nonspecific and mimics various other infective fevers common in the tropics, as mentioned above, from which it has to be differentiated **(Table 1)**. Therefore, one has to rely on laboratory tests for a diagnosis **(Table 2)**. Unfortunately, many of these tests are either not readily available, or are expensive. Comparison of the various diagnostic tests in terms of availability, costs, and their diagnostic accuracy is shown in **Table 3**. The Weil–Felix agglutination test, which is easily available and most extensively used, has poor sensitivity and is nonspecific. The highly sensitive and specific tests are either not readily available in primary care setting where it is most necessary, require sophisticated infrastructure, and/or are very costly for routine use in government hospitals.

TREATMENT

Doxycycline is the preferred drug in the treatment of scrub typhus **(Table 4)**. A therapeutic response to doxycycline therapy is often used as a diagnostic test. In patients who can take orally, it is given as 100 mg twice a day for 7 days. In critically ill patients, intravenous doxycycline should be used. Intravenous

TABLE 1: Differential diagnosis of scrub typhus from common fevers in the tropics.

Disease	Diagnostic tests
Malaria	PBS, antigen
Arbovirus infections (dengue, chikungunya)	NS1 antigen, IgM, IgG assays; dengue rash finer, more erythematous, marked thrombocytopenia
Leptospirosis	PCR (full blood), culture (blood, CSF)
Meningococcal diseases	Blood and CSF cultures
Typhoid	Appropriate sample culture, serology
Relapsing fever (lice or ticks)	*Borrelia* in blood smears, serology, or PCR
Viral fevers (with macular rash): EB, IM, primary HIV	By serology
Other typhus (e.g., SFG, TG)	Distinguished only by specific serological tests with acute and convalescent samples (IFA, IIP, ELISA) or PCR assays tests, same treatment for all

(CSF: cerebrospinal fluid; EB: Epstein–Barr; ELISA: enzyme-linked immunoassay; HIV: human immunodeficiency virus; IFA: immunofluorescent assay; IgG: immunoglobulin G; IgM: immunoglobulin M; IIP: indirect immunoperoxidase test; IM: intramuscular; PBS: peripheral blood smear; PCR: polymerase chain reaction; SFG: spotted fever group; TG: typhus group)

TABLE 2: Different laboratory tests for diagnosing scrub typhus.

Type of test	Name of test
Serology	• Weil–Felix OX-K • Immuno-chromatographic tests (ICTs) • Indirect fluorescent antibody (IFA) test • Indirect immunoperoxidase (IIP)
Orientia tsutsugamushi isolation	• Cell culture • Mouse inoculation
Genetic	Real time PCR

(PCR: polymerase chain reaction)

azithromycin may be used in isolation or combined with oral doxycycline. Azithromycin is also the preferred drug for scrub typhus in pregnancy, where doxycycline is avoided. Rifampicin may be considered when doxycycline resistance is present, but should be avoided in tuberculosis endemic countries. Chloramphenicol is the most common alternative to tetracycline, but is contraindicated in pregnancy.

TABLE 3: Comparison of different diagnostic tests.

Test type	Acute sensitivity	Specificity	Cost/sample	Time	Setting	Comment
Weil–Felix OX-K*	+	++	+	6–18 hours	Primary	Poor sensitivity
ICT	++	+++	+++	<30 minutes	Primary	Rapid simple, quality questionable
IFA/IIP*	++	+++	++++/+++	2 hours	Ref laboratory	Serology gold standard
Real-time PCR	+++	+++++	+++	3 hours	Ref laboratory	Contamination
Cell culture/Mouse Inoculation**	+	+++++	+++++	7–60 days 5–30 days	BSL 3 laboratory	Sophisticated infrastructure
ELISA	+++	+++	++	4–6 hours	Tertiary care setup	Relatively simple, requires infrastructure

(ELISA: enzyme-linked immunoassay; ICT: immunochromatographic test; IFA: immunofluorescent assay; IIP: indirect immunoperoxidase test; PCR: polymerase chain reaction)
*Requires paired samples; retrospective diagnosis
**Retrospective diagnosis
Ref laboratory: Reference laboratory
BSL 3 laboratory: Bio safety level 3 laboratory

TABLE 4: Specific treatment for scrub typhus.

Name of drug	Dose and administration in adults	Comments
Doxycycline	100 mg twice daily for 7 days	• Drug of choice • Intravenous preferred for sick patients • Rapid defervescence within 48 hours
Tetracycline	500 mg 4 times daily for 7 days	Efficacy same as doxycycline, but more side effects
Azithromycin	*Mild infections:* 500 mg single dose *Severe infections:* 500 mg once daily × 3–5 days ± 1 g loading dose	• Preferred drug in pregnancy • In mild cases symptom duration similar when compared with doxycycline • Recommended when doxycycline resistance is present
Chloramphenicol	500 mg every 6 hours for 7 days	• Most common alternative to tetracycline • Contraindicated in pregnancy
Rifampicin	600–900 mg daily for 7 days	• In mild scrub typhus, combination with doxycycline not more efficacious than either drug alone • Caution in tuberculosis endemic areas

■ INDIAN PERSPECTIVE

Is Scrub Typhus Re-emerging in India?

Studies in the 1960s and 1970s have documented the endemicity of scrub typhus in various parts of India. However, the disease was virtually lost from the radar of the scientific community until the beginning of the last decade. The possible causes for this disappearance are the widespread use of insecticides for other vector-borne diseases, the empirical treatment of febrile illnesses with tetracyclines and chloramphenicol and the changes in lifestyle.

However, of late, there has been an increase in the incidence of the disease across the country. It was earlier prevalent in the foothills of Himalayas—in the states and union territories of Jammu and Kashmir, Himachal Pradesh, Sikkim, West Bengal, Assam, Manipur, Nagaland, Meghalaya, and sporadically in Tamil Nadu and Kerala. However, samples are now being tested positive even from Delhi, Chandigarh, Haryana, Rajasthan, Maharashtra, Uttarakhand, and Chhattisgarh. Further, a clear re-emergence has been documented from several states in India, including Himachal Pradesh, Tamil Nadu, Kerala, Maharashtra, Bihar, Karnataka, Jammu and Kashmir, Uttaranchal, Rajasthan,

West Bengal, and Meghalaya. This increase in the incidence of the disease in India since the last decade can be due to two possible reasons: (1) Actual re-emergence of the disease and (2) improved diagnosis.

Some of the possible theories for an actual re-emergence of the disease in recent times are:
- Change in the habitat of mites from shrubs of hilly terrains to urban locales
- Unplanned urbanization in the hitherto forestlands
- Deforestation
- Human behavioral changes, e.g., camping in forests
- Rapid transport leading to displacement of vectors and rodents from one place to another.

Though it is evident that ecological factors have contributed to the re-emergence, the role of improved diagnostic facilities also cannot be ignored. The outbreaks of scrub typhus occur mainly in the post-monsoon seasons, coinciding with other acute febrile illnesses such as dengue and malaria, with similar clinical features. This actually necessitates the need for laboratory tests to confirm the diagnosis. Unfortunately, the diagnostic test widely used earlier, the Weil–Felix agglutination test, lacks both sensitivity and specificity. Therefore, the possibility of underdiagnosis was high. Results may be negative during early stages of disease because agglutinating antibodies are detectable only during second week of illness. However, the newer enzyme-linked immunoassay (ELISA) tests has 90% sensitivity and specificity, allowing detection of immunoglobulin G (IgG) and immunoglobulin M (IgM) antibodies, and provides positive results within 3–4 days after the onset of illness. The rapid immunochromatographic test (ICT) has made diagnosis easier in resource-constrained settings. Confirmatory tests including immunofluorescence assay (IFA) and molecular diagnostics including polymerase chain reaction (PCR) have further aided in confirmation of cases. These possibilities of underdiagnosis in the last decade can be indirectly assessed from the different tests used to diagnose scrub typhus in various Indian studies over the years **(Table 5)**. While most available studies done in first decade of the 21st century used the Weil–Felix test, the studies done subsequently have been using the newer tests, namely IgM ELISA and PCR, which are more sensitive and specific in diagnosing scrub typhus.[7]

RICKETSIAL DISEASES

Rickettsial diseases are a group of important re emergent infections that is gradually coming in the forefront of differentials for acute undifferentiated fevers.

In the past cases have been reported from Assam and Burma army barracks during the Second World War along with malaria. Scrub typhus and Indian tick typhus are the common rickettsial infections reported from

TABLE 5: Tests used to diagnose scrub typhus in various Indian studies.

Year	Region	Authors	Diagnostic tests used
2005	Himachal Pradesh	Sharma et al.	Weil–Felix test
2006	Himachal Pradesh	Mahajan et al.	Weil–Felix test, PCR, IFA
2010	Pondicherry	Vivekanandan et al.	Weil–Felix test
2013	Vellore	Varghese et al.	PCR, IgM ELISA
2013	Delhi	Prakash et al.	IgM ELISA
2014	Foot hills of Himalayas	Kumar et al.	PCR, IgM ELISA
2014	Uttarakhand	Singh et al.	IgM ELISA
2014	Vellore	Varghese et al.	IgM ELISA, PCR
2016	North India	Sharma et al.	IgM ELISA
2020	Meghalaya	Bhattacharya et al.	IgM ELISA

(ELISA: enzyme-linked immunoassay; IFA: immunofluorescent assay; IgM: immunoglobulin M; PCR: polymerase chain reaction)

TABLE 6: Rickettsial diseases

Disease	Species (vector)
1. Typhus fever	
a. Epidemic typhus	Prowazekki (louse)
b. Endemic typhus	R. typhi (flae)
c. Scrub typhus	Tsutsugamushi (mite)
2. Spotted fever	
a. Indian tick typhusb.	R.conorii (tick)
b. Rocky Mountain spotted fever	R.rickettsii (tick)
c. Rickettsial pox	R.akari (mite)
3. Others	
a. Q Feverb.	C. Brunetti (nil)
b. Trench fever	Rochalimaea Quintana (louse)

India so far. Rickettsial diseases are zoonotic bacterial infections in the Indian subcontinent.[8] However, there is under reporting of cases as there is a paucity of proper diagnostic tests, poor awareness among clinicians and vague symptomatology, Different varieties (around 6-10) of Rickettsioses, of which scrub Typhus is the commonest, has been reported from several states in India including Jammu and Kashmir, Himachal Pradesh, Uttaranchal (now known as Uttarakhand), Bihar, West Bengal, Meghalaya, Rajasthan, Maharashtra, Karnataka, Tamil Nadu and Kerala. In some areas scrub typhus constitutes upto 50% of undifferentiated fever Rickettsia belong to a group of obligate intracellular, gram-negative bacteria from the genera Rickettsia, Orientia, Ehrlichia, Neorickettsia, Neoehrlichia, and Anaplasma. They divided into the typhus group and spotted fever group. **(Table 6)**

Orientia spp. makes up the scrub typhus group. Rickettsial diseases are zoonoses where human beings become accidental hosts through between trombiculid mites (chiggers), ticks or fleas and animals (most commonly rodents).

Commonly reported Rickettsial diseases in India are scrub typhus, murine flea-borne typhus, Indian Tick Typhus and Q fever. The increase in the outbreaks reported after the year 2000 may be attributed to human behavioral changes, urbanization, deforestation, and rapid transport leading to the displacement of vectors.

Clinical Features

Outbreaks were observed after the monsoon. The commonest rickettsial infection is scrub typhus which has been described in detail. The clinical presentation of rickettsial infections ranges from mild fever to life-threatening organ dysfunctions if there is delay in diagnosis and management. In most of the outbreaks the presentation is acute febrile illness with nonspecific symptomatology. Rash is very common in spotted fever and uncommon in scrub typhus. Rash usually appears after 3-5 days initially they are discrete maculae which subsequently becomes maculopapular, petechial or hemorrhagic Vomiting, headache, abdominal pain, breathlessness, and lymphadenopathy are other signs and symptoms associated with fever in many cases.[9]

■ DIAGNOSIS

The clinical signs and symptoms including eschar formation are not diagnostic of rickettsial diseases. Epidemiological indicators such as geographical distribution, occupation, animal contact, travel history to forest, and endemic areas may give clues to diagnosis so as to start timely management.

The Weil Felix Test is not performed practically. ELISA IgM is used as a low-cost alternative test to immune fluorescence assay (IFA) in developing countries with poor resources The gold standard test is IFA but not easily accessible in our centres. Four-fold rise in titer is demonstrated in paired sera to confirm the diagnosis of rickettsial infection[10] PCR Test is available only in selected laboratories in India.

■ TREATMENT

The treatment modality is similar to scrub typhus namely Doxycycline 200 mg/day for 7 days, IV may be used in complicated cases for 10-14 days. Azithromycin 500 mg/day is an alternative drug for 5 days specially pregnant women.

TAKE HOME MESSAGE

Scrub typhus is a serious acute febrile illness associated with significant morbidity and mortality, but is treatable, if diagnosed early in the course of the disease. The nonspecific and variable presentations of the disease have made its clinical diagnosis difficult, leading to dependence on laboratory diagnosis. Unfortunately, the diagnostic tests are either too costly and/or not easily accessible in the primary care settings, where these are required most. Due to paucity of resources, the disease remains under-reported, especially in rural areas; the reported incidence may, in fact, be the tip of the iceberg. During the last decade, there has been a significant increased reporting of the disease from across the country, which is possibly mainly due to re-emergence as well as improved diagnostic facilities. In the Indian scenario, scrub typhus should be considered as one the most important differential diagnosis of acute febrile illness which is negative for malaria and dengue.

REFERENCES

1. Kumar D, Raina DJ, Gupta S, Angurana A. Epidemiology of scrub typhus. JK Sci. 2010;12(2):60-2.
2. Bhattacharya PK. "Scrub Typhus: prevalence and profile in India". In: Pareek KK, Wander GS. (eds). Medicine Update 2016 (Progress in Medicine 2016), Volume 26(2), Section 12. New Delhi: Association of Physicians of India. pp. 744-7.
3. Phongmany S, Rolain JM, Phetsouvanh R, Blacksell SD, Soukkhaseum V, Rasachack B, et al. Rickettsial infections and fever, Vientiane, Laos. Emerg Infect Dis. 2006;12(2):256-62.
4. Gurung S, Pradhan J, Bhutia PY. Outbreak of scrub typhus in the North East Himalayan region-Sikkim: an emerging threat. Indian J Med Microbiol. 2013;31(1):72-4.
5. Government of India. (2009). Monthly Newsletter of National Centre for Disease Control, Directorate General of Health Services. Scrub typhus and other rickettsioses. [online] Available from: https://ncdc.gov.in/WriteReadData/linkimages/May%20June-20098604739980.pdf. [Last accessed May 2022].
6. Bhattacharya PK, Murti VS, Jamil M, Barman B. Clinical profile and determinants of scrub typhus presenting with sepsis based on Sepsis-3 criteria. J Vector Borne Dis. 2020;57(4):307-13.
7. Kala D, Gupta S, Nagraik R, Verma V, Thakur A, Kaushal A. Diagnosis of scrub typhus: recent advancements and challenges. 3 Biotech. 2020;10(9):396.
8. Kalal BS, Puranik P, Nagaraj S, Rego S, Shet A. Scrub typhus and spotted fever among hospitalised children in South India: Clinical profile and serological epidemiology. Indian J Med Microbiol. 2016;34:293-8.
9. Thomas R, Puranik P, Kalal B, Britto C, Kamalesh S, Rego S, et al. Five-year analysis of rickettsial fevers in children in South India: Clinical manifestations and complications. J Infect Dev Ctries. 2016;10:657-61.
10. Kamarasu K, Malathi M, Rajagopal V, Subramani K, Jagadeeshramasamy D, Mathai E. Serological evidence for wide distribution of spotted fevers and typhus fever in Tamil Nadu. Indian J Med Res. 2007;126:128-30.

Leptospirosis

Chapter 8

*Subhra Sankar Sen, Biva Bhakat,
Manali Chandra, Purbasha Biswas*

■ INTRODUCTION

Leptospirosis, a (re-)emerging global zoonotic disease, is a cause for serious concern in tropical countries. With the use of geographical information science in health field, more complete understanding of the occurrence of leptospirosis is now possible.[1]

It is caused by spirochaetes, *Leptospira*. It is mainly divided into two types: Pathogenic and nonpathogenic. Pathogenic *Leptospira* are divided into 260 serovars based on antigenic composition. Currently, *Leptospira* is classified based on 16s RNA sequencing analysis and DNA–DNA hybridization techniques, into three types: Pathogenic, intermediate, and saprophytic. The different serovars have different survival times in water, for example, in cattle urine (diluted), the laboratory strain of *Leptospira kirschneri* serovar grippotyphosa could survive for 72 hours at 15°C, *L. interrogans* serovar Hardjo could survive in diluted cattle urine at 4°C for 48–984 hours, however, they cannot survive the high water flow of hose system.

Leptospirosis has led to 1.03 million cases [95% confidence interval (CI) 434,000–1,750,000] and 58,900 deaths (95% CI 23,800–95,900) annually worldwide. Morbidity and mortality were highest in South, South-East Asia, Caribbean, central and tropical Latin America, and in the East sub-Saharan Africa.

The outbreaks are mainly seasonal and related to rainfall. It has been seen that pathogenic *Leptospira* colonize the kidney (renal tubule) of the hosts, such as cattle, rodents, pigs, horses, and wild animals. Human beings, the accidental host, get infected if they come in contact with contaminated (with urine of infected animals) water, soil, or food. Thus, people involved in occupations such as farmers, butchers, rodent control workers, and people engaged in swimming and water recreational activities are at high risk.

■ CLINICAL FEATURES

Leptospirosis has myriad presentation that ranges from subclinical or mild-to-life threatening illness. The incubation period is 2–20 days. The clinical course is mainly biphasic. The initial septicemic phase, characterized by

leptospiremia, is followed by an immune phase in which antibody formation and leptospiruria occurs.
- *Anicteric syndrome:* Leptospirosis usually present as sudden onset febrile illness characterized by high-grade fever with chills. The fever may be biphasic and it may recur after 3-4 days of remission. Fever is associated with myalgia. The myalgia is intense and mainly involves the lower part of the body such as lower back, thigh, and calves. Excruciating headache (sometimes retro-orbital), skin rash, and conjunctival suffusion are seen. The rashes are macular or maculopapular eruption associated with erythematous, urticarial, petechial, or desquamative lesions. It is transient and lasts for <24 hours. Aseptic meningitis may occur especially in younger patients.
- Icteric leptospirosis is the severe form having rapidly progressive clinical course. The hepatic involvement is not associated with hepatocellular necrosis usually. In about 16-40% cases, renal involvement occurs. Most commonly, it presents as nonoliguric renal dysfunction. Oliguria is a significant predictor for high mortality. Transient thrombocytopenia may be present. Respiratory system is also involved. This is unrelated to the presence of jaundice. It manifests as cough, shortness of breath, and hemoptysis. Severe cases may present as adult respiratory distress syndrome. Some patients may develop pleural effusion. Pulmonary infiltrates associated with dyspnea is an indicator of high mortality. Cardiovascular system involvement manifests in the form of heart failure and arrhythmias (due to underlying myocarditis). Ocular involvement occurs in the form of conjunctival suffusion, scleral icterus, and uveitis (chronic uveitis may persist even after recovery). Gastrointestinal system involvement leads to anorexia, nausea, vomiting, abdominal pain, constipation, or diarrhea.

The severe form of leptospirosis is characterized by profound jaundice (hepatic necrosis), renal dysfunction, pulmonary dysfunction, and also hemorrhagic diathesis. It is termed as Weil syndrome.[2]

Leptospirosis in pregnant patients may lead to spontaneous abortions. It sometimes mimics HELLP syndrome (hemolysis, elevated liver enzymes and low platelets), AFLP (acute fatty liver of pregnancy), and pre-eclampsia.

In various literature, some rare presentation of leptospirosis is reported such as acute acalculous cholecystitis, pancreatitis, rhabdomyolysis, erythema nodosum, Guillain-Barré syndrome, and thrombotic thrombocytopenic purpura.

PATHOGENESIS

The bacteria penetrate skin and mucosa and enter the bloodstream. They evades innate immunity and continue to multiply. *Leptospira* due to its complement H activity is resistant to alternative complement pathway and it also binds and inactivates C3b and immunoglobulin G (IgG), therefore

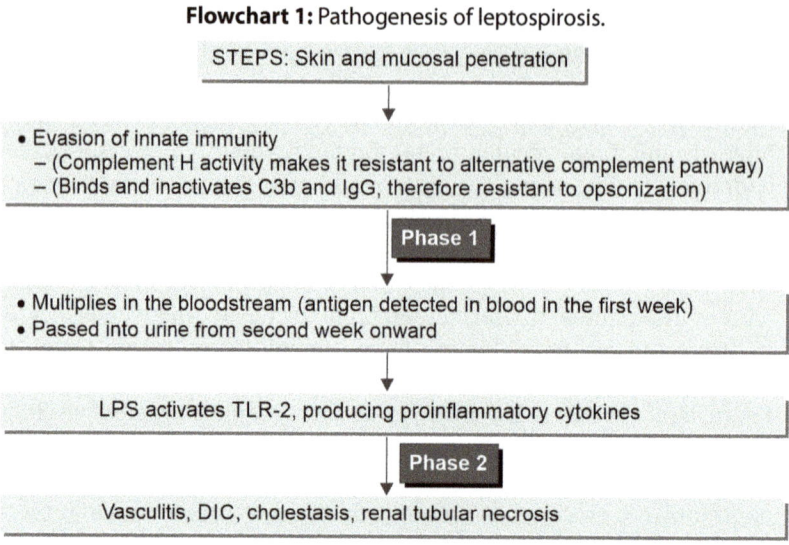

Flowchart 1: Pathogenesis of leptospirosis.

(DIC: disseminated intravascular coagulation; IgG: immunoglobulin G; LPS: lipopolysaccharide; TLR-2: toll-like receptor 2)

becoming resistant to opsonization. *Leptospira* antigen is detected in blood in the first week and in cerebrospinal fluid (CSF) and urine from second week onward. Lipopolysaccharide (LPS) activates toll-like receptor 2 (TLR-2), producing proinflammatory cytokines which results in vasculitis, the key pathogenic mechanism. Eventually organ dysfunction in form of cholestasis, renal tubular necrosis, and disseminated intravascular coagulation (DIC) ensues. This is explained in **Flowchart 1**.

The initial septicemia explains the first febrile phase, whereas the vasculitis occurs in the second febrile, i.e., the immune phase, when the antigens are cleared from the bloodstream and specific antibodies start appearing. Very mild and severe fulminant disease may not reach the second febrile phase.

■ DIFFERENTIAL DIAGNOSIS

Leptospirosis has multiple nonspecific clinical features common to many tropical diseases. The close differentials can be divided as per syndromes as stated below.

- *Acute undifferentiated febrile illness:* Malaria, dengue, scrub typhus, and enteric fever
- *Acute febrile illness with hemorrhage:* Dengue hemorrhagic fever, meningococcemia, and Hantavirus
- *Acute febrile illness with respiratory symptoms:* COVID, influenza, and scrub typhus
- *Acute febrile illness with hepatorenal syndrome:* Dengue, malaria, scrub typhus, and hepatitis A.

Diagnosis

Diagnosis is predominantly based on clinical approach. Since neither clinical nor laboratory findings are specific, high degree of suspicion based on epidemiology (endemic area and rainy season) and clinical manifestations (fever, jaundice, oliguria, and bleeding manifestations) is mandatory before we send for investigations. To guide our diagnosis, modified Faine's criteria **(Table 1)** can be used.

TABLE 1: Modified Faine's criteria.

Part A: Clinical data	
Questions	Score
Headache	2
Fever	2
Temperature >39°C	2
Conjunctival suffusion	4
Meningism	4
Muscle pain	4
Conjunctival suffusion +Meningism +Muscle pain	10
Jaundice	1
Albuminuria/nitrogen retention	2
Total score	
Part B: Epidemiological factor	
Questions	Score
Rainfall	5
Contact with contaminated environment	4
Animal contact	1
Total score	
Part C: Bacteriological and laboratory findings	
Isolation of leptospira in culture–diagnosis certain	
Positive serology	*Score*
ELISA IgM positive*	15
SAT—positive	15
MAT—single high titer*	15
Rising titer (paired sera)	25
Total score	

*Any one of the tests only should be scored. By modified Faine's criteria a score of ≥26 when using Part A, Part A+B or ≥25 using part A+B+C can be considered as current leptospirosis.
(ELISA: enzyme-linked immunoassay; MAT: microscopic agglutination test; SAT: serum agglutination test)

The laboratory features found in this disease are leukocytosis and thrombocytopenia, raised erythrocyte sedimentation rate (ESR) and C-reactive protein (CRP). Liver function test (LFT) shows characteristic dissociation between slight elevation of transaminase and alkaline phosphatase despite exceedingly high bilirubin levels. Anuric phase has rapid rise in urea, creatinine requiring dialysis in the first 3–4 days followed by gradual normalization of creatinine with polyuria. Hyperkalemia initially, hypokalemia later on may happen. CSF study may show lymphocytic pleocytosis with slightly elevated protein and normal glucose. Imaging of the chest may show diffuse patchy opacity like acute respiratory distress syndrome (ARDS).

■ DIAGNOSTIC TOOLS

The available diagnostic tools are molecular tests, serology, culture, and antigen detection.
- *Molecular tests:* Test methods available are reverse transcription polymerase chain reaction (RT-PCR) and loop-mediated isothermal amplification. It comes positive in the first week itself helping in early diagnosis. Blood, urine, and CSF any of these can be tested by this technique.
- *Serology:* It can be done by MAT (microscopic agglutination test), IgM ELISA (enzyme-linked immunosorbent assay), and point-of-care rapid lateral flow assays (kit tests).
- *MAT:* It is considered positive if there is fourfold rise in antibiotic titer between acute and convalescent samples, or a single value comes to >1:800. It was earlier considered the gold standard test. High false positive (syphilis, relapsing fever, lyme disease, and legionellosis) and false negative (first week, infection with serovar not included in testing panel of organisms), and background positivity are a problem with this assay.
- *Culture:* It is done in appropriate media prior to antibiotic administration. However, this test is insensitive, takes several weeks, and urine culture may remain positive long after disease resolution.
- *Antigen detection:* In future, it expected to be a cost-effective alternative to PCR. Ag detection is done using monoclonal anti-LipL32.

■ TREATMENT

Supportive Care

Leptospirosis-related severe illness may also necessitate *supportive care,* including renal replacement therapy, ventilatory support, and blood products.[3]
- *Acute kidney injury (AKI):* Individuals with significant kidney damage may benefit from kidney replacement treatment (KRT), which is recommended for patients with AKI.

CHAPTER 8: Leptospirosis

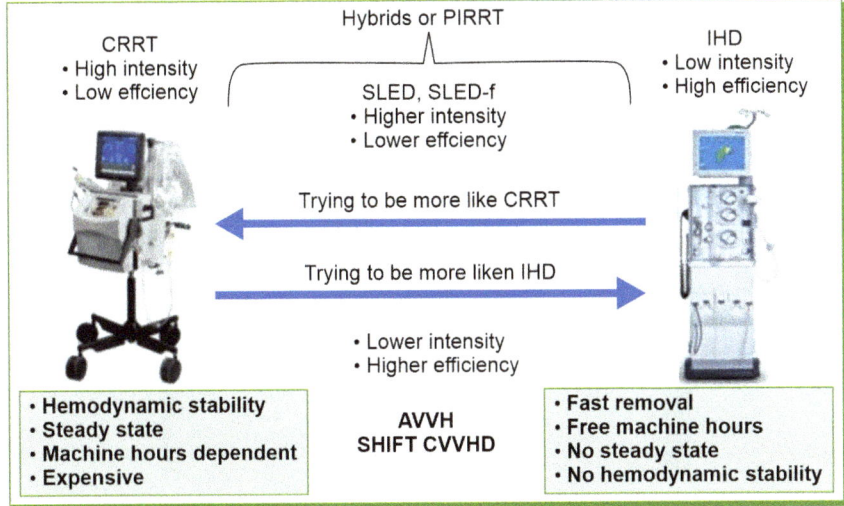

Fig. 1: Different forms of dialysis.
(AVVH: accelerated venovenous hemofiltration; CRRT: continuous renal replacement therapy; CVVHD: continuous venovenous hemodialysis; IHD: intermittent hemodialysis; PIRRT: prolonged intermittent renal replacement therapy)

There are numerous KRT methods available:
- Continuous kidney replacement treatments (CKRTs)
- Prolonged intermittent kidney replacement therapies (PIKRT)
- Sustained low-efficiency dialysis (SLED)
- Extended-duration dialysis
- Intermittent hemodialysis (IHD) **(Fig. 1)**.

Even with these many approaches, mortality in individuals with AKI is still significant, topping 40–50% in those who are very sick.[4]

- Acute respiratory distress syndrome **(Fig. 2)**:
  - Noninvasive ventilation
  - *Invasive ventilation:* Lung protective ventilation (CPV)
    - Assist control volume control mode
    - *Tidal volume:* 4–8 mL/kg body weight
    - Plateau pressure (Pplat) <30 cmH$_2$O
    - High positive-end expiratory pressure
    - Low tidal volumes (VT) are hypothesized to reduce alveolar overdistension brought on by mechanical ventilation, which can increase lung damage and death in ARDS patients.
- *Judicious use of intravenous fluids* depending on urine output, hydration status, invasive blood pressure monitoring, and adjustment as per renal parameters.
- Treatment of underlying *arrhythmias*

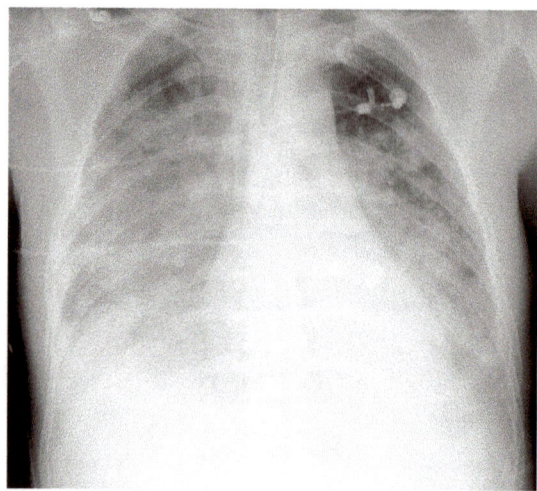

Fig. 2: Chest X-ray showing acute respiratory distress syndrome (ARDS) in a case of leptospirosis.

- Treatment of *coagulopathy*, if any
- *Avoid steroids:* In patients with severe leptospirosis, the administration of steroids has been linked to an increased risk of nosocomial infections.

Antimicrobial Treatment

- Mild disease:
    - Azithromycin 500 mg once daily for 3 days:
        - *Children:* 10 mg/kg orally on day 1 (maximum dose 500 mg/day) followed by 5 mg/kg/day orally once daily on subsequent days
    - Doxycycline 100 mg orally twice daily for 7 days:
        - *Children:* 2 mg/kg per day in two equally divided doses (not to exceed 200 mg daily) for 7 days
- Severe disease:
    - Ceftriaxone (1–2 g IV once daily)
    - Doxycycline (100 mg IV twice daily)
    - Cefotaxime (1 g IV every 6 hours)

    Treatment for serious illnesses typically lasts *7 days*.
- Pregnant women:
    - Azithromycin, ceftriaxone, penicillin, and cefotaxime
    - *Doxycycline* should be taken into consideration if the diagnosis of leptospirosis is uncertain and murine typhus is a potential alternate diagnosis because it seems to be safer during pregnancy than other tetracyclines.[5]

Other Options
- *Intravenous corticosteroid therapy* has been suggested; however, there is currently insufficient data to support routine corticosteroid administration.[6]
- *Plasmapheresis* is beneficial for treating severe leptospirosis, according to some studies, but there is not enough high-quality randomized data to support routine use.[7]

> **TAKE HOME MESSAGE**
> - Leptospirosis, a re-emerging global zoonotic disease, is caused by a spirochete.
> - The pathogenesis involves septicemic and vasculitic phases.
> - Management is based on antimicrobials with supportive therapy, however early clinical suspicion and prompt intervention are imperative.

REFERENCES
1. Bharti AR, Nally JE, Ricaldi JN, Matthias MA, Diaz MM, Lovett MA, et al. Leptospirosis: a zoonotic disease of global importance. Lancet Infect Dis. 2003;3(12):757-71.
2. Gouveia EL, Metcalfe J, Carvalho ALF, Aires TSF, Villasboas-Bisneto JC, Queirroz A, et al. Leptospirosis-associated severe pulmonary hemorrhagic syndrome, Salvador, Brazil. Emerg Infect Dis. 2008;14:505-8.
3. Andrade L, Cleto S, Seguro AC. Door-to-dialysis time and daily hemodialysis in patients with leptospirosis: impact on mortality. Clin J Am Soc Nephrol. 2007;2:739.
4. Herath NJ, Kularatne SA, Weerakoon KG, Wazil A, Subasinghe N, Ratnatunga NVI, et al. Long term outcome of acute kidney injury due to leptospirosis? A longitudinal study in Sri Lanka. BMC Res Notes 2014;7:398.
5. Cross R, Ling C, Day NP, McGready R, Paris DH. Revisiting doxycycline in pregnancy and early childhood—time to rebuild its reputation? Expert Opin Drug Saf. 2016;15:367.
6. Azevedo AF, Miranda-Filho Dde B, Henriques-Filho GT, Leite A, Ximenes RAA. Randomized controlled trial of pulse methyl prednisolone × placebo in treatment of pulmonary involvement associated with severe leptospirosis. [ISRCTN74625030]. BMC Infect Dis. 2011;11:186.
7. Trivedi SV, Vasava AH, Bhatia LC, Patel TC, Patel NK, Patel NT. Plasma exchange with immunosuppression in pulmonary alveolar haemorrhage due to leptospirosis. Indian J Med Res. 2010;131:429.

Chapter 9

Zika and Chikungunya

Anivita Agarwal, Animesh Ray, Tanuka Mandal

■ INTRODUCTION

Zika virus (ZIKV) is an arbovirus belonging to the genus *Flavivirus* and *Flaviviridae* family. This positive sense single-stranded ribonucleic acid (RNA) virus is transmitted by the bite of infected mosquitoes. The disease usually presents as an acute febrile illness with rash arthralgia and conjunctivitis. Zika virus infection has been associated with significant neurological complications as well as congenital microcephaly.

Chikungunya is also an arthropod borne single-stranded RNA virus, presenting as Alphavirus febrile illness with rash. The virus belongs to the family *Togaviridae*, genus alphavirus, and causes characteristic debilitating joint pains. Though usually a self-limiting illness, a substantial proportion of the population develops chronic disease in the form of characteristic incapacitating polyarthralgia and inflammatory arthritis lasting for months to years. Millions of cases across the globe and the association with severe disease with multiorgan failure have been lately been a major public health concern.

Overlapping clinical features of acute onset fever with rash and joint pains with other arboviral disease pose a diagnostic challenge for both these viral fevers in tropical countries **(Table 1)**. Currently there are no therapeutic drugs available, and vaccines are under trial.

■ ZIKA VIRUS

Epidemiology

Zika virus was first isolated from non-primate hosts in 1947, then from *Aedes africanus* mosquito in 1947 and later described in a human case from Nigeria in 1954. The virus was further isolated periodically from various serosurveys across Asia and Africa. However, major outbreaks in the Western Pacific Islands of Yep (2007), French Polynesia in the South Pacific (2013-2014), and Brazil (2015-2016) brought focus due to the large numbers of affected population. Based on genomic sequencing of NS-5 encoding gene and phylogenetic studies, ZIKV has been classified into three lineages: East African, West African, and Asian, having varied clinical presentations.

TABLE 1: Clinical features, laboratory parameters, and diagnostic tests to differentiate dengue fever, chikungunya fever with Zika fever.

Differentiating parameter	Zika	Chikungunya	Dengue
Clinical features:			
• Fever	++	+++	+++
• Rash	+++	++	+
• Arthralgias	++	+++	+
• Conjunctivitis	++	+	–
• Hemorrhage	–	–	++
• Shock	–	–	+
Laboratory parameters:			
• Leukopenia	–	+	+
• Thrombocytopenia	–/+	+/–	+
Diagnostic tests	RT-PCR if <2 weeks, IgM if >2 weeks	PCR if <5 days, IgM if >5 days	NS1 antigen if <3–5 days, dengue IgM if >5 days

(IgM: immunoglobulin M; RT-PCR: reverse transcription polymerase chain reaction)

Indian outbreaks in 2017–2018, ascribed to the Asian lineage and the recent outbreak in Kerala in 2021, were not reported to have any zika-associated microcephaly. **Figure 1** illustrates the geographical distribution of outbreaks of ZIKV in India. With growing globalization and travel, over 86 countries and territories have reported cases of ZIKV as per World Health Organization (WHO).

Pathogenesis

The primary mode of transmission of ZIKV is by *Aedes* (*Aedes aegypti, Aedes albopictus*, etc.) mosquito bite which is also shared by the Dengue and Chikungunya viruses. Recently described, alternative modes of transmission include spread via transplacental route, sexual intercourse, blood transfusion, organ transplant, and breast milk. Zika virus RNA has also been found to be shed in urine, semen, saliva, blood, female genital tracts, breast milk, amniotic fluid, and cerebrospinal fluid (CSF), etc. for prolonged periods of time.

The virus is transmitted via the bite of an infected mosquito harbouring the virus in its salivary glands after a blood meal from another infected vertebrate (extrinsic incubation period of 8–12 days). Humans are accidental hosts, whereas animals are reservoirs. The exact pathogenesis remains largely unknown, but the virus is believed to replicate in dendrites at the site of mosquito bite. After an (intrinsic) incubation period ranging from 3 to 12 days, it spreads to the regional lymph nodes and distant organs such as the nervous system along hematogenous route. In pregnant females, it

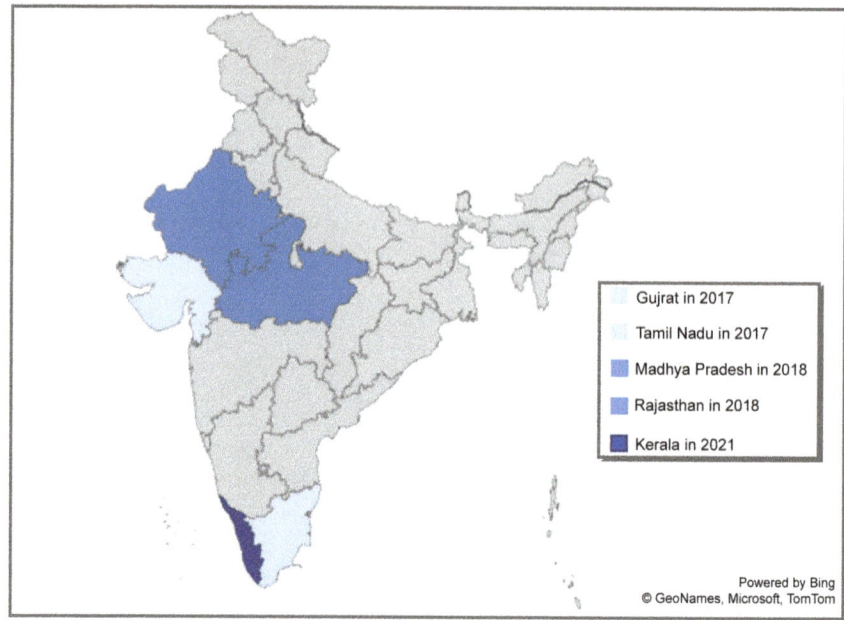

Fig. 1: Geographical distribution of outbreaks of zika virus in India.

may infect the foetus through transplacental transmission. Zika virus may persist in whole-blood, immune-sanctuary sites, semen and urine for weeks to months.[1]

Clinical Features and Complications

Incubation period from the bite of mosquito to symptom onset may vary between 3 and 12 days. Over 75–80% infected are likely to develop asymptomatic disease. Historically symptoms were believed to be mild self-limiting disease, with low case fatality rate. However, in recent past, many cases of severe disease with multiorgan failure requiring intensive care and mortality have also been seen. Predominant feature is fever (72%) which is typically low grade, usually resolving within 1–2 weeks. Maculopapular pruritic rash spreading proximally to extremities, including face palms and soles, which spontaneously resolves in 1–4 days is a characteristic finding. Associated symptoms such as arthralgias and myalgias (65%), and nonpurulent conjunctivitis (63%) are also commonly noted.[2] Other reported symptoms include headache, retro-orbital pain, and rarely of pericarditis, myocarditis facial puffiness, and uveitis.

The Brazil ZIKV outbreak (2015) was notable for the dreaded complication of the disease in pregnant women resulting in infants born with microcephaly was reported in 20/10,000 live births compared to a background rate of 0.5/10,000 live births). Pregnant women are susceptible to ZIKV infection in all trimesters with maternal-foetal transmission. The severe form commonly arises due to infection in the first or second trimester. Congenital zika syndrome could present as foetal losses, microcephaly, facial dysmorphism, sensorineural hearing loss, and ocular abnormalities. Studies have demonstrated the incidence of microcephaly as <7%.[3]

Severe neurological manifestations, first noticed in the French Polynesia outbreak (2013-2014), have also been described such as Guillain-Barré syndrome, meningitis, and meningoencephalitis.[4] Other neurological manifestations include transverse myelitis, encephalitis, neuropsychiatric and cognitive symptoms.

Acute febrile illness such as dengue, chikungunya, malaria, leptospirosis, scrub typhus, enteric fever must be considered as a differential diagnosis in India due to significant overlap of clinical features.[5] Zika fever should be suspected in patients with clinical manifestations as well as epidemiological exposure (travel to an area where ZIKV infection has been reported, or unprotected sexual contact with a person who meets these criteria).

Diagnosis

The Centre for Disease Control and Prevention (CDC), National Health Service (NHS), and WHO have classified it as a level 2 pathogen requiring biosafety level 2 laboratory for sample handling.

Reverse transcription polymerase chain reaction (RT-PCR) in serum, whole blood, or urine sample within weeks of symptom onset can be used to diagnose ZIKV. A positive RT-PCR confirms the diagnosis, a negative test however, does not rule it out and should be followed by serology testing. Urine RT-PCR is found to have higher sensitivity.

Immunoglobulin M (IgM) capture enzyme-linked immunoassay (ELISA) serology/CSF analysis performed after 1-2 weeks of illness has good specificity. However, structural similarities between Dengue virus and ZIKV can lead to cross reactivity of antibodies produced against *Flaviviruses*, hence must be interpreted with caution. Testing for neutralizing antibodies via PRNT (plaque reduction neutralization test) can be performed to determine false positivity.

Treatment and Prevention

Being essentially a self-limiting disease, management is primarily supportive. Symptomatic management with rest, intake of fluids, antipyretics, and analgesics are to be provided. Zika virus could lead to immune-mediated thrombocytopenia (ITP), hence nonsteroidal anti-inflammatory drugs (NSAIDs) should be avoided to prevent the risk of bleeding. Currently there is no approved drug or vaccine against ZIKV, although several are being investigated. Vector control and prevention from mosquito bites remains the sole preventive and most effective strategy against *Flaviviruses*.

CHIKUNGUNYA VIRUS

Epidemiology

Chikungunya was first isolated in 1952 from an outbreak in Tanzania, in patient having severe rheumatological manifestations. The disease was named in their Kimakonde language as chikungunya meaning "to bend over", referring to the patients' posture assumed with disabling joint pains. Across the globe various outbreaks have occurred in tropics and subtropics, causing millions of human infections and serious public health concerns.

Reported in India first in 1963, the illness re-emerged in 2005 (The Indian Ocean lineage) and subsequently resulted in periodic outbreaks all over the country making the disease endemic. A notable mutation, E1-A226V, among many others has been identified that has led to its enhanced fitness, survival adaptability (to *Aedes albopictus*), and severity, causing numerous Indian outbreaks.[6]

As Dengue, Zika and Chikungunya viruses are all transmitted via the same vector, it is often difficult to differentiate these epidemiologically. Dengue and Chikungunya coinfections have also been frequently reported. **Table 1** delineates the differentiating features between Dengue, Zika and Chikungunya.

Pathogenesis

Being an arbovirus, CHIKV (Chikungunya virus) is primarily transmitted by the bite of its vectors *Aedes aegypti* and *Aedes albopictus* mosquitoes. Mosquito replicates the CHIKV in its midgut and reaches the salivary glands during the extrinsic incubation period (of 10 days). After the bite of the infected mosquito, it replicates within dermal fibroblasts at the site of inoculation and then spreads via the bloodstream to various organs. Animal models suggest that the virus directly infects the synovium and replicates in the joints causing production of proinflammatory cytokines and chemokines.

Chikungunya virus is also transmitted to the eggs from adult mosquitos through vertical transmission. Mother-to-child transmission, although very rare, has also been reported in pregnant women who developed chikungunya fever in their last trimester of gestation, potentially leading to poor pregnancy outcomes.[6] Occasionally, it may also be transmitted via blood products.

The transmission is via two types of cycles: (1) Sylvatic cycle, where there is enzootic transmission between non-primates (which acts as both host and reservoir) and mosquitoes; (2) urban cycle where *Aedes* mosquitoes spread the disease to human hosts.[7]

Clinical Features and Complications

After an incubation period of 2–6 days from the bite of a mosquito, clinical presentations may range from asymptomatic to severe disease.

Acute phase (first three weeks of illness) of chikungunya fever is characterized by acute high-grade fever, characteristic intense join paint, myalgias, headache, and rash, which subsequently resolve within 1–2 weeks. Polyarthralgia, seen in over 70% patients, is bilaterally symmetrical affecting small and large joints typically with swelling and morning stiffness. Skin manifestations in the form of maculopapular erythematous rash often start on days 2–5 and lasts a few days, affecting extremities, truck, and face. Atypical manifestations such as skin hyperpigmentation with predilection for the tip of the nose, chondritis involving ear pinna, and cervical lymphadenopathy may be seen in a few. Myalgias commonly noted may be a frequent confounder with dengue fever. The common laboratory abnormalities seen are lymphopenia and thrombocytopenia.

Relapsing or intermittent debilitating joint pain and progression to chronic disease is seen in 25–75% of the patients. It could last weeks to months and known as post-chikungunya chronic polyarthralgia (lasting >3 months), causing significant morbidity and loss of quality of life. Nerve compression syndromes, osteoarthritis, arthralgia, arthritis, synovitis, tendinitis, bursitis, tenosynovitis, etc. could occur due to the ongoing inflammation. Chronic arthritis is proposed to be due to persistent viral replication, persistent viral RNA initiating inflammatory responses or autoimmunity, usually affecting patients over 45 years of age or pre-existing osteoarthritis.

Complications including neurological manifestations such as encephalitis, meningitis, Guillain–Barré syndrome; cardiovascular features such as myocarditis and tachyarrhythmias have been also reported in elderly and patients with underlying medical conditions. Deaths have been reported during chikungunya outbreaks in India and other countries.

Diagnosis

Based on clinical manifestations and epidemiological clues, the diagnosis of chikungunya must be suspected. Laboratory diagnosis can be based on viral isolation, RT-PCR, or serological testing (IgG and IgM antibodies) using ELISA or rapid immunochromatographic assays. RT-PCR, not widely available, has very high sensitivity and specificity for the detection of CHIKV and can be performed on blood or CSF samples within first week of illness. ELISA/immunochromatographic assays for IgM antibodies are used for detection after five days from illness. These persist for weeks to three months and must be correlated with IgG antibodies, clinical features, and epidemiological setting.

In endemic areas, many acute febrile illnesses may be misdiagnosed on the basis of serological tests due to cross reactivity of IgM and coinfection with other arboviruses. Hence, physicians must keep a high index of suspicion for alternative etiologies.

Treatment and Prevention

There is no specific antiviral therapy or effective vaccine available for chikungunya fever. Management is essentially supportive including rest, fluids, antipyretics, and anti-inflammatory or analgesics. NSAIDs must be carefully administered after ruling out dengue fever in acute phase due to risk of bleeding manifestations. Polyarthritis usually resembles inflammatory arthritis on imaging and typically responds to conventional anti-inflammatory drugs. However, for persistent symptoms or nonresponsiveness after even two weeks of NSAID therapy, with elevation of inflammatory markers, corticosteroid administration may be considered. For patients with post-chikungunya polyarthralgia, disease-modifying antirheumatic drug (DMARD, e.g., methotrexate or sulfasalazine) can be initiated.

Vector control in the form of insecticide sprays, biological control, and personal protections from bites of mosquitos are the most useful steps that are essential for prevention of arboviral diseases such as chikungunya.

TAKE HOME MESSAGE

- Zika virus (ZIKV) leads to a relatively uncommon arboviral disease in India transmitted via the bite of *Aedes* mosquito.
- The most dreaded complication due to ZIKV infection is microcephaly occurring due to disease in pregnant females typically in their first or second trimesters.
- Chikungunya disease, caused by the same vector, leads to an acute febrile illness with severe joint pain.
- In some patients, Chikungunya can lead to relapsing or intermittent disabling joint pain which requires treatment in the line of inflammatory arthritis.
- The management of both Zika and Chikungunya is essentially supportive while vector control and personal protection forms the backbone of preventive strategy.

■ REFERENCES

1. Pierson TC, Diamond MS. The emergence of Zika virus and its new clinical syndromes. Nature. 2018;560(7720):573-81.
2. Musso D, Bossin H, Mallet HP, Besnard M, Broult J, Baudouin L, et al. Zika virus in French Polynesia 2013-14: anatomy of a completed outbreak. Lancet Infect Dis. 2018;18(5):e172-82.
3. Brasil P, Pereira JP, Moreira ME, Ribeiro Nogueira RM, Damasceno L, Wakimoto M, et al. Zika virus infection in pregnant women in Rio de Janeiro. N Engl J Med. 2016;375(24):2321-34.
4. Cao-Lormeau V-M, Blake A, Mons S, Lastère S, Roche C, Vanhomwegen J, et al. Guillain-Barré Syndrome outbreak associated with Zika virus infection in French Polynesia: a case-control study. The Lancet. 2016;387(10027):1531-9.
5. Gupta N, Kodan P, Baruah K, Soneja M, Biswas A. Zika virus in India: past, present and future. QJM. 2019;hcz273.
6. Sunil S. Current status of chikungunya in India. Front Microbiol. 2021;12:1497.
7. Cunha MS, Costa PAG, Correa IA, de Souza MRM, Calil PT, da Silva GPD, et al. Chikungunya virus: an emergent arbovirus to the south american continent and a continuous threat to the world. Front Microbiol. 2020;11:1297.

Chapter 10

Viral Respiratory Illness

J Rajkumar, Subramanian Swaminathan, Arkaprava Hati

INTRODUCTION

Acute respiratory illnesses are the most frequently occurring illness worldwide affecting all ages uniformly. Though the disease is mostly limited to the upper airways in the initial stages and is self-limiting, a small percentage can progress to lower respiratory tract infections (RTIs) presenting as bronchiolitis and pneumonia.[1] Viruses are the most common pathogens causing these illnesses with a considerable overlap of clinical syndromes.

ETIOLOGY

A range of different viruses can cause RTIs[2]; the most common viruses implicated are:

- *Orthomyxoviridae:* Influenza viruses
- *Paramyxoviridae:* Respiratory syncytial virus (RSV), parainfluenza virus (PIV) 1-4, and human metapneumovirus (hMPV)
- Coronavirus
- *Picornaviruses:* Enteroviruses and parechoviruses.

The incubation period and seasonality of these individual viruses vary **(Tables 1 and 2)**.[3] These viruses are predominantly transmitted by droplet

TABLE 1: Viruses and incubation period.

Virus	Incubation period (in days)
Adenovirus	4.8–6.3
Coronavirus	2–5
Influenza A	1.3–1.5
Influenza B	0.5–0.6
Metapneumovirus	3–6
Parainfluenza	2.1–3.1
RSV	3.9–4.9
Rhinovirus	1.4–2.4

(RSV: respiratory syncytial virus)

TABLE 2: Seasonality of viruses.

Season	Viruses
Winter	- Influenza - Coronavirus - RSV
Summer	Rhinovirus
All year	- Adenovirus - Parainfluenza - Human metapneumovirus - Rhinovirus

(RSV: respiratory syncytial virus)

transmission and by fomites. Airborne transmission is possible particularly in ventilated patients and patients undergoing aerosol-generating procedures (e.g., influenza).

■ CLINICAL MANIFESTATIONS

Influenza

Influenza viruses are the most common respiratory viruses causing major outbreaks of varying severity leading on to excess morbidity and mortality.[4] There are two types of viruses, types A and B that cause the illness. Influenza is usually associated with a U-shaped epidemic curve, with attack rates being highest in young and mortality more among elderly. Patients with underlying medical conditions, pregnancy, and obesity are at increased risk.

Typical uncomplicated influenza often begins with an abrupt onset of symptoms after an incubation period of 1-2 days. Systemic symptoms such as fever, chills, headache, myalgia, malaise, and anorexia predominate and persist for 3 days. Respiratory symptoms include a dry cough, severe pharyngeal pain, nasal obstruction, and discharge. The patient appears toxic with flushing of face. The mucous membranes of nose and throat are hyperemic and nasal discharge is clear. Crackles and wheeze may be found occasionally. Then, a convalescent period of 1 or more weeks to full recovery ensues.

Bacterial superinfection is a well-recognized complication of influenza and accounts for a substantial proportion of the morbidity and mortality of the disease. The continuous evolution and reassortment of these viruses remain a cause for concern warranting continuous monitoring and surveillance.

Respiratory Syncytial Virus

Respiratory syncytial virus is the major cause of lower respiratory tract illness in young children. Essentially all persons get infected with RSV within the first few years of life. RSV is also of concern in the elderly people >65 years and particularly in people with cardiopulmonary disease.

Respiratory syncytial virus is the most frequent cause of bronchiolitis constituting 40–90% of the hospitalized cases and 50% of the pneumonia in infants. Croup and tracheobronchitis are the other clinical manifestations. Preterm gestation, with or without underlying chronic lung disease or congenital heart disease, is clearly a major risk factor for more severe RSV disease. In young children, it is confined to the upper respiratory tract and otitis media can occur. Recurrent wheeze is a known sequelae in children.

Among healthy adults, following RSV infection, 84% were symptomatic and 22% had lower respiratory tract manifestations similar to influenza. Among older individuals, RSV is remarkably similar to influenza with respect to clinical manifestations and as a cause of hospitalization. Though reinfections are common in all age groups, they tend to be less severe.

Parainfluenza

Human PIVs cause predominantly a mild and self-limiting illness; however, life-threatening lower RTIs do occur, particularly in the elderly and immunocompromised. Parainfluenza is the second most common viral cause of hospitalization in children. Human PIV are of four types. PIV-1 and PIV-2 cause seasonal outbreaks in winter and PIV-3 causes epidemics in summer.

Parainfluenza viruses cause a variety of upper and lower respiratory tract illnesses, ranging from mild cold-like syndromes to life-threatening pneumonias. Infections in children are limited to the upper respiratory tract, with otitis media and sinusitis occurring in 30–50% and 15% having a lower respiratory tract involvement. In children, PIV-1 and PIV-2 are associated with croup, or laryngotracheobronchitis, PIV-3 with pneumonia and bronchiolitis and PIV-4 with mild upper respiratory infections. In adults, PIV-3 causes influenza-like illness. PIV is also increasingly associated with exacerbations of asthma and chronic bronchitis. Meningitis, myocarditis, pericarditis, and Guillain–Barré syndrome are rare extrapulmonary complications.

Human Metapneumovirus

Human metapneumovirus more commonly occurs as a coinfection with other viral and bacterial respiratory pathogens. Seroprevalence studies indicate that 50% are seropositive by 2 years and 100% by 5 years of age. Outbreaks of hMPV usually alternate with RSV activity.

Most young children with hMPV infection exhibit fever, cough, and rhinorrhea. Fever appears to be more common and febrile seizures is noted in 16% of patients. Apart from conjunctivitis, pharyngitis, and laryngitis, wheezing and acute otitis media do occur. Neurologic complications, such as seizures, ataxia, and encephalitis, appear to be 10 times more common in children with hMPV. Maculopapular rash and diarrhea are the other manifestations. In healthy adults, hMPV generally presents with mild influenza-like illness and common cold syndromes. Hoarseness of voice is more common and occasionally a mononucleosis-like syndrome have been reported.

Laboratory findings are nonspecific. Lymphopenia and elevated hepatic transaminases have been described. Radiographic findings include peribronchial cuffing, perihilar infiltrates, patchy opacities, and hyperinflation. In adults, patchy, multilobe infiltrates associated with small pleural effusions are noted in 50% of cases.

Coronavirus

Coronaviruses are subclassified into four genera, among which human coronavirus (HCoVs) belong to two groups: Alpha coronaviruses (HCoV-229E and HCoV-NL63) and beta coronaviruses [HCoV-HKU1, HCoV-OC43, Middle East respiratory syndrome coronavirus (MERS-CoV), the severe acute respiratory syndrome coronavirus (SARS-CoV), and SARS-CoV-2].

Coronavirus accounts to 5–10% cases of common cold. Asymptomatic infection does occur. It is also implicated as a cause of acute otitis media. Coronavirus causes pneumonia similar to or somewhat lower than other respiratory viruses such as influenza, RSV, and rhinovirus. They have been found to cause exacerbations of chronic obstructive pulmonary disease and also temporally linked to acute asthma attacks in both children and adults. SARS was characterized by fever and myalgia rapidly progressing to a respiratory syndrome of cough and dyspnea followed by acute respiratory distress syndrome. More mild and asymptomatic cases are observed with MERS, and mortality is strongly associated with age and comorbidities. SARS-CoV-2 has similar clinical picture with initial upper respiratory or gastrointestinal symptoms along with fever and myalgia progressing to pneumonia in selected patients.

Adenovirus

Adenovirus usually causes a mild, self-limiting disease. Infections are more common in childhood and by 10 years of age, many are serologically positive. Almost 50% of individuals may have a subclinical infection and sporadic outbreaks being more common.

There are several subtypes. Children may present with mild pharyngitis or tracheitis. It is usually associated with types 1, 2, 5, and 6 and rarely 3 and 7. It is at times indistinguishable from Group A streptococcal pharyngitis. Types 1–5, 7, 14, and 21 are associated with pneumonia. Severe, complicated pneumonia is reported with virus types 3, 7, 14, and 21. Pharyngoconjunctival fever is a common presentation characterized by benign follicular conjunctivitis, fever, pharyngitis, and cervical adenitis caused by adenovirus types 3 and 7.

Other clinical manifestations include acute gastroenteritis, mesenteric adenitis, and hemorrhagic cystitis. Extrapulmonary complications occur rarely and include meningoencephalitis, hepatitis, myocarditis, nephritis, neutropenia, and disseminated intravascular coagulopathy particularly in the immunocompromised patients.

Rhinovirus

The rhinoviruses are among the most common of the pathogens that infect humans. They are the most important cause of common cold and implicated in 30–50% of all cases of acute respiratory disease.

Rhinovirus colds frequently begin as a sore or "scratchy" throat that is followed closely by development of nasal obstruction and rhinorrhea. Cough occurs in one-third cases and frequently appears after the onset of nasal symptoms and often persists longer. The clinical features are similar in adults and children with absence of fever in adults. Rhinovirus causes up to 40% of exacerbations of chronic bronchitis and occasionally complicated by bacterial sinusitis and acute otitis media.

■ DIAGNOSIS

Though clinical history and examination may give important clues toward establishing the specific viral diagnosis, they are still nonspecific. Etiologic diagnosis can only reliably be made by detection of virus, antigens, or nucleic acids in respiratory or other specimens or by retrospectively by demonstrating an immune response in paired serum samples.[5]

Culture

Detection of viruses by observing the cytopathic effect and hemadsorption in cell culture has been considered the "gold standard" for diagnosis of respiratory viral pathogens for decades. Viruses such as adenovirus, influenza A/B, RSV, and human PIVs are the most common respiratory viruses that are isolated and detected by cell culture. Modified cell culture methods such as the centrifugation-enhanced shell-vial method has reduced the turnaround time from 5 to 10 days to 24 hours. Shell-vial culture using combination cell lines also allows simultaneous detection of multiple respiratory viruses. As compared to conventional culture, has similar sensitivity for parainfluenza 1–3 (87% vs. 83%) and influenza A/B (78% vs. 75%), and significantly higher sensitivity for RSV (73% vs. 42%). Despite these advantages, many clinically relevant viruses are difficult to grow in culture (such as rhinovirus and coronavirus) and may produce variable results.

Rapid Antigen Detection Method

Multiple rapid direct antigen detection tests are widely available and are used by most laboratories. The direct and indirect immunofluorescent assays are both sensitive (93–98%) and specific (92–97%) but require several hours and skilled laboratory personnel. Other methods available are the enzyme immunoasay (EIA) method and, to a lesser extent, the optical immunoassay (OIA), which has a sensitivity of 88–95% and specificity of 97–100% when compared with culture.

Serological Tests

Serological tests are useful in detecting pathogen specific antibodies. These antibodies typically appear about 2 weeks after initial infection and is useful in detecting most respiratory pathogens such as RSV, adenovirus, influenza A and B, and parainfluenza 1–3 virus. However, they are still less sensitive when compared to molecular methods such as reverse transcription polymerase chain reaction (RT-PCR). They are still useful for epidemiological studies, as it increases the probability of identifying acute viral infections.

Nucleic Acid Amplification Tests

Detection of respiratory pathogens by nucleic acid amplification tests (NAATs) such as polymerase chain reaction (PCR), nucleic acid sequence-based amplification (NASBA), transcription-mediated amplification (TMA), strand displacement amplification (SDA), loop-mediated isothermal amplification (LAMP), and rolling circle amplification (RCA) has gained immense popularity over the past decade.

Several types of specimens can be used for detection of respiratory viruses, including: Bronchoalveolar lavage (BAL), throat swab, nasopharyngeal (NP) washes, NP aspirates, lung aspirates, and NP swabs, although the appropriate specimen type depends on the specific patient population. For optimal results, specimens should be collected within 3–5 days after onset of symptoms to ensure high concentration of virus particles and should be transported with an appropriate transport media at 2–8°C and testing performed within 48 hours. Studies have reported increased diagnostic yield (60% vs. 35%) and considerably higher sensitivity (80–100%) and specificity (82–100%) for these assays when compared to conventional diagnostic methods such as direct fluorescent antibody (DFA), viral isolation, and immunoassays. Molecular testing has considerably improved the diagnosis of respiratory pathogens and is being considered as the new "gold standard."

■ PREVENTION

Despite the huge health impact caused by these viruses, vaccines are available only for few. Influenza and SARS-CoV-2 are the viruses for which vaccines are currently available.

Influenza virus is remarkable for its high mutation rate, compromising the ability of the immune system to protect against new variants. Hence, vaccines are produced biannually for both the Northern and Southern hemispheres based on prevalent strains that are detected by surveillance. The vaccines usually cover for the predominant lineages of H3N2, H1N1 and B viruses and are available as trivalent or tetravalent vaccines based on the number of strains.

Vaccines to prevent SARS-CoV-2 infection are considered the most promising approach for curbing the COVID-19 pandemic. Several COVID-19 vaccines are available globally. mRNA vaccines (BNT162b2 and mRNA-1273) and the adenovirus vector vaccines (Ad26.COV2.S) are commonly used. All the available vaccines are highly effective, substantially reduce the risk of COVID-19, especially severe/critical disease, thereby reducing COVID-19-associated hospitalizations and deaths.

■ TREATMENT

Despite the varied presentation and severity of illness following viral infections, the treatment options are mainly supportive. Antiviral agents are available for selected viruses and are recommended only in specific populations. Cidofovir is available for severe adenovirus infections and should be administered with probenecid simultaneously. Ribavirin is available as oral or aerosolized formulations for the treatment of RSV infections; however, its use is not routinely recommended except in selected patients such as extreme preterm, neonates with underlying heart or lung disease. Humanized anti-RSV immunoglobulins (palivizumab) are available for the prevention of RSV infection in these high-risk groups.

Neuraminidase inhibitors such as oseltamivir and zanamivir, which inhibit influenza virus neuraminidase, are effective for treatment and prophylaxis of influenza. For uncomplicated influenza, treatment is generally not required, but if at all, neuraminidase inhibitors need to be given within 48 hours of onset for any clinical benefit. For severe influenza, influenza in the immunocompromised, and avian influenza, benefit can still be found when administered after 48 hours, and treatment should not be withheld in these cases. Amantadine and rimantadine have become obsolete due to development of resistance.

Several drugs have been studied for SARS-CoV-2 following the epidemic. Antiviral agents such as remdesivir, antibody-based therapies such as casirivimab and imdevimab, glucocorticoids, drugs like tocilizumab and baricitinib, and anticoagulants are found to be effective depending upon the time of onset and severity of the disease.

■ INDIAN PERSPECTIVE

Various studies have been done to look at the prevalence of viruses causing respiratory infections in India. In a recent study among adults with acute respiratory infection (ARI), influenza accounted for the maximum number of cases (27.6%) followed by RSV (5.2%), hMPV (3.7%), and parainfluenza-3 virus (3%).[6] Earlier studies have shown a similar pattern with influenza A being predominant (17%) followed by influenza B (6.5%), RSV (5.2%), and HMPV (3.7%). Among children with ARI, a recent study reported RSV (25.8%) as the predominant virus followed by rhinovirus (21.9%), influenza (21%), and adenovirus (12.5%).[7] The study results have been similar in comparison with the past, where RSV and influenza A reported more commonly followed by parainfluenza and metapneumovirus in variable proportions.

> **TAKE HOME MESSAGE**
> - Viruses are the major cause of respiratory infections.
> - Influenza and RSV cause significant illness among young children and the elderly.
> - Rapid antigen detection tests and NAATs are useful in the diagnosis.
> - Vaccines against specific viruses are helpful in prevention and antiviral drugs are available for selected viruses in selected situations.

REFERENCES

1. Bennett JE, Dolin R, Blaser MJ. Mandell, Douglas, and Bennett's Principles and Practice of Infectious Diseases E-Book. Philadelphia: Elsevier Health Sciences; 2019.
2. Park CE. Diagnostic methods of respiratory virus infections and infection control. Korean J Clin Lab Sci. 2021;53(1):11-8.
3. Lessler J, Reich NG, Brookmeyer R, Perl TM, Nelson KE, Cummings DA. Incubation periods of acute respiratory viral infections: a systematic review. Lancet Infect Dis. 2009;9(5):291-300.
4. Van Doorn HR, Yu H. Viral respiratory infections. In Hunter's Tropical Medicine and Emerging Infectious Diseases. Philadelphia: Elsevier; 2020. pp. 284-8.
5. Das S, Dunbar S, Tang YW. Laboratory diagnosis of respiratory tract infections in children-the state of the art. Front Microbiol. 2018;9:2478.
6. Palani N, Sistla S. Epidemiology and phylogenetic analysis of respiratory viruses from 2012 to 2015-A sentinel surveillance report from union territory of Puducherry, India. Clin Epidemiol Glob Health. 2020;8(4):1225-35.
7. Mishra P, Nayak L, Das RR, Dwibedi B, Singh A. Viral agents causing acute respiratory infections in children under five: a study from Eastern India. Int J Pediatr. 2016;2016:7235482.

Chapter 11

Enteric Fever

Pritam Roy

■ INTRODUCTION

Enteric fever is a common tropical disease manifested by fever and yet preventable. The term "enteric fever" comprises of typhoid and paratyphoid fevers. Typhoid fever is caused by a Gram-negative organism, *Salmonella enterica* subspecies *enterica serovar typhi* (*Salmonella typhi*), while paratyphoid fever is due to any of the three serovars of *Salmonella enterica* subspecies enterica, namely *Salmonella paratyphi A*, *Salmonella schottmuelleri* (also called *Salmonella paratyphi B*), and *Salmonella hirschfeldii* (also called *Salmonella paratyphi C*). In the beginning, it was called typhoid fever because of its clinical resemblance to typhus. In the first half of 1800s, typhoid fever was obviously defined pathologically as an inimitable illness based on its connotation with enlarged Peyer's patches and mesenteric lymph nodes. In 1869, given the anatomic site of infection, the term enteric fever was put forward as an alternate designation to differentiate typhoid fever from typhus. However, to this day, the two names are used interchangeably.[1,2]

Enteric fever is very frequent in the South East Asian region, especially in India; and it can deteriorate quite rapidly to present with complications that can be both intestinal and extraintestinal. Hence, there is a need for the treating doctors to stay alert when managing such cases.

■ PATHOPHYSIOLOGY

The virulence of *Salmonella* is determined by:
- Typhoid toxin
- *Vi antigen (polysaccharide capsule):* Acts as an antiphagocytic agent preventing the action of macrophages, thus shielding the O antigen from antibodies that confer the serum resistance. The attack rate is double in strains positive for Vi antigen than that of Vi negative strains, in spite for the equal dose of microorganisms.
- Liposaccharide O antigen
- *Flagellar H antigen:* Delivers bacterial mobility and adherence upon the gut wall mucosa. Invasion of the gut wall is aided by flagella, and the

type III secretion system is capable of transferring bacterial protein into enterocytes and M cells or by direct penetration of mucosa.

Bacteria attach to M cells and are absorbed by pinched off cytoplasm containing bacteria. This is then extruded into the luminal space. During this, the basal lamina is exposed as M cells are damaged. The clinical condition worsens as it offers easy entry to pathogens for the invasion.

For the uptake of *Salmonella*, the cystic fibrosis transmembrane conductance regulator (CFTR) is said to be important. Thus, patients with abnormal CFTR protein are resistant to typhoid. The transferred proteins stimulate the host cell Rho guanosine triphosphatase (GTPases), which induces the actin rearrangement. This helps the bacteria to grow by uptaking bacterial protein in the phagosomes. This singular characteristic of the bacteria benefits them to endure viable in a pool of host immunity. The bacteria also produces a molecule that excites the epithelial release of chemoattractant eicosanoid, which sequesters neutrophils into the lumen. Mucosal damage is mainly caused by this phenomenon.[3]

Proliferation of Peyer patches, induced by bacteria, causes necrosis and finally, ulceration that complicates the symptoms. Bacteria reach the reticuloendothelial system (RE system) via both lymphatic system and bloodstream, along with other multiple organs, most commonly gallbladder. The early bacteremia phase (24–72 hours) is asymptomatic and transient as these bacteria are phagocytosed by macrophages and monocytes in the RE system called *primary bacteremia*. The capacity of pathogens to grow in these immune cells makes them characteristic, and intracellular multiplication of bacteria in the RE system enforces them to re-enter the bloodstream causing continuous bacteremia for several days and weeks known as *secondary bacteremia*. Secondary bacteremia is the phase in which disease symptoms manifest. Like in other Gram-negative bacteria, an endotoxin has an important role in the pathogenesis. The lipopolysaccharide induces the shock-like reaction, and endotoxemia leads to vascular hyperactivity and catecholamine release, which causes focal necrosis and hemorrhage.[3]

■ CLINICAL DEFINITION[1]

- *Confirmed enteric fever:* Fever ≥38°C for at least 3 days, with a laboratory-confirmed positive culture (blood, bone marrow) of *S. typhi*
- *Probable enteric fever:* Fever ≥38°C for at least 3 days, with a positive serodiagnosis or antigen detection test but without *S. typhi* isolation.

■ CLINICAL FEATURES

Insidious onset of disease but may be abrupt with chills and high fever (especially among children).

Fever

Prolonged fever [38.8–40.5°C (101.8–104.9°F)] which may continue up to 4 weeks in subjects not receiving antibiotic therapy. Relative bradycardia at the peak of high fever may hint toward enteric fever diagnosis. Fever usually ascends in *"step-ladder fashion"* i.e., the temperature rises over the course of each day and dips by the next morning. The peaks and troughs upsurge gradually. Fever typically attains a plateau (39–40°C) after a week when the subject appears toxic, exhausted, and often prostrated. Stepladder fever pattern is characteristically seen in less than one-fifth of cases and there the fever has a steady insidious onset.

Other prominent features are:
- Headache mostly followed by chills, cough, sore throat, sweating, myalgias, malaise, and arthralgia—mainly during prodromal stage.
- Gastrointestinal manifestations included anorexia, abdominal pain, nausea, or vomiting. Initially, there is marked constipation followed by diarrhea.

Physical findings included dry and coated tongue, relative bradycardia (most important clinical sign), hepatosplenomegaly, and abdominal distention and tenderness. In fact, the presence of *fever with hepatosplenomegaly* should make one think of this condition as one of the differential diagnoses. Usually, liver becomes palpable first and then spleen becomes palpable only after a week.

"Temperature–pulse dissociation" (relative bradycardia) occurs in typhoid fever (may be also noted in brucellosis, leptospirosis, some drug-induced fevers). Dicrotic pulse—double beat, the second beat weaker than the first is also noted.

Enteric fever may have typical rash [*"rose spots"*, pinkish maculopapules of around 3 mm diameter which fade on pressure (blanching) and usually appear during the second week of disease around the trunk and finally disappear within next 4 days]. However, it is rarely seen in clinical practice.

Third week of illness is comparatively serious. The typical typhoid state characterized by apathy, confusion, and psychosis is observed along with thready pulse and tachypnea. There is increase in toxemia, crackles over lung base. Severe abdominal distension, anorexia, weight loss, and sometimes foul, green-yellow, liquid diarrhea (pea-soup diarrhea) is observed. Bowel perforation and peritonitis occur due to necrosis in Peyer's patches. Death may occur due to severe toxemia, myocarditis, or intestinal hemorrhage **(Fig. 1)**.

Complications of typhoid fever (in less than one-third of hospitalized cases) are associated with (1) prolonged period of symptoms before hospitalization, (2) host genetics, (3) immunosuppression, (4) using proton

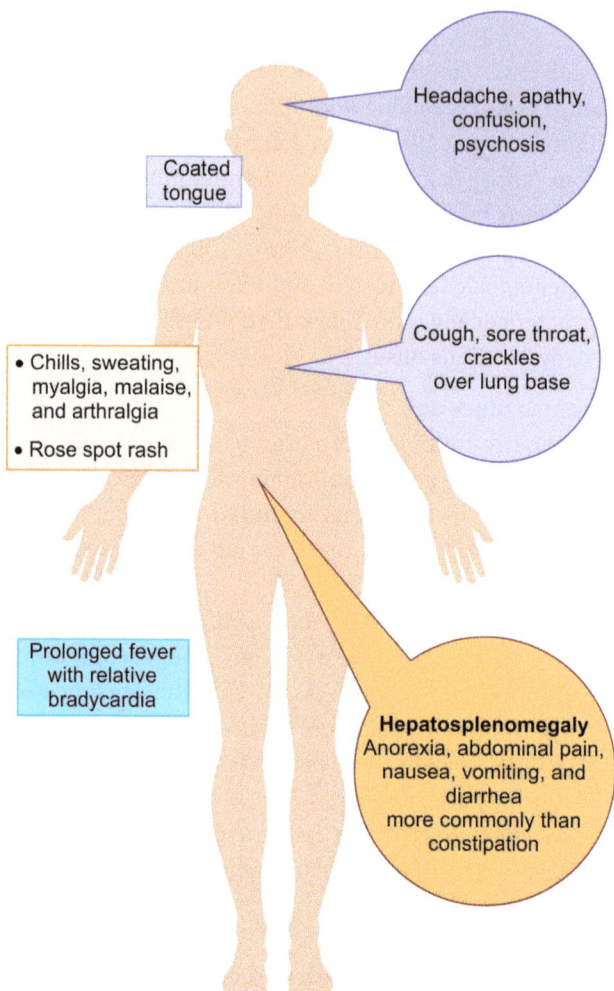

Fig. 1: Summary clinical features.

pump inhibitors (PPIs) for long duration, (5) strain virulence and inoculum, and (6) choice of antibiotic therapy.

Gastrointestinal bleeding (6%) and intestinal perforation (1%) most commonly occur in the third and fourth weeks of illness. Mild relapse develop maximum up to 10% of patients, usually within 2–3 weeks of fever resolution. Nearly 2–5% develop chronic asymptomatic carriage, shedding *S. typhi* in either urine or stool for >1 year. Women, infants, and persons who have biliary abnormalities or concurrent bladder infection with *Schistosoma haematobium* are more prone toward being chronic carriers. Estimated case fatality ranges below 5% but may go up to 20% in cases if not treated **(Fig. 2)**.

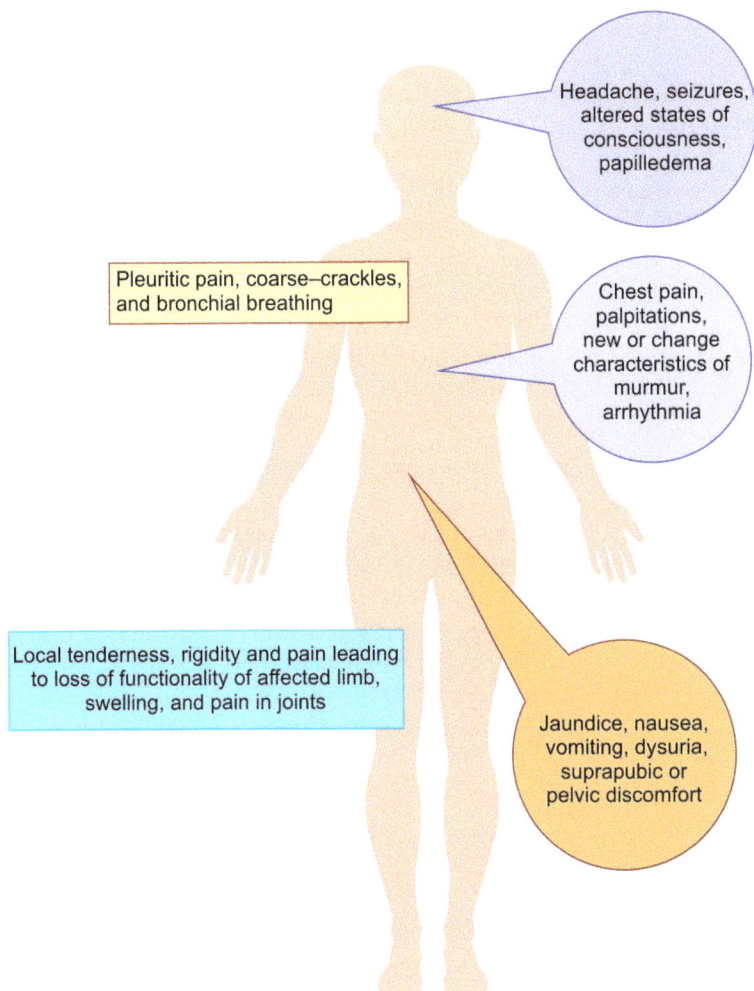

Fig. 2: Red flag symptoms in enteric fever.

LABORATORY EVALUATION (TABLE 1)

TABLE 1: Laboratory evaluation.

Test	Findings
Complete blood count	- *Hemoglobin:* Mild anemia - *Total leukocytic count (TLC):* Low to normal. Monocytosis is also a usual finding. Eosinopenia - *Platelets:* Low to normal - The presence of both eosinopenia and thrombocytopenia is strongly suggestive of enteric fever

Contd...

Contd...

Test	Findings
Blood culture	The specificity of a blood culture is 100%. Direct blood culture followed by microbiological identification remains the gold standard in the diagnosis of enteric fever
Stool culture	Stool culture can help in detecting typhoid carriers
Nested polymerase chain reaction	Due to its high sensitivity and specificity, nested PCR can serve as a useful tool to diagnose clinically suspected, culture negative cases of enteric fever
Widal test	In acute enteric fever, therefore, the anti-O antibody titer is the first to rise, followed by a gradual increase in anti-H antibody titer. The anti-H antibody response persists longer than the anti-O antibody. Difficult to pinpoint a definite cut-off for a positive result since it varies between areas and between times in given areas. A fourfold rise in antibody titer in a paired serum is considered more diagnostic
Typhidot	Detection of IgM signifies acute enteric in the early phase of infection while detection of both IgG and IgM indicates acute enteric in the middle phase of infection, sensitivity (95%), specificity (75%)

(IgG: immunoglobulin G; IgM: immunoglobulin M; PCR: polymerase chain reaction)

■ TREATMENT

Majority of the patients having uncomplicated enteric fever can be treated at home with oral antibiotics and antipyretics. Patients with persistent vomiting, diarrhea, and/or abdominal distension must be admitted and given supportive therapy as well as a parenteral third-generation cephalosporin, a fluoroquinolone, or carbapenem depending on the susceptibility profile. Treatment should be continued for at least 10 days or for 5 days after resolution of febrile episodes.

Antibiotic Therapy for Enteric Fever in Adults (Table 2)

Antibiotic preferences in clinical practice:
- Third-generation cephalosporins are recommended for first-line treatment. While cefixime and cefpodoxime proxetil are administered orally, ceftriaxone, cefotaxime, and cefoperazone are given parenterally. Of these, ceftriaxone is the most convenient to use. Oral third-generation cephalosporins need to be given in higher doses to treat enteric fever.
- Azithromycin is a preferred alternative agent in uncomplicated enteric fever.
- Aztreonam is a potential second-line drug.

TABLE 2: Antibiotic therapy for enteric fever in adults.[2]

Indication	Antibiotic of choice	Dosage	Note
Empirical treatment	• Ceftriaxone • Azithromycin	• 2 g/day IV for 14 days • 1 g/day orally for 5 days	
Fully susceptible	• Ciprofloxacin • Azithromycin • Cefixime • Cefpodoxime proxetil	• 500 mg orally twice a day for 7 days • 1 g/day orally for 5 days • 400 mg twice a day orally for 14 days • 200 mg twice a day orally for 14 days	
Multidrug resistance, fluoroquinolone susceptible	• Ceftriaxone • Cefotaxime • Azithromycin	• 2 g/day IV for 14 days • 100–150 mg/kg/day intravenously in four divided doses • 1 g/day orally for 5 days	• Preferred • To be given till the patient was afebrile for 7 days • Azithromycin is associated with lower rates of treatment failure and shorter durations of hospitalization than are fluoroquinolones
Ceftriaxone resistant	• Aztreonam • Meropenem • Ciprofloxacin	• 1 IV every 8–12 hours • 1 g IV 8 hourly for 14 days • 500 mg twice a day for 28–42 days	• Second line
Carrier	• Amoxicillin	• 2 g orally thrice a day for 28–42 days	• 2–5% of patients who develop chronic carriage of *Salmonella* can be treated with an eradication rate of ~80% • Oral amoxicillin is associated with lower eradication rates than fluoroquinolones but can be considered in persons with fluoroquinolone-resistant strains that are susceptible to ampicillin

- For life-threatening infections resistant to all other recommended antibiotics, fluoroquinolones may be used.
- People infected with enteric fever, or exposed to someone infected with enteric fever, must not be permitted to work if their work involves food handling or caring for children, patients, or the elderly, and should not prepare food for others.
- As enteric fever can be carried on the hands, it is very important to wash hands thoroughly after using the toilet and before handling food. Hands should be washed with soap and water for at least 15 seconds, rinsed and dried well.

CHRONIC CARRIER STATE

A chronic carrier is a person who continues to excrete *S. typhi* for more than a year, either in stool or urine. They may have repeated positive bile or duodenal string cultures. Sometimes, *S. typhi* may be excreted in patients giving no history of enteric fever. The 2–5% of patients who progress to chronic carriage of *Salmonella* should be managed with 4–6 weeks of oral ciprofloxacin or other fluoroquinolones, with an eradication rate of ~80%. Oral amoxicillin is linked with lesser eradication rates than fluoroquinolones but can be prescribed in subjects with fluoroquinolone-resistant strains that are susceptible to amoxicillin. In cases of anatomic abnormality (e.g., biliary or kidney stones), eradication often requires both antibiotic therapy and surgical correction.

Besides, the chronic carrier state is the single most important risk factor for development of hepatobiliary carcinomas, as salmonella carriers with gallstones have been shown to carry an 8.47-fold higher risk of developing cancer of the gallbladder. It is for these reasons that the eradication of carriage is of prime importance.[4]

IMMUNIZATION

Enteric fever can mainly be controlled through improved sanitation, personal and domestic hygiene, safe water for drinking and cooking, and avoiding foods having potential of contamination. Another practical approach of prevention is immunization which is a specific protective measure. Killed whole-cell vaccine was effective but produced strong side effects. Hence, two effective and safe vaccines are now licensed and used in India.

Typhoid Fever Vaccines

The typhoid fever vaccination and revaccianation are summarized in **Table 3**.

TABLE 3: Typhoid fever vaccines.

Vaccine	Age	Route	Dosage	Confers protection	Revaccination	Safety issues
Vi polysaccharide vaccine	≥2 years	Subcutaneously Or Intramuscular	Single dose (0.25 μg); 0.5 mL	7 days after injection	Every 3 years	• Can be coadministered with other vaccines relevant for international traveler. • No serious adverse events and a minimum of local side events are associated.
Ty21 a, live	≥5 years	Oral	1 enteric coated capsule every other day; on 1, 3, and 5th day; total of three-dose regimen	7 days after the last dose	Every 3 years	• Can be coadministered with other vaccines including polio, cholera, yellow fever, and MMR • Proguanil and antibacterial drugs should be stopped from 3 days before until 3 days after giving vaccine • Not to be given during ongoing diarrhea • Well tolerated and low rates of adverse events

(MMR: measles, mumps, and rubella)

> **TAKE HOME MESSAGE**
> - Early diagnosis, complete treatment, and appropriate management of enteric fever reduce both morbidity and mortality.
> - More than 90% of enteric fever cases can be managed at home with proper oral antibiotics and good care.
> - Supportive management such as the use of antipyretics, hydration maintenance, nutritional support, and prompt recognition of complications through red flag signs and managing that ensures a favorable outcome. Electrolyte imbalances, anemia, and thrombocytopenia also need to be corrected if detected.
> - Close follow-up is necessary to detect complications or failure to therapy.
> - Many patients will get suboptimal or inappropriate antibiotic therapy even for suboptimal duration for acute illness with fever prior to proper therapy. This may change the clinical course of the disease, diminish the sensitivity of diagnostic tests, and effect on final patient management.

■ REFERENCES

1. Upadhyay R, Nadka MY, Muruganathan A, Tiwaskar M, Amarapurkar D, Banka NH, et al. API recommendations for the management of typhoid fever. J Assoc Physicians India. 2015;63(11):77-96.
2. Pegues DA, Miller SI. Salmonellosis. In: Locsalzo J, Fauci AS, Kasper DL, Hauser S, et al. (Eds). Harrison's Principles of Internal Medicine, 21st edition. New York: The McGraw-Hill Companies, Inc.; 2022.
3. Bhandari J, Thada PK, DeVos E. Typhoid fever. In: StatPearls. Treasure Island (FL): StatPearls Publishing; 2022.
4. Kalra SP, Naithani N, Mehta SR, Swamy AJ. Current trends in the management of typhoid fever. Med J Armed Forces India. 2003;59(2):130-5.

Chapter 12

Japanese B Encephalitis

*Muralidharan K, Sowmini PR,
Mugundhan K, Pranabananda Pal*

■ INTRODUCTION

Japanese encephalitis (JE) is the most common epidemic encephalitis in the world and is found throughout South and Southeast Asia. The estimated world incidence of JE cases is 30,000–50,000 cases per year, mostly in children. Approximately 25% die and around 50% are left with permanent neurological and psychiatric sequelae. Genetic studies reveal that Japanese encephalitis virus (JEV) originated from an ancestral virus in the area of Malay of Archipelago. Clinical recognition dates back to the 19th century.[2] First case was reported in 1871, in Japan. The disease then spread to Korea, China, Pakistan, India, Northern Australia, and several other countries. Japanese encephalitis virus was isolated from the infected brain tissue in 1924 and *Culex* was found as the vector in 1938. In India, it was first recognized in 1955, when cases from North Arcot district of Tamil Nadu and Andhra Pradesh were admitted in Christian Medical College (CMC), Vellore. JE affected districts in India are Tamil Nadu, Andhra Pradesh, West Bengal, Uttar Pradesh, Assam, Bihar, Pondicherry, Karnataka, Kerala, Maharashtra, and Goa.[1]

■ CAUSATIVE AGENT

It is a zoonotic disease caused by arthropod borne virus, the JE virus, which is an enveloped, positive sense single-stranded RNA virus belonging to *Flaviviridae* group. It is spherical, 40–60 nm in diameter. Its outer envelope is formed by envelope (E) protein and is the protective antigen, which aids in the entry of virus to the inside of the cell.[11] The genome also encodes many nonstructural proteins—NS1, NS2a, NS3, NS4a, NS4b, and NS5 **(Fig. 1)**.

It is transmitted to humans through the bite of infected *Culex* mosquitoes—*Culex tritaeniorhynchus, Culex vishnui,* and *Culex pseudovishnui.* Other mosquitoes such as *Aedes* and *Anopheles* are also considered vectors for JE, but it is very rare. Mosquitoes are responsible for birds-mosquito-birds cycle as well as pig-mosquito-pig cycle. Natural hosts of JE virus are the water birds of *Ardeidae* family, mainly pond herons and cattle egrets. Pigs act as amplifier host, which allows manifold virus multiplication without getting the disease and maintain prolonged viremia. Humans are the end host due to low and transient viremia. Man-to-man transmission does not occur and

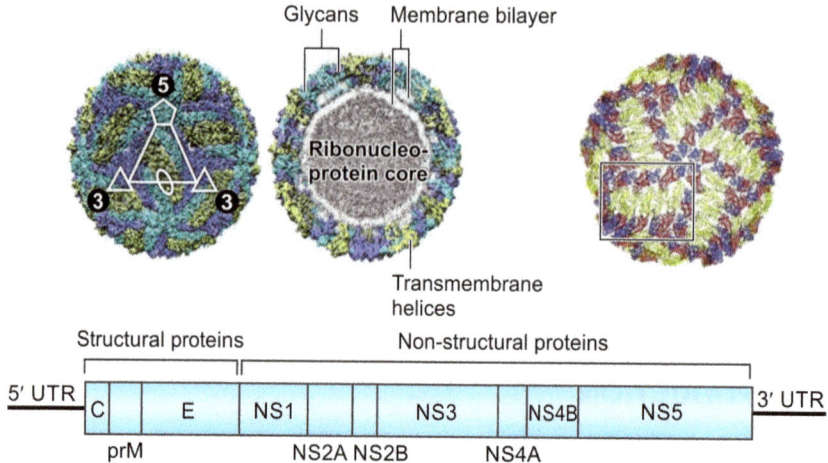

Fig. 1: The structure of Japanese encephalitis virion.[11]

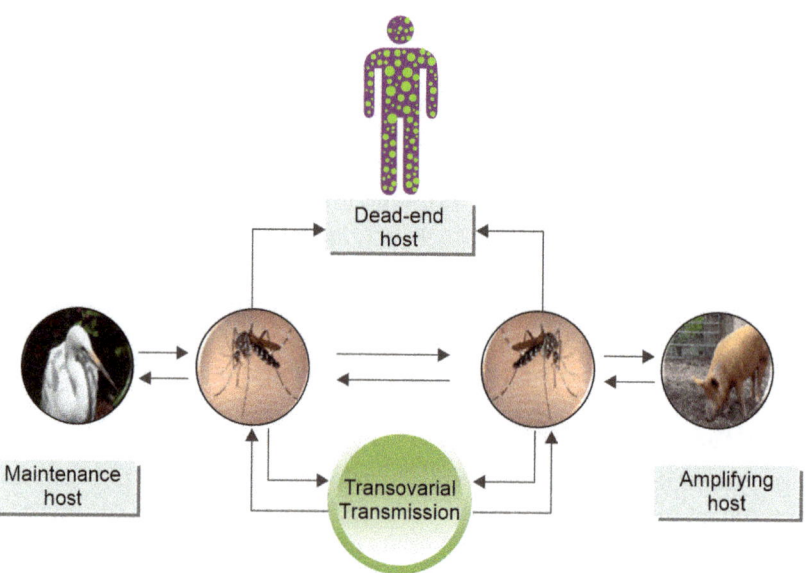

Fig. 2: Vectors and transmission of Japanese encephalitis.[12]

infection does not spread from humans to the mosquitoes. In highly endemic area, vector mosquitoes and their reservoirs—pigs, pond herons, and cattle egrets **(Fig. 2)**—are found in abundance in agricultural areas, particularly rice fields.[12] In temperate areas of Asia, JE transmission is seasonal. Human disease peaks in summer and fall. In the subtropics and tropics, transmission can occur year round often with a peak during the rainy season. Nonvector transmission of JEV between pigs via respiratory secretions has also been described under experimental conditions, but the relevance of this process to the natural cycle of the virus is unclear.

■ PATHOPHYSIOLOGY[3]

Following the bite of an infected mosquito, local replication of virus takes place at the site of the bite, which is followed by lymphatic and hematogenous spread. Replication beyond the primary site leads to secondary viremia, leading to central nervous system (CNS) involvement. The virus gains entry by absorption of viral envelope spikes on to the plasma membrane, subsequently leading to virion production and release by exocytosis. Majority of the infections are subclinical because they are cleared by the immune system before the virus reaches the CNS. The JE virus infects the endothelium of capillaries of the brain. An inflammatory response happens and glial nodules are formed which consists of foci of degenerating neurons surrounded by inflammatory cells **(Fig. 3)**. The predominant cell type in cerebrospinal fluid (CSF) as well as in the brain tissue is the helper/inducer CD4 T-cells. B lymphocytes are predominantly confined to the perivascular space. Circulating antibodies play a vital role in modulation of infection by limiting the viremia in pre-neuroinvasive stage.

On gross pathology, there is mild leptomeningeal reaction and diffuse edema of the brain. The lesions are restricted mainly to the gray matter. The thalamus, substantia nigra, anterior horn of the spinal cord, the cerebral cortex, and the cerebellum are most severely affected. Histopathological changes include loss of Nissl substance in the affected neurons. They become hyaline and eosinophilic, surrounded by predominantly neutrophils microglial phagocytes which ingest the dead neurons. Cuffs of mononuclear lymphocytes distend the Virchow Robin spaces. Microglia hypertrophy and microglial lipid phagocytes appear in response to necrosis.

■ CLINICAL FEATURES

The incubation period is between 5 and 15 days. Mostly the disease is asymptomatic or mildly symptomatic. Patient present with a febrile headache syndrome, aseptic meningitis, or encephalitis. In the encephalitic form, there is prodrome of headache, fever, nausea, vomiting, malaise, and abdominal symptoms, which last for 2-4 days. Prodromal stage may be abrupt (1-6 hours), acute (6-24 hours), or more commonly subacute (2-5 days). Fever is usually high grade and abrupt.[7] In half of the cases, it is more gradual. It is followed by the encephalitis stage, which is characterized by signs of cortical, subcortical, extrapyramidal, bulbar, cerebellar, and spinal cord involvement. Seizures and psychosis are more common in children, while headache and meningismus are more common in adults. Convulsions may be generalized or focal. Status epilepticus is not common. Decerebration and decortication can be seen in severe cases. Focal neurological signs such as hemiplegia, quadriplegia, and cerebellar signs all have been reported. Parkinsonian features such as mask-like blank staring facies and tremors suggest involvement of basal ganglia. Movement disorders such as lip-smacking, bruxism, choreoathetosis,

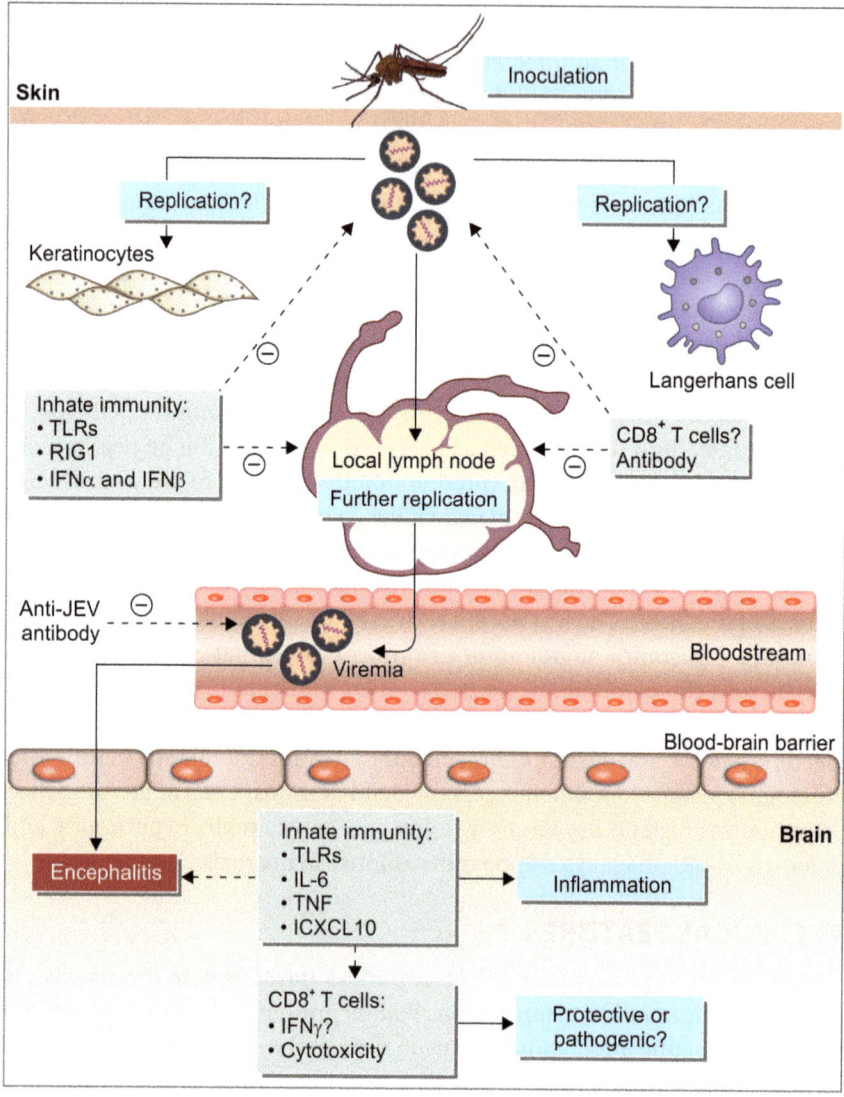

Fig. 3: Pathogenesis of Japanese encephalitis.[3]
(IFN: interferon; IL: interleukin; TLR: toll-like receptor; TNF: tumor necrosis factor)

dystonia, and hemiballismus are also seen.[5] Poliomyelitis like acute flaccid paralysis indicates damage to anterior horn cells. It has also been occasionally associated with Guillain–Barré syndrome, transverse myelitis, acute disseminated encephalomyelitis, and N-methyl-D-aspartate (NMDA) receptor encephalitis. Brainstem involvement is evidenced by conjugate deviation of eyes, pupillary abnormalities, and abnormal breathing patterns. Non-neurological signs during acute illness are pulmonary and urinary symptoms, gastric hemorrhage, hypertension or hypotension, bradycardia or tachycardia, and pericarditis. During the convalescent phase, fever and features of raised intracranial pressure (ICP) subside. There may be complete improvement or patients may be left with severe residual deficits such as movement disorders, neuropsychiatric symptoms, muscle weakness, or cerebellar signs.[6]

DIAGNOSIS

The core of encephalitic syndrome constitutes acute febrile illness with meningeal involvement and various combinations of the following signs and symptoms: Hemiparesis with asymmetry of deep tendon reflexes, mutism or aphasia, Babinski sign, and involuntary movements. For clinical clues to JE, we should look for abnormal posturing, typical facies, focal deficits, and involuntary movements.[7]

Clinical Suspect

Febrile illness of variable severity associated with neurological symptoms ranging from headache to meningitis or encephalitis. Symptoms can include headache, fever, meningeal signs, stupor, disorientation, coma, tremors, paralysis, hypertonia, and loss of coordination.

Probable Case

A suspected case with presumptive laboratory results—detection of an acute phase antiviral antibody response through immunoglobulin M (IgM) or elevated and stable JE antibody titers in serum through enzyme-linked immunosorbent assay (ELISA)/ hemagglutination inhibition (HI)/ neutralizing assay.

Confirmed Case

A suspect case with confirmed laboratory result—JE IgM in CSF or fourfold or greater rise in paired sera (acute and convalescent) through IgM/IgG ELISA, HI, neutralization test or detection of virus, antigen, or genome in tissue, blood or other body fluid by immune-chemistry, immunofluorescence, or polymerase chain reaction (PCR).

INVESTIGATIONS[9]

Routine Hematology

Polymorphonuclear leukocytosis and elevated erythrocyte sedimentation rate (ESR).

Cerebrospinal Fluid Study

In cerebrospinal fluid, pleocytosis is seen, with cell count ranging from 10 or less to 1,000 cells/cu mm. It is polymorphonuclear in the early stage, followed by mononuclear cells in the later phase. Cerebrospinal fluid protein is mildly elevated and it is usually <100 mg/dL.

Electroencephalogram

Electroencephalogram changes are often nonspecific, showing diffuse slowing in the delta or theta range. Alpha coma and epileptiform discharges can also be seen.

Electrophysiology

Motor evoked potentials (MEPs) show various abnormalities such as unrecordable MEP, prolongation of central motor conduction time (CMCT), and normal CMCT. These abnormal MEP is attributed to the involvement of spinal cord, brainstem, subcortical white matter, and cerebral cortex. Somatosensory evoked potential (SEP) and brainstem evoked response audiometry (BERA) are usually normal. Electromyography may show a high frequency of positive sharp waves and fibrillation, consistent with anterior horn cell involvement.

Neuroimaging[8]

Computed tomography (CT) of the brain shows hypodense lesions in the thalami and basal ganglia **(Fig. 4A)**. Computed tomography is abnormal in 56% of the patients. Magnetic resonance imaging (MRI) shows more prominent changes in the thalami, basal ganglia, cerebellum, pons, substantia nigra, cerebral cortex, and spinal cord. In an endemic area, bilateral thalami involvement in an encephalitis patient is suggestive of JE. The lesions are hypointense on T1 and hyperintense on T2 **(Fig. 4B and C)**. In the subacute stage, lesions may be of mixed intensity on T1 and T2, reflecting the hemorrhage.

Virology and Serology

Definitive diagnosis needs virological or serological confirmation. It is very difficult to isolate the virus from blood cultures since the viremia is very shorter and transient. It can be recovered from the CSF in one-third of the cases. The most reliable serological test is IgM capture ELISA. It detects the antibodies in about 75% of patients within four days after onset of illness and in nearly all the cases by the end of a week. Demonstration of fourfold rise in the titer of IgG antibody by hemagglutination, neutralizing, or complement fixing tests in convalescent sera is also diagnostic.[9]

■ TREATMENT

There is no specific antiviral medicine available against JEV. Clinical management of JE is supportive and is directed at maintaining fluid and electrolyte balance and control of convulsions. High-dose steroids are found

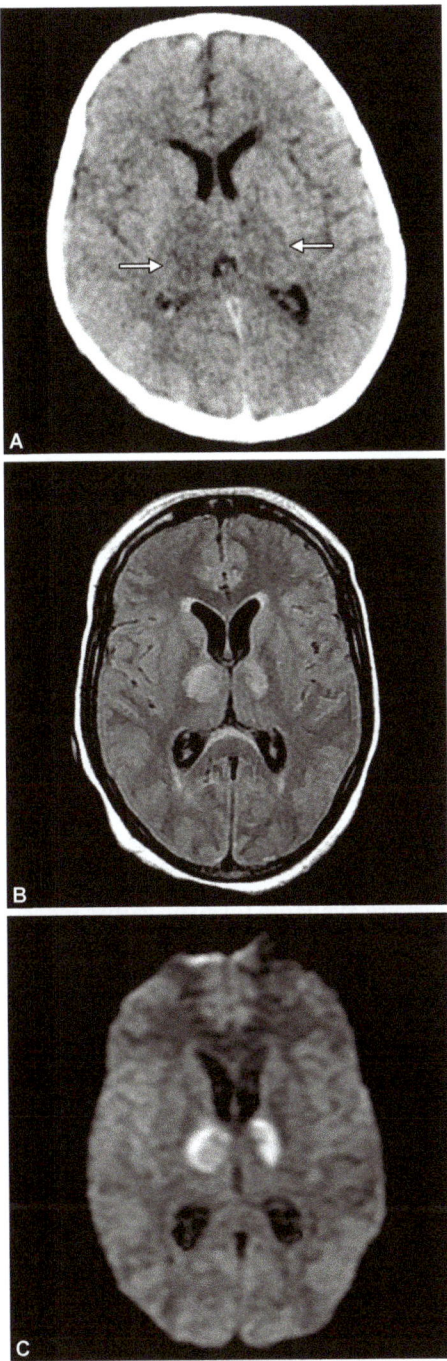

Figs. 4A to C: (A) Computed tomography (CT) of the brain showing bilateral thalamic hypodensity; (B and C) Magnetic resonance imaging (MRI) of the brain showing hyperintense fluid-attenuated inversion recovery (FLAIR) signal and restricted diffusion in the thalami bilaterally.[8]

to have no demonstrable benefit. No drugs are available to arrest or minimize the damage after the symptom onset. Treatment is structured to provide symptomatic relief in the milder cases and prevention of complications in severe cases by means of good nursing care, adequate nutrition, and fluid intake.[10] Raised ICP is managed by airway management and hyperventilation and by use of mannitol. Other diuretics such as acetazolamide and furosemide are of uncertain benefit. In a randomized double blind trial, interferon alpha-2a has not reduced either the mortality or the long-term neurological sequelae. Other clinical trials involving ribavirin, intravenous immunoglobulin (IVIg), minocycline, pentoxifylline, fenofibrate, etanercept, and nitazoxanide also did not yield satisfactory results.

■ CONTROL MEASURES

It involves control of the reservoir and the vector. It is practically impossible to take care of reservoirs. Pig rearing should be discouraged in areas where rice cultivation is widespread. Piggeries should be kept away (4–5 km) from human dwellings. With respect to vector control, insecticide spray is not feasible as vector breed in paddy fields. Eco-management of paddy fields such as alternate wetting and drying can be done instead of irrigation systems. Ultra-low volume insecticide spray by fogging and sterile male technique are other available options. Mosquito bite should be prevented by use of mosquito nets and repellents, especially after dusk, as the biting period of mosquito lasts from dusk to early morning.

■ PREVENTION[10]

Four type of vaccines are available for use against JE: Mouse brain-derived killed vaccine, cell culture-based killed vaccine, live-attenuated vaccine, and live chimeric vaccine. In mouse brain-derived killed vaccine, Nakayama and Beijing strains are used. The Nakayama vaccine is given subcutaneously in two doses, each 1 mL 1–4 weeks apart, to children 1–3 years of age. Booster dose is given after 1 year and after 3 years. The vaccine produced from Beijing virus contains higher antigen concentration and is used in 0.5 mL dose. Three doses are given on days 0, 7, and 30 or days 0, 7, and 14. JE vaccines available in India are as follows:
- Live-attenuated SA-14-14-2 from China (Chengdu)
- Vero cell-derived inactivated SA-14-14-2 vaccine (JEEV in India and internationally available as IXIARO)
- Vero cell-derived inactivated vaccine based on Indian Kolar strain (JENVAC).

Vaccination is recommended for children till 15 years living in JE endemic areas and for travelers to endemic/epidemic areas, provided expected stay is for a minimum of four weeks.

Japanese encephalitis vaccination has mass vaccination and routine vaccination. For mass vaccination (1-15 years), one dose JE vaccine. For routine vaccination, it will be two doses schedule—0.5 mL subcutaneous with first dose at 9-12 months and second dose at 16-24 months.

■ CONCLUSION

Japanese encephalitis is still a devastating disease since no specific treatment are available other than the best supportive care. In spite of availability of vaccines, 69,000 cases of JE are estimated to occur every year in Asia, and this figure is also probably an underestimate. Given the paradoxical role of the immunity in JE, with evidence of both pathological and protective elements, strong consideration must be given to trials involving combination therapy which test the treatment regimens consisting of both antiviral and anti-inflammatory drugs. Some potential treatments, such as JEV-specific monoclonal antibody, may provide a clinical proof of principle to develop treatments for other arboviral encephalitides and could hasten up the development of treatments for other newly emerging *Flaviviruses* in the future.

> **TAKE HOME MESSAGE**
> - Japanese encephalitis (JE) is caused by arthropod borne virus, the JE virus, belonging to *Flaviviridae* group. It is transmitted to humans through the bite of infected *Culex* mosquitoes—*C. tritaeniorhynchus, C. vishnui,* and *C. pseudovishnui*.
> - Natural hosts of JE virus are the water birds of *Ardeidae* family, mainly pond herons and cattle egrets. Pigs act as amplifier host, which allows manifold virus multiplication without getting the disease and maintain prolonged viremia. Humans are the end host due to low and transient viremia. Man-to-man transmission does not occur.
> - The incubation period is 5-15 days. It has a prodrome phase, encephalitis phase, and convalescence phase. Patient can present with seizures, psychosis, meningismus, headache, altered sensorium, Parkinsonism, movement disorders such as lip-smacking, bruxism, choreoathetosis, dystonia, and hemiballismus, poliomyelitis-like acute flaccid paralysis, and focal deficits.
> - Cerebrospinal fluid pleocytosis is seen. MRI shows more prominent changes in the thalami and basal ganglia. In an endemic area, bilateral thalami involvement in an encephalitis patient is suggestive of JE. The most reliable serological test is IgM capture ELISA.
> - There are no specific antiviral medicine available against JEV. Clinical management of JE is supportive. Vaccine is given as two doses schedule—0.5 mL subcutaneous with first dose at 9-12 months and second dose at 16-24 months.

■ REFERENCES

1. Rodrigues FM. Epidemiology of Japanese encephalitis in India, A brief overview. In: National conferences on Japanese encephalitis. New Delhi: Indian Council of Medical Research; 1984. pp. 1-9.
2. Igarashi A. Epidemiology and control of Japanese encephalitis. World Health Stat. 1992;45(23):299-305.

3. Myint KS, Kipar A, Jarman RG, Gibbons RV, Perng GC, Flanagan B, et al. Neuropathogenesis of Japanese encephalitis in a primate model. PLoS Negl Trop Dis. 2014;8(8):e2980.
4. Ricklin ME, García-Nicolás O, Brechbühl D, Python S, Zumkehr B, Nougairede A, et al. Vector-free transmission and persistence of Japanese encephalitis virus in pigs. Nature Commun. 2016;7:10832
5. Misra UK, Kalita J. Movement disorders in Japanese encephalitis. J Neurol. 1997;244(5):299-303.
6. Kumar R, Tripathi P, Singh S, Bannerji G. Clinical features in children hospitalized during the 2005 epidemic of Japanese encephalitis in Uttar Pradesh, India. Clin Infect Dis. 2006;43(2):123-31.
7. Sarkari NB, Thacker AK, Barthwal SP, Mishra VK, Prapann S, Srivastava D, et al. Japanese encephalitis (JE). Part I: clinical profile of 1,282 adult acute cases of four epidemics. J Neurol. 2012;259(1):47-57.
8. Dung NM, Turtle L, Chong WK, Mai NT, Thao TT, Thuy TT, et al. An evaluation of the usefulness of neuroimaging for the diagnosis of Japanese encephalitis. J Neurol. 20090;256(12):2052-60.
9. Ravi V, Vanajakshi S, Gowda A, Chandramuki A. Laboratory diagnosis of Japanese encephalitis using monoclonal antibodies and correlation of findings with the outcome. J Med Virol. 1989;29:221-3.
10. Indian Academy of Pediatrics, Advisory Committee on Vaccines and Immunization Practices (acvip); Vashishtha VM, Kalra A, Bose A, Choudhury P, Yewale VN, et al. Indian Academy of Pediatrics (IAP) recommended immunization schedule for children aged 0 through 18 years, India, 2013 and updates on immunization. Indian Pediatr. 2013;50(12):1095-108.
11. Turtle, L., Solomon, T. Japanese encephalitis — the prospects for new treatments. Nat Rev Neurol 14, 298–313 (2018).
12. Shailendra K. Saxena et al. Japanese Encephalitis: A Neglected Viral Disease and Its Impact on Global Health. Trends in infectious disease. March 2014.

Chapter 13

Filariasis

Shantanu Kumar Kar, Md Karimulla

■ INTRODUCTION

Filariasis is caused by roundworms of the *Filarioidea* type and belongs to a group of diseases called helminthiases. Being parasites, they are transmitted by blood-feeding insects such as black flies and mosquitoes and exists in the wild in subtropical parts of Asia, Africa, the South Pacific, and some parts of South America. Out of eight known filarial worms, where humans are definitive hosts, are broadly divided into three groups according to the body parts they affect:

1. Lymphatic filariasis (LF) caused by parasites of *Wuchereria bancrofti*, *Brugia malayi*, and *Brugia timori* that primarily affect lymphatic system.
2. Subcutaneous form of filariasis is caused by Loa Loa that affects eye, *Mansonella streptocerca*, and *Onchocerca volvulus* cause river blindness.
3. Serous cavity filariasis is caused by *Mansonella perstance* and *Mansonella ozzardi* that occupy serous cavity of abdomen.

Lymphatic filariasis poses a major health problem globally and affects 863 million people in 50 countries including India. Being a debilitating parasitic disease, it is associated with social stigmas and poor health. Next to leprosy, it is the most common cause of physical disability globally. The clinical disease manifestations have a wide range starting from acute filarial fever, acute adeno lymphangitis, tropical pulmonary eosinophilia (TPE), to chronic features such as hydrocele, lymphedema, and grotesque elephantiasis. The infection is caused mostly due to parasitic *W. bancrofti*, (90%) transmitted by mosquito species Culex quinquefasciatus. *B. malayi* is called *Brugian filariasis* which is transmitted by *Mansonia* mosquito species.[1]

Around 40% of global filarial infections in humans, i.e., 450 million account for infected and affected people in India is mainly due to filariasis. Besides this, approximately, 450 million people are at risk of infection. Currently, the disability adjusted life years (DAYLs) lost due to LF is nearly 2.06 million that is equivalent to 8.11 million in dollars due to wage loss.

Lymphatic filariasis has been targeted by World Health Assembly for global elimination as a public health problem.[2] The infection is prevalent in both urban and rural areas. The rural areas of several states of Uttar Pradesh,

Andhra Pradesh, Bihar, Odisha, Kerala, Tamil Nadu, and West Bengal are affected by filariasis. Bihar has the highest endemicity of filariasis (17%), followed by Kerala (15.7%), and Uttar Pradesh (14.6%). Both Andhra Pradesh and Tamil Nadu have (10%) endemicity, while Lakshadweep (1.8%) and Goa (<1%) showed lower rates. Madhya Pradesh (>3%) and Assam (5%) exhibited moderate endemicity. Around 97% of cases with disease and 86% of mf. carriers are contributed by few states such as Andhra Pradesh, Bihar, Kerala, Odisha, West Bengal, and Uttarakhand. *W bancrofti* causing filariasis is considered as one of the major vector-borne disease and exhibited as the leading cause of disability globally due to manifestation lymphoedema, hydrocele, and elephantiasis. While recognizing the impact of filarial disease on economy, disability and associated stigmas and near availability of various strategies to prevent the filarial infection and possible effective management of associated morbidity, global program was launched by the World Health Organization (WHO) for elimination of lymphatic filariasis (GPELF) in the year 2000 that includes two major objectives: (1) Interruption of transmission of parasite by repeated programs of Mass Drug Administration (MDA) annually and (2) prevention of LF-related morbidity management and disability prevention (MMDP).

Mass Drug Administration was targeted to reduce both prevalence of infection and density of microfilaria (mf). In order to maintain the density of microfilaria to a very low level, MDA was envisaged annually, since it can eventually lead to elimination of infection. This strategy was based on two pillars: (1) MDA and (2) preventive chemotherapy by using a combination therapy of diethylcarbamazine citrate (DEC) with albendazole in *Bancrofti* endemic filariasis with morbidity management tools for those already affected. In different areas of Africa, combination of ivermectin (IVM) with albendazole is used where onchocerciasis or river blindness is coendemic.

Based on WHO published new guidelines, an alternative to new MDA regimen recommended to eliminate LF is combination of treatment with ivermectin, DEC, and albendazole (IDA) to accelerate the impact of transmission of parasite. In India, in 2019, IDA was used to treat around 41 million people in 4–16 districts. Recently, reports have shown the global decline of transmission of LF after MDA program was initiated. Accordingly, 16 countries have been acknowledged to have achieved elimination of LF as a public health problem.

Global program of lymphatic filariasis's target to eliminate LF as a public health problem globally by 2020 will not be achieved by then. Despite this setback due to COVID-19, WHO will accelerate work to achieve target by 2030.[3]

■ PATHOPHYSIOLOGY

To maintain the life cycle, filarial worms require a vertebrate host as well as a blood-sucking arthropod vector to pick up mf from the human infected host to propagate through the vector. These microfilariae lose their sheath inside the intermediate host, the vector mosquito. After desheathing, these migrate to thoracic muscle of mosquito where these develop into first-stage larvae and then to second-stage and subsequently, the third-stage larvae when they migrate to hemocoel to proboscis of mosquito. For further development, they require human host and enter the host during blood meal by an infected mosquito and penetrate the host skin and reach lymphatic vessels of human host. Within the lymphatic vessels, they develop into adult worms that take around 6 months. The adult worm resides in lymphatics for 6-8 years as per their life span. The active reproductive phase lasts 4-6 years; when the mature female and male mate and produce very small millions of larvae called mf that enters host's blood circulation. The mf measures 244-296 μm by 7.5-10 μm, get sheathed, and get their characteristic nocturnal periodicity.[1] During night time, the mf of both *W. bancrofti* and *B. malayi* get distributed in blood circulation in an even manner and are available for ingestion and transmission by mosquitoes. The microfilarial 24 hours cycle follows the host's 24-hour cycle and some rhythmic change of the host acts as a cue to the mf.

Both *W. bancrofti* and *B. malayi* mf. are dependent on absolute size of the arterial (venous–arterial) difference in their oxygen tension called oxygen barriers that is lower at night, i.e., 40 mm Hg, compared to its day, i.e., 55 mm Hg, thereby, mf passes through lungs at night, but gets accumulated there by day. To promote transmission at night, the mf behavior is adopted in the blood circulation, when large number of mf came to peripheral blood circulation, and the arthropod vector mosquito is likely to bite human host.

When the mosquito bites a healthy person, the L3 of larval worm traversing the integument, reaches the lymph vessels, where they develop into adult worm. This arrangement is carried out by the vector to achieve 24-hour rhythm is called the classic periodicity. A person who is micro-filaremic can serve as a source of infection to other healthy people through mosquito bites.[4]

Adult worm after entering lymph vessels of human hosts initially cause lymphatic flow dysfunction due to lymphangiectasia as well as inflammatory reaction due to damage caused by worm. The worms reside in the afferent, efferent, and hilar lymphatics that may cause blockage or obstruction to lymph flow exhibited by the subclinical lymphangiectasia. The *Wolbachia* bacteria residing in the mf after release cause damage due to inflammatory reaction causing lymphatic damage.[5]

Based on host's immune response, the disease progression varies between the infected subjects. Suppression of Th 1 and Th 2 immune response of the host can lead to chronicity of the disease. During asymptomatic carrier stage of the host, synergistic interplay occurs between natural immunoglobulin G4 (IgG4), in blocking the pathogenesis. However, genetic predisposition of the host can lead to lymphedema. In endemic areas also, prenatal exposure play important role.

CLINICAL FEATURES

Clinically, as per disease spectrum, individuals can be classified in the following in endemic areas:
- *Endemic normal (EN):* Endemic population who neither exhibit microfilaremia nor any disease symptom
- *Chronic (CH):* Subjects manifesting clinical features such as elephantiasis, hydrocele, or both exceeding 4 years
- *Asymptomatic carriers (AS):* Subjects who have both microfilaremia and antigenemia without any clinical symptoms.
Clinical manifestation of the disease can be seen as acute or chronic.

Manifestation in acute stage:
- Adenolymphangitis occurs due to host immune response to antigen released by parasites while dying. It exhibits bouts of fever with sudden onset accompanied by painful lymphadenopathy. Epididymitis occurs in males which is painful.

DIAGNOSIS

Detailed history taking like travel to endemic areas, onset, and duration of illness is important for diagnosis. The laboratory examination of complete blood count showing eosinophilia, a peripheral thick blood smear collected at night and stained in Giemsa showing microfilariae in blood is essential and clinches the diagnosis. This method has now been replaced by more specific (100%) and sensitive (97%) test like detection of circulating filarial antigen test which can be performed in daytime. This is dipstick in nature and can diagnose also of negative condition. Besides, other tests include visualization of adult worm in tissue specimens, membrane filtration technique, ultrasonography demonstrating filarial dance sign, lymphoscintigraphy, molecular tests such as in situ hybridization, immunochromatography, and polymerase chain reaction (PCR) serologic and enzyme assay and tests for detection of IgG1 and IgG4 provide alternative to earlier used microscopic method for diagnosis of mf. Routine assays can detect elevated levels of IgG4 in blood. Assays for detecting filarial antigen can also be used to indicate filarial infection.[5]

TREATMENT

Adults and children, >18 years, affected by active filarial infection can be treated either by 1 day or 12-day regimen of DEC (6 mg/kg/day) treatment. 1 day is generally as effective as 12-day regimen. In TPE cases, a prolonged regimen with DEC is given for 14–21 days. DEC is well tolerated.

ANTIPARASITIC TREATMENT

The goal of antiparasitic treatment in LF is for killing adult worms as the disease pathology like hydrocele and lymphoedema are primarily driven by adult parasite. DEC is considered as the drug of choice as it works as both microfilaricidal and active against adult worm. The side effects are limited and depend upon microfilarial density in blood. Common side reactions are dizziness, fever, muscle pain, or pain in joints, which are transient and reversible. The potent microfilaricidal drug, ivermectin, is effective against mf of both *B. malayi* and *W. bancrofti* but no effect in parasite adult stage.

The symbiosis of filarial nematodes and intracellular *Wolbachia* bacteria was exploited as target for antibiotic therapy of LF that results in sterility and inhibits larval development and adult LF. Doxycycline could in addition acts to the effect in worm sterility or viability, prevents the onset of development of filarial pathology. Even adult worms killing with doxycycline in dosage of 200 mg/day for 4-6 weeks have shown good results in some studies. The disease in its late stage does not get benefit from pharmacologic therapy.

MANAGEMENT OF CHRONIC FILARIAL INFECTION

Response to DEC treatment in acute forms of filariasis is excellent. Those cases exhibit chronic stage of the disease such as lymphedema or elephantiasis respond poorly. Patients with hydrocele respond to surgery such as hydrocelectomy, but recurrences are seen in some cases.

Chronic forms such as lymphoedema and elephantiasis are very debilitating which makes the subject incapable of carrying out regular routine work. With longstanding filarial infection presenting with complication such as elephantiasis is the grimmest. These cases may be subjected to appropriate surgical techniques such as lymphovenous anastomosis (LVA) or other techniques that can yield good result in reducing limb size; but needs postsurgical management and compressive stockings. An interprofessional approach by trained team is required for achieving optimal result in patients.

The lymphoedema subjects can be managed by role of basic principle of patient care such as hygiene, elevation of limb, exercising regularly, besides wound care, and wearing appropriate shoes and stockings.

Restricting a fatty acid diet is extremely useful to overcome chyluria cases.

Disabilities arising from lymphoedema, elephantiasis, and hydrocele cause significant public health problem.

Medical measures that can be one like treatment of acute attack (ADL) while reducing its frequency and severity with hygiene measures washing and basic skin care can help in preventing lymphoedema progression to elephantiasis stage. Usually, bouts of ADL can be treated with use of antibiotics as recommended with supporting measures.

> **TAKE HOME MESSAGE**
> - LF is transmitted by mosquito bite infected by filarial nematode *W. bancrofti*.
> - Globally, it constitutes the second most common cause of disability.
> - The most debilitating complication of the disease is manifestation of elephantiasis.
> - DEC constitutes the mainstay of treatment worldwide.
> - GPELF advocates an annual dose of DEC and albendazole for elimination of LF. Recently, a combination of a single dose of triple-drug therapy (ivermectin + DEC + albendazole) has been recommended and is being implemented, given annually for a few years is advocated for elimination along with package for MMDP.

REFERENCES

1. Suma T. Krishnasastry, Charles D. Mackenzie and Rajeev Sadanandan. Scaling-up flariasis lymphoedema management into the primary health care system in Kerala State, Southern India: a case study in healthcare equity. Infectious Diseases of Poverty (2022) 11:9 https://doi.org/10.1186/s40249-022-00936-6.
2. Wahied Khawar Balwan, Neelam Saba. Elimination of Lymphatic Filariasis: A Neglected Disease of India. EAS Journal of Parasitology and Infectious Diseases. Infectious Diseases of Poverty (2022) 11:9.https://doi.org/10.1186/s40249-022-00936-6.
3. Eliza T. LupenzaID1, Dinah B. Gasarasi, Omary M. Minzi2. Lymphatic filariasis elimination status: Wuchereria bancrofti infections in human populations and factors contributing to continued transmission after seven rounds of mass drug administration in Masasi District,Tanzania.(2022) PLoSONE 17(1): e0262693.
4. P. L. Joshi. Epidemiology of Lymphatic Filariasis. Lymphatic Filariasis(2018), https://doi.org/10.1007/978-981-13-1391-2_1.
5. Hassam Zulfiqar; Ahmad Malik. Bancroftian Filariasis. Treasure Island (FL): StatPearls Publishing; 2022 Jan.

Fungal Infections in the Tropics

Chapter 14

Shreya Singh, Arunaloke Chakrabarti, Md Karimulla

■ INTRODUCTION

The tropics are characterized by high average daily temperatures, consistent rainfall, and high humidity making their environment ideal for the growth of the fungi.[1,2] Tropical mycoses can be encountered not just by the residents of tropical countries but also by travelers visiting these regions.[1,2] Tropical fungal infections range from superficial, subcutaneous to systemic disseminated infections, affecting both immunocompromised and apparently healthy individuals.

One of the most commonly encountered superficial tropical mycosis is dermatophytosis, caused by fungi that thrive in keratinized host tissue. Increased hyperhidrosis in tropical conditions is also associated with another superficial infection of pityriasis versicolor.[3] Implantation mycoses due to transcutaneous trauma, manifesting as subcutaneous infections comprises a group of heterogenous fungal diseases including entomophthoromycosis, phaeohyphomycosis, sporotrichosis, eumycetoma, lobomycosis, and chromoblastomycosis.[4] Certain endemically restricted dimorphic fungal diseases are also reported mainly in tropical countries. These include paracoccidioidomycosis in South America from Mexico to Argentina; talaromycosis in South-east Asian countries and emergomycosis (formerly called disseminated emmonsiosis) from China, India, and South Africa.[5]

■ PATHOPHYSIOLOGY

The common tropical fungal infections, their associated pathogens, their ecology, and mode of transmission are summarized in **Table 1**.

■ CLINICAL FEATURES

The commonly encountered clinical manifestations of tropical mycoses are shown in **Figures 1A to F**.

Superficial Infection

Dermatophytosis, commonly called Tinea, is a common pruritic fungal infection caused by dermatophytes of genus *Microsporum, Trichophyton,*

TABLE 1: The geographic distribution, ecology, and mode of transmission of common tropical fungal infections.

Fungal infection (pathogen)	Geographic distribution	Host and ecology	Mode of transmission
Superficial mycoses			
Dermatophytosis (*Dermatophytes*)	Worldwide, majority in tropical zones	Contact with infected humans, pet cats and dogs, cattle, guinea-pigs, etc.	On exposure to arthroconidia present in superficial lesions
Pityriasis versicolor (*Malassezia* spp.)	Worldwide, majority in tropical zones	*Malassezia* spp. commensal of healthy skin, and it is most common in oily areas such as the face, scalp, and back	Conversion to pathogenic form due to genetic predisposition, environmental conditions, immunodeficiency, pregnancy, and application of oily lotions
Subcutaneous mycoses			
Sporotrichosis, "rosebush mycoses," or the "gardener's mycoses" (*Sporothrix* spp.)	Worldwide, majority in tropical zones (Brazil, China, India, Japan, Mexico, Peru, and Uruguay)	Leisure and occupational activities, such as floriculture, agriculture, mining, and wood exploitation. Cats and armadillos are potential sources of zoonotic transmission	Traumatic inoculation or inhalation of infective fungal propagules
Chromoblastomycosis (*Fonsecaea pedrosoi, Phialophora verrucosa, Cladosporium carrionii, Rhinocladiella aquaspersa,* or *Fonsecaea compacta, Exophiala* spp.)	Worldwide, majority in tropical zones (Madagascar island in Africa, Brazil in South America, and China, India, Malaysia, Sri Lanka, Thailand in South-east Asia)	• Strong association with agricultural, labor activities, gardeners, lumberjacks, etc. • In India reported among workers of black tea cultivation farms in Assam, and rubber plantations in Kerala and Western Ghats	Traumatic inoculation
Lobomycosis (*Lacazia loboi*)	Tropical rain forest of South America	In soil, vegetation and aquatic mammals such as dolphins	• Traumatic inoculation/direct contact with infected animals • Accidental direct human-to-human transmission

Contd...

Contd...

Fungal infection (pathogen)	Geographic distribution	Host and ecology	Mode of transmission
Eumycetoma (*Madurella mycetomatis, Madurella grisea,* and *Pseudallescheria boydii* are common agents)	Worldwide, majority in tropical zones (Africa, Latin America, and India)	Soil and vegetation	Traumatic inoculation
Systemic mycoses			
Talaromycosis (*Talaromyces marneffei*)	Southeast Asia including Hong Kong, Myanmar, north-eastern part of India, Southern part of China, Thailand, and Vietnam	Common among patients living with HIV/AIDS, primary immunodeficiency, autoimmune diseases, malignancy, and solid organ and bone marrow transplantations underlying structural lung disease at risk for pulmonary infection. Bamboo rats and dogs are reservoir endemic areas	Inhalation of spores
Emergomycosis (*Emergomyces africanus, E. pasteurianus, E. orientalis*)	Reported from tropical regions of China, India, South Africa	Disease associated with occupational dust exposure	Inhalation of spores
Entomophthoramycosis (*Conidiobolus coronatus, Conidiobolus incongruus,* and *Basidiobolus ranarum*)	Worldwide, majority in tropical zones (Egypt, India Iran, Saudi Arabia, and Thailand)	Plant debris, soil, gastrointestinal tract commensal in bats, fish, amphibians, and reptiles	Inhalation of spores, minor trauma, insect bites (in *Basidiobolus* spp.) and iatrogenic routes
Paracoccidioidomycosis, South American blastomycosis (*Paracoccidioides brasiliensis* and *Paracoccidioides lutzii*)	Latin America from Mexico to Argentina	• Male preponderance, endemicity near waterways and certain agricultural crops (e.g., coffee, tobacco) • The natural habitat is also not precisely known, but it is found in soil near armadillo burrows	Inhalation of spores

(AIDS: acquired immunodeficiency syndrome; HIV: human immunodeficiency virus)

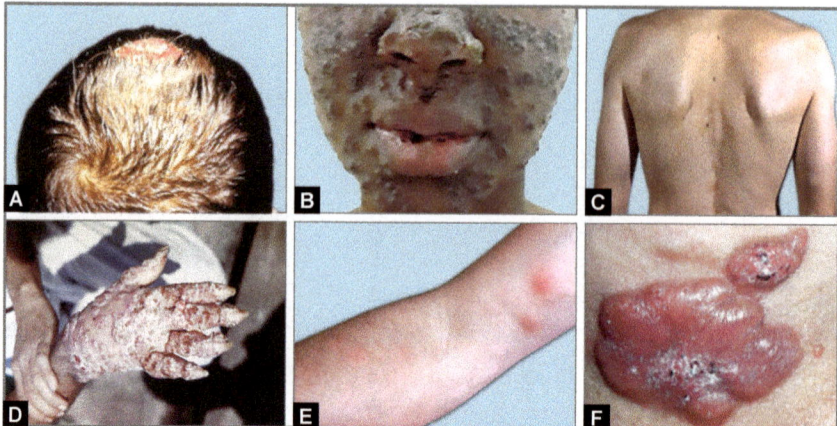

Figs. 1A to F: Clinical images showing (A) superoposterior view tinea capitis; (B) *Emergomyces africanus* infection, with ulcerated and crusted facial plaques and nodules; (C) posterior view of a man's torso with pityriasis versicolor; (D) patients hand with chromoblastomycosis; (E) patient's right arm, with erythematous, papulosquamous lesions, involving the arm's lymphatics due to sporotrichosis; and (F) keloidal skin lesion in lobomycosis.
Source: Images reproduced from the Public health image library, Centre for Disease control and prevention and reference (5) published under the commons attribution non-commercial-no-derivative 4.0 International license.

and *Epidermophyton* (**Table 2**). In India, an increase in dermatophytosis especially antifungal drug resistant infection has been seen over the past 4–5 years with a change in its clinical pattern due to irrational use of both oral antifungals and topical fixed drug combination (FDC) creams.[6] Atypical presentations with ill-defined or multiple bordered lesions, which slowly increase in size, developing unusual shapes are reported.[7]

Another common superficial infection, *pityriasis versicolor*, presents as various, well-demarcated, oval, scaling patches, hyper- or hypopigmented papules or macules usually over the trunk, neck, and proximal extremities. It is seen mostly among teenagers and young adults perhaps due to the more sebum production.[8]

Subcutaneous Infection

The most common clinical manifestation of *sporotrichosis* is cutaneous (lymphocutaneous, fixed cutaneous, multiple inoculation) followed by mucosal (ocular, nasal, or other sites), systemic (osteoarticular, pulmonary, neurological, etc.), and immunological (erythema nodosum, erythema multiforme, reactive arthritis, etc.). Typical lesions are papulonodular at the site of fungal inoculation into the skin, ulcers, or erythematous-scaly, papulopustular, infiltrative, or crusty lesions or fistula progressing along the regional lymphatic channels.[9]

TABLE 2: Clinical presentation of common dermatophytic infections.

Fungal infection (site) (common name)	Clinical presentation
Tinea pedis (foot) (Athlete's foot)	Interdigital subtype—maceration or scales between toes chronic hyperkeratotic (moccasin-type)—chronic plantar erythema with scaling over lateral and plantar foot vesiculobullous or inflammatory subtype
Tinea unguium (nail) (onychomycosis)	Yellowish or brownish discoloration associated with onycholysis and subungual hyperkeratosis or white spots on the nail plate
Tinea capitis (scalp)	Scaly patches, alopecia with black dots at the follicular opening, and subtle hair loss. Severe form called kerion with tender plaque with pustules and crusting
Tinea corporis (body) (ringworm)	Skin infection on the skin of sites other than face, hands, feet, or groin. Annular plaques with central clearing and leading scale
Tinea cruris (groin) (Jock itch)	Infection in groin fold. Annular plaques with central clearing and leading scale
Tinea incognito	Infection misdiagnosed and inappropriately treated with topical corticosteroids or other immunosuppressants. Attenuated scale and erythema, as well as a less well-defined border of lesions

Rhinofacial involvement is common in *entomophthoromycosis* due to *Conidiobolus* spp. with facial deformity, fixed subcutaneous nodules, lymphadenopathy, cellulitis, visual impairment, periorbital swelling, and headaches.[10] *Basidiobolus* spp. infection on the other hand is associated with mobile subcutaneous nodules, hyperpigmentation, and ulceration of skin over the limbs, buttocks, back with lymphedema, and constipation or rectal bleeding in case of gastrointestinal involvement. Gastrointestinal basidiobolomycosis is seen in Middle-East Asian countries. Cases are also reported from India.[10]

Mycetoma is a subcutaneous infection characterized by localized swelling, draining sinuses, and grains (which are aggregates of infecting organisms). It commonly affects the foot.

Chromoblastomycosis lesions are clinically polymorphic and often misdiagnosed. The lesions are erythematous macular, or papulosquamous and spread locally assuming varying grades of severity. There is no involvement of fascia, tendons osteoarticular sites like seen in sporotrichosis and mycetoma, however lymphatic involvement can result in lymphedema. Secondary bacterial infection may occur leading to further disability. One of the most disabling complication is malignant transformation leading to squamous cell carcinoma.[4]

Mycetoma and chromoblastomycosis are reported as neglected tropical disease by World Health Organization.

Lobomycosis or "keloid blastomycosis" lesions are typically red, hard, and shiny keloidal plaques and this disease is seen in South American countries.

Systemic Infection

Paracoccidioidomycosis can have a subclinical form which may last for years and later evolves to clinically manifested disease. The acute/subacute form comprises of fever, weight loss, lymphadenopathy, hepatosplenomegaly, and skin or mucosal lesions. In chronic form, pulmonary infiltrates on chest radiographs and skin or mucosal lesions are seen. Adrenal insufficiency is commonly reported.

Emergomycosis is generally reported in immunocompromised patients with human immunodeficiency virus (HIV) infection, solid organ transplantation, or hematological malignancies and presents as skin lesions with papules, nodules, ulcers, or more invasive forms as pulmonary or disseminated disease.[5]

Talaromycosis (penicilliosis) also primarily affects individuals with advanced HIV disease and other immunosuppressive conditions. It is characterized by molluscum contagiosum type cutaneous lesions mainly on the face and extremities. However, involvement of lungs, liver, spleen, gastrointestinal tract, bloodstream, skin, and bone marrow can be seen especially in immunocompromised patients. Primary pulmonary talaromycosis is described even in apparently healthy people.

■ DIAGNOSIS

Diagnosis of tropical fungal infections is dependent on the logical association between the clinical appearances, radiological findings, and appropriate laboratory tests such as conventional histopathology, microscopy, and culture or immunopathological and molecular techniques.

Direct examination: For direct examination, the specimens are usually observed in the presence of 10% potassium hydroxide (KOH). To digest keratin from samples of hair or nails, up to 20% KOH with or without dimethyl sulfoxide, 10% sodium hydroxide, Amann's chloral lactophenol, and detergents such as sodium dodecyl sulfate (SDS) can also be used.[11] In case of mycetoma, the grains (0.2–5 mm) may be observed grossly in the specimen and microscopic evaluation of crushed grains with KOH or stained with Gram stain is useful in differentiating fungal from bacterial causes. The color of mycetoma grains can also give a clue of the etiological agent as black grains are seen in *Madurella* spp., *Curvularia* spp., *Exophiala* spp., etc., while pale white grains are seen in *Pseudallescheria boydii*, *Acremonium* spp., *Fusarium* spp., etc. Yellow, brown, and red grains are typically seen in bacterial actinomycetoma.

Histopathological examination: Hematoxylin and eosin (H&E) stain, other special stains such as Gomori methenamine silver (GMS) or periodic acid-Schiff (PAS) stain, can be employed to enhance fungal detection. Tissue reaction must be also evaluated in histopathological examinations from patients. Chronic inflammation and tissue destruction with *"Splendore-Hoeppli* phenomenon" is seen in sporotrichosis and entomophthoromycosis. "Asteroid body" or an aggregate of macrophages with epithelioid and multinucleate giant cells, plasma cells, lymphocytes, eosinophils, and surrounded an eosinophilic, PAS-positive extracellular material can also be seen. In chromoblastomycosis, polyhedral cells with a thick pigmented wall along with transverse and longitudinal cross-walls called "medlar bodies" or "copper pennies" or "sclerotic or meristematic" cells can be seen along with hyperkeratosis, acanthosis, and atrophy.[4]

Culture: Definitive diagnosis is based on the isolation and identification of the etiological agent in culture after inoculating the clinical specimens on Sabouraud agar with antibiotic with incubation at 25 and 37°C. In case of dimorphic fungi, for demonstration of dimorphism subculturing, the fungus on enriched media such as brain heart infusion agar, chocolate agar, and blood agar is needed. To detect *Talaromyces marneffei* in blood circulation, automated blood culture system is used so as other fungemia detection. As for other mycelial fungi, sporulation patterns observed on lactophenol cotton blue stained mounts from culture are essential for the morphological identification. Dermatophytes take a longer time to sporulate and to induce spores, sporulation media, which stimulates conidiation and pigment production of dermatophytes, may be used.[11] Biochemical test panels, matrix-assisted laser desorption ionization time of flight (MALDI-TOF) mass spectrometry, or molecular methods can be used for species level characterization. The microscopic and culture findings in common tropical fungal infections are summarized in **Table 3** and **Figures 2A to F**.

Molecular detection: Identification of an organism is achieved using variety of primers such as species specific primer (amplify only the genus/species of interest), or pan fungal primer [amplifies the DNA of any fungal agent which usually targets internal transcribed region (ITS) or 28S region of ribosomal DNA sequence or gene encoding topoisomerase II, or chitin synthase I (CHS I)]. Real-time polymerase chain reaction (PCR) is a rapid and sensitive approach to detect an organism directly from clinical samples. Molecular studies are used to diagnose new infections such as emergomycosis; however, *Emergomyces* spp. can cross react with commercial DNA probes for *Blastomyces dermatitidis* and this should be borne in mind.[5]

Serology: Antigen and antibody detection from serum samples can be used for diagnosis of fungal infections. In talaromycosis, although definitive diagnosis

TABLE 3: Microscopic and culture findings in common tropical fungal infections.

Fungal infection	Microscopy	Culture
Dermatophytosis	Thin septate hyphae can be seen in clinical specimens	Mycelial growth with pigment production in some species
Sporotrichosis	• Small (2–6 µm) budding yeast cells (rare in human, abundant in infected cats) • Cigar-shaped buds (2 by 3 to 3 by 10 µm) rare • Asteroid bodies, the Splendore–Hoeppli reaction on HPE	• Thermally dimorphic • *Mycelial phase at 25–30°C:* Filamentous hyaline • *Yeast phase at 35–37°C:* Creamy colonies with yellow to tan color
Entomophthoromycosis	Broad, thin-walled, sparsely septated, ribbon-like hyphae coupled with acute and chronic inflammatory infiltrate	• *Conidiobolus* spp.: Beige to brown colonies with white aerial hyphae. Spores may have hair-like, villous projections • *Basidiobolus* spp.: Beige waxy colonies with club-shaped spores with knoblike tip that are forcibly discharged. Zygospores have beak-like appendage
Chromoblastomycosis	Single or cluster of muriform cells (chestnut like) 5–12 µm in diameter	Slow growing dark pigmented mycelial colonies (*Exophiala* spp. show initial black yeast phase)
Lobomycosis	Typical globose lemon-shaped cells (about 9 µm in diameter), either singly or in short chains	Cultivation of *Lacazia loboi* in culture medium has not been achieved
Paracoccidioidomycosis	Small and large budding yeasts 2–30 µm in diameter that resembles a "mariner's or pilots wheel"	• Thermally dimorphic • *Mycelial phase at 25–30°C:* glabrous leathery, brownish, flat colony with a few tufts of aerial mycelium to a wrinkled, folded, floccose form, to velvety, white, pink, and beige forms • *Yeast phase at 35–37°C:* Yellowish-beige color and a creamy texture

Contd...

Contd...

Fungal infection	Microscopy	Culture
Talaromycosis	Pleomorphic, sausage-like shape, and cross-wall yeasts, approximately 2.5–4.5 um in diameter, with elongated forms being 1–2 × 3–6 um. Presence of a centrally located transverse septum (e.g., "cross wall") differentiates it from *Histoplasma capsulatum*	• Thermally dimorphic • *Mycelial phase at 25–30°C:* Initially cream-colored, smooth, and moist but turn brown/black after a few weeks. On microscopy of culture growth delicate branching septate hyphae with short tapering conidiophores and surrounding pyriform conidia in a flower-like arrangement seen • *Yeast phase at 35–37°C:* Beige, creamy colonies
Emergomycosis	Small (2–5 μm) yeasts with narrow-based budding, best seen with fungal stains	• *Mycelial phase at 25–30°C:* Yellowish white to tan, initially glabrous, becoming powdery, slightly raised, and furrowed. On LCB, slender conidiophores with "florets" of short secondary conidiophores bearing single small subspherical conidia are seen • *Yeast phase at 35–37°C:* Yellowish-white to tan, pasty, cerebriform colonies

(HPE: Histo-pathological examination; LCB: lactophenol cotton blue)

is usually made by fungal culture of blood, skin biopsy, bone marrow, or lymph nodes, antigen detection is an active area of research. The commercial assay for the detection of *Aspergillus galactomannan* has also shown good sensitivity for detecting *T. marneffei*. Recently, mannoprotein Mp1p enzyme-linked immunosorbent assay (ELISA) and a urine immunochromatographic strip test (ICT) using yeast phase specific monoclonal antibody 4D1 for detection of *T. marneffei* have been reported. In *Sporothrix* spp., the immunodominant antigen is not well established yet, although research groups have found promising accurate serological tests of which, ConA-binding factor is a good candidate as a biomarker.

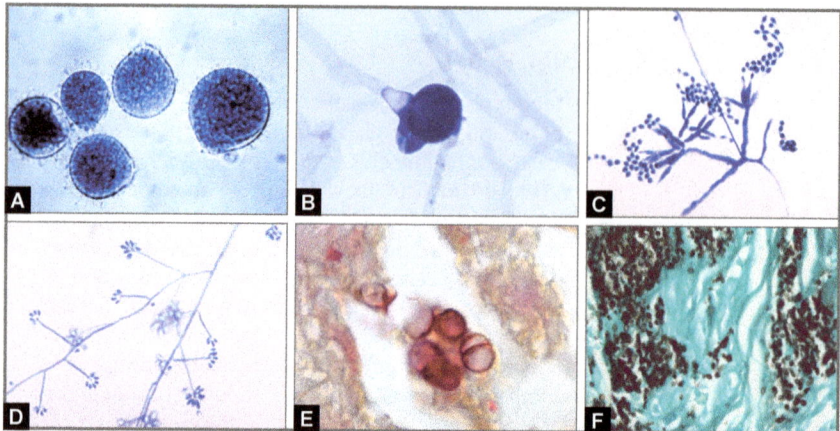

Figs. 2A to F: Photomicrograph depicting ultrastructural morphology of (A) globose-shaped, primary conidia, of *Conidiobolus coronatus* with hair-like appendages projections; (B) *Basidiobolus ranarum* zygospore, prior to its germination into a spore-containing sporangium; (C) Mycelial phase of *Talaromyces marneffei*; (D) Mycelial phase of *Sporothrix schenckii*, showing "flower-petal" arrangement of oval-shaped conidia; (E) "Medlar bodies" or muriform cells seen in chromoblastomycosis; and (F) *Emergomyces africanus* under Grocott stain.
Source: Images reproduced from the Public health image library, Centre for Disease control and prevention and reference (5) published under the commons attribution non-commercial-no-derivative 4.0 International license.

Antibody-based serodiagnosis of fungal infections using different techniques of immunoelectrophoresis, agglutination, immunodiffusion, and ELSIA with crude antigenic fractions or recombinant antigens are also in use. These are commonly used for paracoccidioidomycosis, sporotrichosis, and talaromycosis. Sera from patients suspected of paracoccidioidomycosis should be tested against the traditional exoantigen and purified gp43 of *Paracoccidioides brasiliensis* and circulating free antigen from *Paracoccidioides lutzii*. Results from antibody detection tests provide a presumptive diagnosis and require clinical and epidemiological correlation for an accurate evaluation and determination of the final diagnosis.

▣ TREATMENT

Treatment options for tropical mycoses include topical and systemic antifungal therapy, surgical intervention, and other adjuvant therapies.
- *Antifungal therapy:* For decades, most tropical mycoses have been treated successfully with antifungal agents such as potassium iodide, triazole compounds such as fluconazole, itraconazole, voriconazole, and more recently, isavuconazole, polyenes such as amphotericin B, and allylamines such as terbinafine. Antifungal susceptibility testing as a part of management is now gaining importance, especially in the context of dermatophytosis as drug-resistant infections are rising. Unfortunately,

for dermatophytes, the clinical breakpoints of the minimum inhibitory concentrations of drugs on performing the antifungal susceptibility testing have not been established. However, epidemiological cutoff values can be used to guide therapy. Additionally, most treatment recommendations in India are experience driven rather than evidence-based highlighting the need for more systematic comparative trials. The antifungal regimens used for treating the common tropical mycosis are summarized in **Table 4**.

TABLE 4: Antifungal regimens used for treating the common tropical mycosis.

Fungal infection	Antifungal regimen	Other comments
Dermatophytosis	• Topical cream/gel/shampoo etc. 2–3 times per day • Efinaconazole 10% solution for onychomycosis • *Oral terbinafine:* 250 mg/day for 2–4 weeks • *Oral itraconazole:* 100 mg/day for 2 weeks or 200 mg/day for 1 week • *Oral griseofulvin:* 0.5–1 g/day for 2–8 weeks	Susceptibility testing if patients fail to respond
Pityriasis versicolor	• Ketoconazole, clotrimazole, terbinafine, selenium sulfide shampoos, and creams • *Oral itraconazole:* 200 mg/day for 1 week or 400 mg single dose • *Oral fluconazole:* 150–300 mg/week or 400 mg single dose • *Oral pramiconazole:* 200 mg single dose	Longer duration of topical treatment has more favorable outcomes but multiple applications may be inconvenient and limit compliance
Sporotrichosis	• *Oral itraconazole:* 200 mg/once or twice a day depending on the clinical response for 2–4 weeks in cutaneous disease • *In systemic disease:* Liposomal amphotericin B (3–5 mg/kg/day) and then itraconazole 200 mg bid with total treatment for up to 12 months • Supersaturated potassium iodide (SSKI) for skin sporotrichosis	SSKI and azole drugs such as itraconazole should not be used in pregnant women and only severe sporotrichosis should be treated in them with amphotericin B

Contd...

Contd...

Fungal infection	Antifungal regimen	Other comments
Chromoblastomycosis	• Oral itraconazole 200–400 mg/day depending on severity for 6–12 months • *Oral posaconazole:* 800 mg/day for 6–12 months	Oral antifungal therapy with the newer azole, isavuconazole has also shown good efficacy in clinical trials
Lobomycosis	• Combination of clofazimine at 100 mg/day and itraconazole at 100 mg/day for 1–2 years • *Posaconazole:* 400 mg bid for 2 years	Fibrosis in long-standing cases makes the action of medication difficult
Eumycetoma	• Prolonged treatment for 6–12 months is needed • *Oral itraconazole:* 200–400 mg • *Oral ketoconazole:* 400–800 mg • *Oral voriconazole:* 200 mg • *Oral posaconazole:* 400 mg bid	Olorofim targets the pyrimidine biosynthesis, and thus can be used for the treatment and is a promising agent under clinical trial New azole fosravuconazole is also under clinical trials
Talaromycosis	• *Induction:* Liposomal amphotericin B 3–5 mg/kg/day—2 weeks • *Consolidation:* Oral itraconazole, 200 mg every 12 hours—10 weeks • *Maintenance:* Oral itraconazole 200 mg/day till CD4 count rises above 100 cells/mm^3 for ≥6 months	Primary prophylaxis recommended for patients with HIV with CD4 counts <100 cells/mm^3 in the highly-endemic regions who are unable to take or have treatment failure with ART
Emergomycosis	Amphotericin B for 10–14 days followed by itraconazole or another newer azole for 12 months pending immune reconstitution	–
Entomophthoramycosis	• Saturated potassium iodide (30 mg/kg/day) • Amphotericin B, imidazoles, and hyperbaric oxygen have been used with varying success	MICs of fluconazole, posaconazole, and itraconazole against *Basidiobolus* may be within attainable plasma levels for some isolates.

Contd...

Contd...

Fungal infection	Antifungal regimen	Other comments
	• Voriconazole has been used successfully in treatment of basidiobolomycosis	However, the MICs of fluconazole, posaconazole, and itraconazole against *Conidiobolus* usually exceed safely achievable plasma concentrations
Paracoccidioidomycosis	• *Oral itraconazole:* 200 mg/day for 6–18 months depending on severity • *Amphotericin B:* 0.5–1.0 mg/kg/alternate day for severe disease till clinical improvement	Another medicine often used is trimethoprim/sulfamethoxazole (TMP/SMX)

(ART: antiretroviral therapy; bid: two doses per day; HIV: human immunodeficiency virus; mg: milligram; MIC: minimum inhibitory concentration)

- *Thermotherapy/cryotherapy/photodynamic therapy:* These are usually applied for subcutaneous or superficial lesions in chromoblastomycosis and lobomycosis.
- *Surgery:* Surgical management is used early in course of nasofacial conidiobolomycosis disease and in gastrointestinal lesions due to basidiobolomycosis. In chromoblastomycosis, surgical excision is not recommended as surgical manipulation in the area of the lesion may favor the dissemination of the disease. For lobomycosis, surgical approach is the main treatment recommended in the literature, but the difficulty in defining the lesion and aesthetic limitations may compromise final results.

TAKE HOME MESSAGE

- As with other neglected tropical diseases, tropical fungal infections disproportionally affect people living in poverty in the tropical and subtropical regions.
- Mycetoma and chromoblastomycosis are currently recognized as a neglected tropical disease.
- The development of an affordable, accessible, and feasible diagnostic test for these infections should be prioritized to enable the prompt diagnosis and for epidemiological surveillance.
- The tropical mycoses warrant recognition by global entities as well as local, regional, and international clinicians, researchers, funders, and public health organizations for better management and research for early diagnosis and therapy.
- Multilevel efforts can help in substantially reducing the morbidity and mortality associated with these conditions.

REFERENCES

1. Yang HL, Limin W, Esther STN, Eduardo G. Tropical fungal infections. Infect Dis Clin North Am. 2012;26(2):497-512.
2. Charles AJ. Superficial cutaneous fungal infections in tropical countries. Dermatol Ther. 2009;22(6):550-9.
3. Nenoff P, Reinel D, Krüger C, Grob H, Mugisha P, Süß A, et al. Tropical and travel-related dermatomycoses : Part 2: cutaneous infections due to yeasts, moulds, and dimorphic fungi. Hautarzt. 2015;66(7):522-32.
4. Queiroz-Telles F, de Hoog S, Santos DW, Salgado CG, Vicente VA, Bonifaz A, et al. Chromoblastomycosis. Clin Microbiol Rev. 2016;30(1):233-76.
5. Govender NP, Wayne G. Emergomycosis (*Emergomyces africanus*) in advanced HIV disease. Dermatopathol (Basel, Switzerland). 2019;6(2):63-9.
6. Pietro N, Verma SB, Resham V, Anke B, Uta-Christina H, Franziska W, et al. The current Indian epidemic of superficial dermatophytosis due to *Trichophyton mentagrophytes* -A molecular study. Mycoses. 2019;62(4):336-56.
7. Verma S. Steroid modified tinea. BMJ. 2017;356:j973.
8. Karray M, McKinney WP. Tinea versicolor. Treasure Island (FL): StatPearls; 2021.
9. Orofino-Costa R, Macedo PM, Rodrigues AM, Bernardes-Engemann AR. Sporotrichosis: an update on epidemiology, etiopathogenesis, laboratory and clinical therapeutics. An Bras Dermatol. 2017;92(5):606-20.
10. Shaikh N, Hussain KA, Petraitiene R, Schuetz AN, Walsh TJ. Entomophthoramycosis: a neglected tropical mycosis. Clin Microbiol Infect. 2016;22(8):688-94.
11. Rudramurthy SM, Shaw D. Overview and update on the laboratory diagnosis of dermatophytosis. Clin Dermatology Rev. 2017;1(3):3.

Section 3

Syndromic Approach to Fever

- **Acute Undifferentiated Fever**
  Saikat Datta, Sharmistha Bhattacherjee, Atanu Chandra
- **Fever with Rash: Approach**
  Prantiki Halder, Agnibho Mondal, Bibhuti Saha, Soumyadip Chatterjee
- **Hemorrhagic Fever**
  Ketan K Patel, Atul K Patel
- **Fever with Hepatorenal Dysfunction**
  D Suresh Kumar, N Naveen Kumar
- **Fever with Central Nervous System Dysfunction**
  Suba Guruprasad, Ramasubramanian, Prasun Chatterjee
- **Fever with Acute Respiratory Distress Syndrome**
  Chandrasekhar Valupadas
- **Fever with Hepatosplenomegaly/Lymphadenopathy**
  Alladi Mohan, G Bindhu Madhavi
- **Fever in Intensive Care Unit**
  Dhruva Chaudhry, Arpana Chatterjee, Debraj Jash
- **Approach to an Adult with Pyrexia of Unknown Origin**
  Sudhir Mehta, Shaurya Mehta
- **Emerging Tropical Infections in India**
  Anupam Prakash
- **Neglected Tropical Diseases**
  Aritra Kumar Ray
- **Health Policies and Economic Impact of Fever on Indian Society**
  Saswati Chaudhuri, Biswajit Mandal, Swati Pal

Acute Undifferentiated Fever

Chapter 15

Saikat Datta, Sharmistha Bhattacherjee, Atanu Chandra

■ INTRODUCTION

Though acute undifferentiated fever (AUF), also known as acute undifferentiated febrile illness (AUFI), does not have a universally acceptable definition, but conventionally, it is defined as a fever of <2 weeks' duration, and lack localizable or organ specific clinical features at the onset. But few authors opine that the AUF be diagnosed if the fever is <3 weeks, and fever of unknown origin (FUO) if the fever persists >3 weeks.[1] In tropical countries such as India, the AUF holds a special place in clinical practice. The causes can be varied, clinical features overlapping and nonspecific, and the diagnostic approach difficult. When the diagnosis is proven, they are called diagnosed AUFs, when the diagnosis remains unproven, they are termed as undiagnosed undifferentiated fever (UUF)[2] **(Flowchart 1)**.

■ ETIOLOGY AND PATHOPHYSIOLOGY

The pathophysiology of AUF varies depending on the etiology of the fever. The most important cause of AUF in tropics is malaria. Hence, malaria, as a cause of the fever, should be excluded before embarking for any other cause of AUF, when they are diagnosed as nonmalarial AUF.[3] When AUF persist for >3 weeks, they are termed as fever of unknown origin.

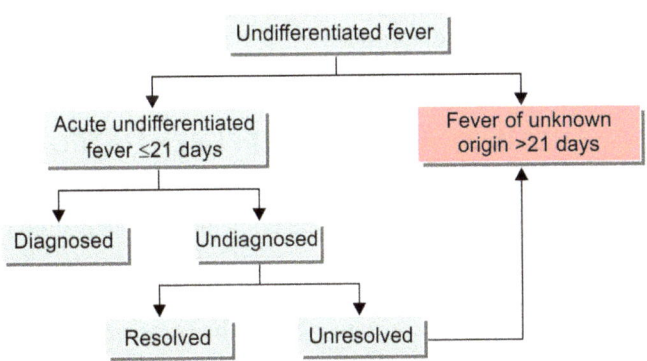

Flowchart 1: Evaluation of undifferentiated fever.[2]

Flowchart 2: Classification of acute undifferentiated fever (AUF) into malarial and nonmalarial fever.

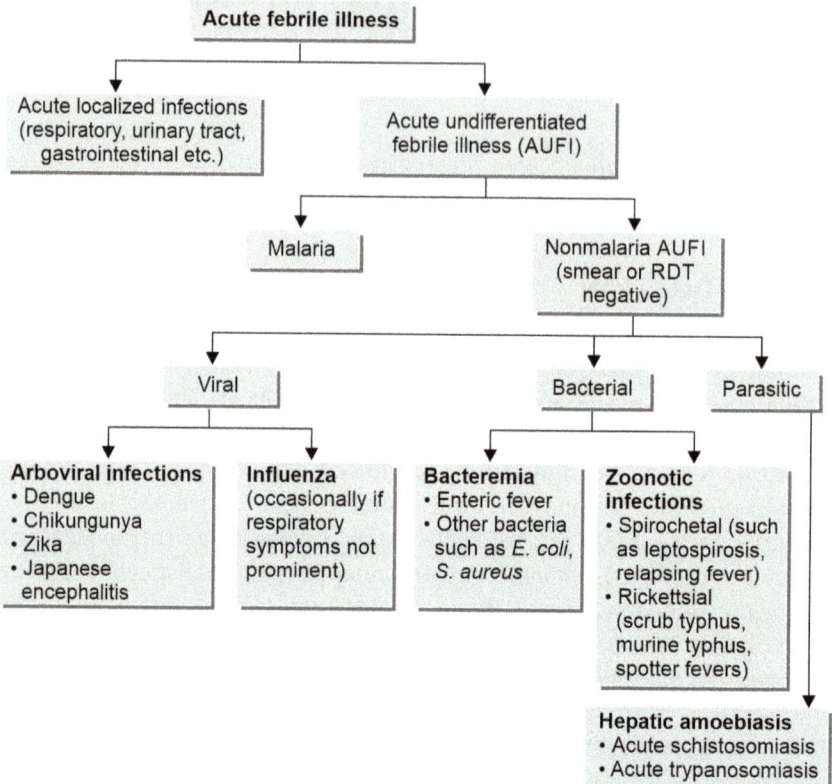

(*E. coli: Escherichia coli; S. aureus: Staphylococcus aureus*)
(*Reproduced from:* Bhargava A, Ralph R, Chatterjee B, Bottieau E. Assessment and initial management of acute undifferentiated fever in tropical and subtropical regions. BMJ. 2018;363, copyright notice year 2022 with permission from BMJ Publishing Group Ltd.)

In India, apart from malaria, other causes of AUF include dengue, chikungunya, enteric fever, leptospirosis, or rickettsial infections.[4] But still, about 25–50% of the AUF in Asia remain undiagnosed.[2,5]

Flowchart 2 depicts the approach to AUF based upon the classification into malaria and nonmalarial AUF.

PATHOGENESIS OF ACUTE UNDIFFERENTIATED FEBRILE ILLNESS

The presence of various pathogens in the body induces activation of various pyrogens which induce cytokines. These cytokines activate febrile response from the thermoregulatory center of hypothalamus. The various cytokines are proposed to be playing important roles in the fever include interleukin 1 (IL-1) and tumor necrosis factor (TNF). Finally, the major cytokine is IL-6.[6]

Dengue virus, a single-stranded RNA virus, targets dendritic cells and macrophages of innate immune system, which activates proinflammatory cytokines.[7] Finally, the cytokines IL-6, IL-8, CXCL10, CXCL11, and chemokine ligand five are the players that induce the inflammatory responses and fever.[8]

Approach to a Patient of Acute Undifferentiated Febrile Illness[9]

- *Step 1:* Severity assessment based upon the history and symptoms: Proper history remains the key to evaluation of any patient of fever. This should include the pattern of fever, duration of symptoms, and the progression of the symptoms. Also, the travel history and history of vaccination remains important. If bacteremia/sepsis is suspected, blood cultures following standard protocol should be sent before initiating any antibiotics.[10]
- *Step 2:* Localization of fever: The clinical features specific of any organ involvement should be diligently searched, though these remain nonspecific and inaccurate. Still, they may give some clues to the etiology. For instance, in dengue, around 30–35% cases present with cough, running nose, and coryza. Similarly, neck rigidity, though classical of meningitis, may also be found in typhoid fever and other infections.[11] The classical signs of severe dengue such as pain in the abdomen, vomiting, prostration, hypotension, and cold clammy extremities are very rare, and usually develop <24 hours prior to hospitalization.[12]

  There may be other clues to approach to the diagnosis. For example, the presence of fever with rash helps in narrowing down the diagnosis based upon the pattern of rash. Varicella, herpes zoster of herpes simplex presents with vesicular rash. Maculopapular rash is found in measles or rubella. Macular rash is characteristic of dengue, and also found in typhoid fever. Arboviral infections such as dengue, zika, or chikungunya present with rash and/or polyarthritis.[13] Scrub typhus has a diagnostic eschar (a well-localized necrotic skin lesion at the site chigger bite).[9] Petechial bleeding may be a manifestation of thrombocytopenia, which is usually a nonspecific finding found in many conditions such as malaria, leptospirosis, or dengue. Jaundice associated with fever points toward the diagnosis of acute viral hepatitis, leptospirosis, or complicated malaria. Although aspartate aminotransferase (AST) and alanine aminotransferase (ALT) may be nonspecifically elevated in AUFI, >25 times elevation of AST and ALT is seen in viral hepatitis.[14]
- *Step 3:* Rapid diagnosis of malaria and dengue: As malaria and dengue are important causes of AUFI in our country, these should always be excluded using rapid diagnostic tests (RDTs) before proceeding for more extensive investigations. The RDT-histidine-rich protein (HRP)-II based test for diagnosis of malaria due to *Plasmodium falciparum* has very high sensitivity and specificity.[15] The plasmodium lactate dehydrogenase

(pLDH) based test for diagnosis of *Plasmodium vivax* infection has a high specificity but has relatively lower sensitivity (75–80%), hence a peripheral smear examination should follow when the RDT is negative.[16]

For detection of dengue, the NS1 antigen based test is used. NS1 usually becomes positive by the first day of fever and continues to remain positive till 9th day. RDT for immunoglobulin M (IgM) antibody against dengue is useful only after the 5th day of illness.[17]

- *Step 4:* Use of antipyretics alone till the 3rd day of fever: Only paracetamol should be used to treat the fever which is <3 days' duration and is negative by RDT for malaria. But proper monitoring, including explaining the red flag signs such as severe weakness, cold clammy skin, severe vomiting, altered sensorium, or convulsions should be explained to the patient and the family members **(Box 1)**. Also, fever persisting for longer duration should ensure a thorough evaluation of signs and symptoms which might suggest organ specific fever or complicated AFU or sepsis.[9]
- *Step 5:* If fever persists for >72 hours, and initial RDTs are negative: Usual causes of the fever lasting for >72 hours are leptospirosis, scrub typhus of typhoid fever. Specific investigations should be ordered to exclude these etiologies. Also, urine analysis to exclude urinary tract infection and other imaging modalities based upon the clinical features should be ordered.[4] Deciding upon a drug in case of AUFI is always a challenge. Many studies have suggested that doxycycline, being a broad-spectrum antimicrobial, may be effective in these situations. This is because of its efficacy in downregulating proinflammatory cytokines.[18] It also inhibits dengue viral

---

BOX 1: Red flag signs in acute undifferentiated febrile illness (AUFI) which needs immediate hospitalization.

- *Prostration:* Unable to stand, sit, or walk without support
- *Temperature:* Hyperpyrexia (temperature >41.5°C) or hypothermia (temperature <36°C) or rigors
- *Respiration:* Shortness of breath, respiratory rate >22 breaths/minute, cyanosis, arterial oxygen saturation <92% on room air
- *Circulation:* Blood pressure <100 mm Hg systolic, cold clammy extremities, capillary refill >3 seconds
- *Neurological:* Altered mental status (Glasgow coma scale <13), convulsions, positive meningeal signs (such as neck stiffness and Kernig sign)
- *Abdominal pain:* Severe or persistent vomiting
- *Severe conjunctival or palmar pallor*
- *Jaundice on examination of sclera*
- *Petechial or purpuric rash*
- *Bleeding:* From nose, gums, or venepuncture sites; hematemesis, and melena

(*Reproduced from:* Bhargava A, Ralph R, Chatterjee B, Bottieau E. Assessment and initial management of acute undifferentiated fever in tropical and subtropical regions. BMJ. 2018;363, copyright notice year 2022 with permission from BMJ Publishing Group Ltd.)

CHAPTER 15: Acute Undifferentiated Fever

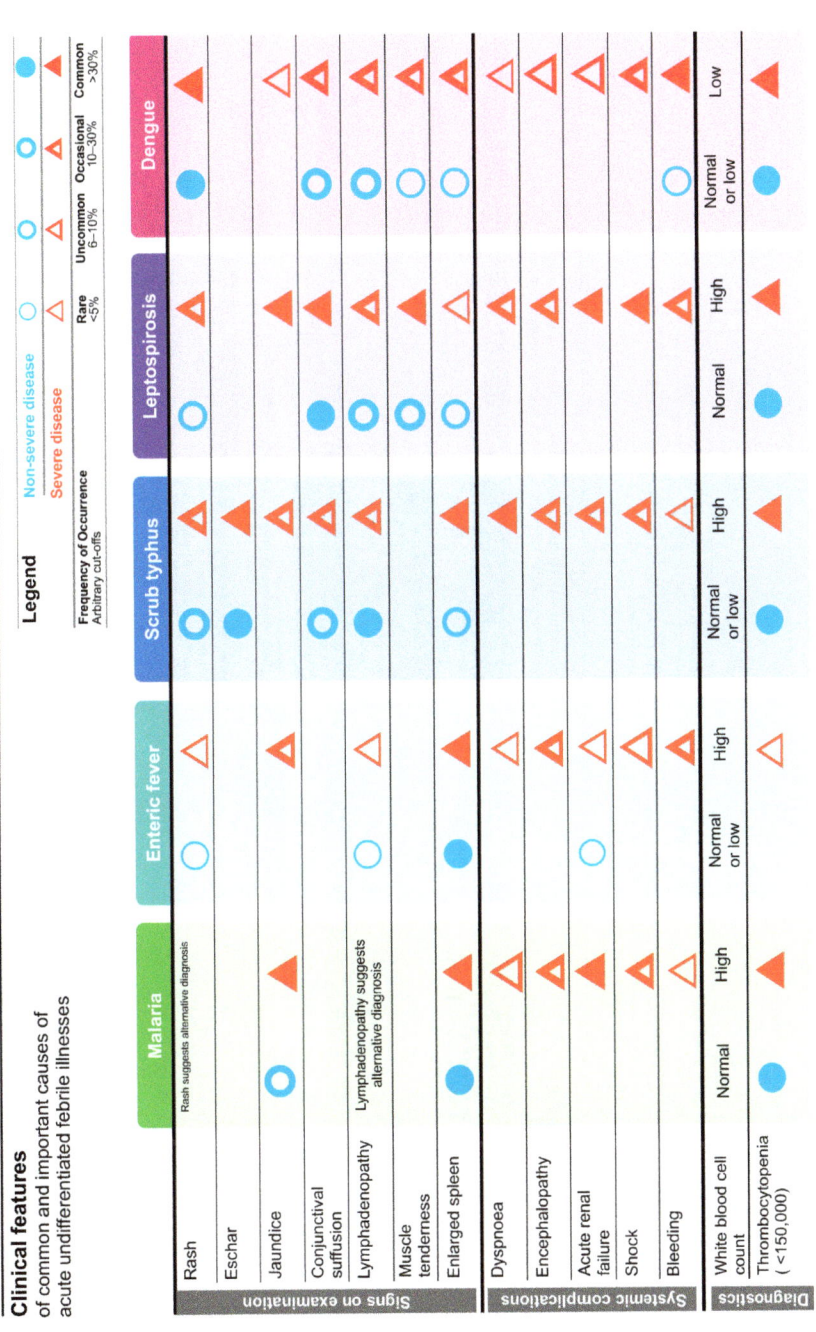

Fig. 1A: Clinical features of common and important causes of acute undifferentiated febrile illness (AUFI). *(Reproduced from:* Bhargava A, Ralph R, Chatterjee B, Bottieau E. Assessment and initial management of acute undifferentiated fever in tropical and subtropical regions. BMJ. 2018;363, copyright notice year 2022 with permission from BMJ Publishing Group Ltd.)

Excluders and predictors
in clinical findings and basic laboratory tests

Rule out features Presence of these features suggests alternative diagnosis	Rash and lymphadenopathy	Generalised rash or generalised lymphadenopathy		Fever >12 days, combination of normal tourniquet test and normal leucocyte count (LR-0.12)
Rule in features Associated with an increase in probability of disease	Fever >40 degrees, Splenomegaly, thrombocytopenia and hyperbilirubinemia are associated with moderate to large increase in probability of disease	Fever in endemic areas >3 days duration and presence of abdominal tenderness is associated with moderate to increase in probability of disease	Eschar virtually pathognomonic for scrub typhus (OR 46). Eschar seen in 17–86% of patients in recent series	Leukopenia and thrombocytopenia. Positive tourniquet test is a good predictor of infection (OR: 4.86) and ascites is a good predictor of severe dengue (OR:13.91)

Confirming a diagnosis
Accuracy and interpretation of specific tests

Serological tests based on antibody detection are confirmatory only on demonstration of fourfold rise in titre in IgG or seroconversion in IgM in paired specimens

Rapid tests Request malarial testing and routine blood tests in all patients	**Malarial antigen test** (ICT format) Sensitivity 95% Specificity 95% for *P. falciparum* ⏱ Minutes		**Specific Immunoglobulin M test** (ICT format) Sensitivity 66% Specificity 92% ⚡ Rapid	**Ns1 antigen test** Sensitivity 66% Specificity 98% ⏱ Minutes
		Antibody test Sensitivity 47–98% Specificity 58–100% ⏱ 2–4 hours	**ELISA for specific Immunoglobulin M using recombinant antigens** Sensitivity variable Specificity 90–100% $$ Medium	**Immunoglobulin M test** Sensitivity 83% Specificity 86% ⏱ Minutes
Confirmatory tests The results of blood culture or serological tests may confirm the diagnosis and guide further therapy	**Microscopy** Detects as few as 5–10 parasites per μL of blood ⏱ 20–30 Minutes $ Inexpensive	**Culture** Sensitivity 40–87% Specificity 100% ⏱ 3–6 days	**Immunofluorescent or Immunoperoxidase assay for antibodies** Sensitivity variable (100% with paired specimens) $$$ Expensive	**Culture** Sensitivity −40% Specificity 100% ⏱ 1–2 weeks $$$ Expensive
		Widal test Sensitivity depends on local prevalence Specificity 100% (paired specimens) $ Inexpensive	**Microscopic agglutination test for antibody** Sensitivity 41% in 1st week 82% in 2nd–4th week Specificity variable $$$ Expensive	**Nucleic acid amplification** Sensitivity 60–100% Specificity >95% $$$ Expensive ⏱ Same day
			Nucleic acid amplification Sensitivity >95% even in 1st week $$$ Expensive	**Serology** Sensitivity 100% Retrospective in severe cases $$ Medium
			Immunoglobulin M test Sensitivity 13–22% in 1st week ~60% in 2nd week ~80% afterward Specificity low ⏱ Hours	
			Well-Felix test Sensitivity variable Specificity high (paired specimens) low (single specimens) $ Inexpensive	
			Culture Sensitivity low Specificity 100% ⏱ Very slow $$$ Expensive	
Malaria		**Enteric fever**	**Scrub typhus** / **Leptospirosis**	**Dengue**

Fig. 1B: Excluders, predictors, and laboratory diagnosis of common and important causes of acute undifferentiated febrile illness (AUFI). (Reproduced from Bhargava A, Ralph R, Chatterjee B, Bottieau E. Assessment and initial management of acute undifferentiated fever in tropical and subtropical regions. BMJ. 2018;363., copyright notice year 2022 with permission from BMJ Publishing Group Ltd). (ELISA: enzyme-linked immunoassay; IgG: immunoglobulin G)

Flowchart 3: Diagnostic and management algorithm for acute undifferentiated febrile illness (AUFI).[4]

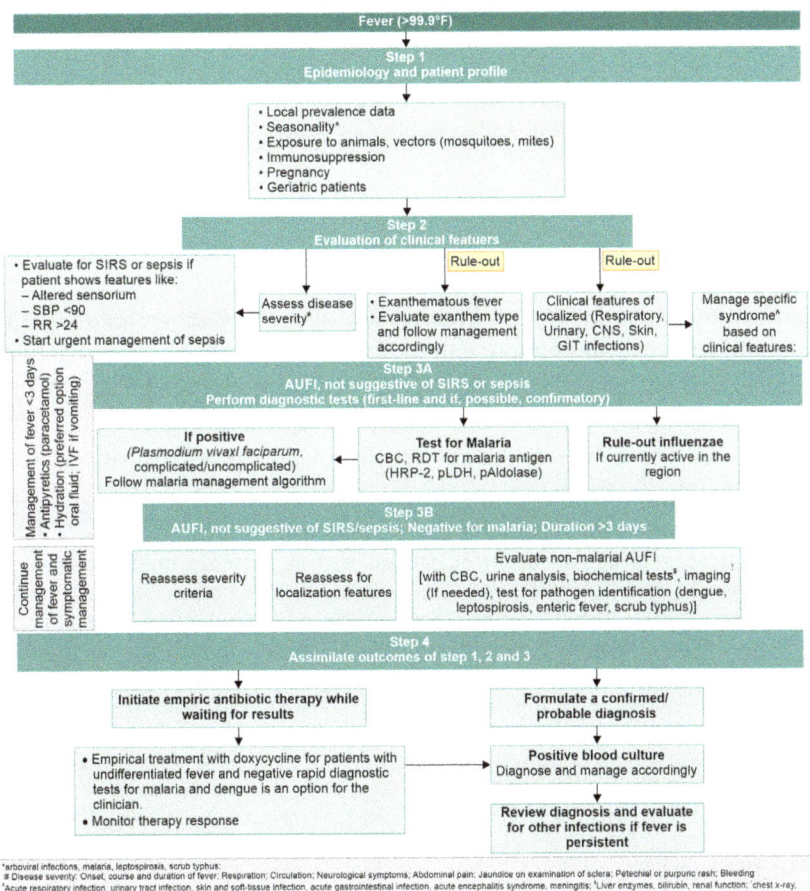

replication by reducing viral protease activity.[19] It is also effective against leptospirosis, scrub typhus, *Mycoplasma pneumoniae*, and *Legionella pneumophilia*.[4] Usage of doxycycline is contraindicated in pregnancy and children because of its effect on discoloration of growing teeth and potential adverse effect upon growing bones.[20]

- *Step 6:* AUFI that persists despite empirical antibiotic therapy: AUF persisting despite empirical antimicrobial therapy is a tricky situation. There are no consensus guidelines for the management of the same. Most clinicians stop antibiotics, re-evaluate the case, reinvestigate with blood and urine cultures, cerebrospinal fluid (CSF) study, human immunodeficiency virus (HIV) serology and imaging. In proper clinical context, connective tissue disorders should also be excluded. A search for hematological malignancies and granulomas in bone marrow should be done. As, by this time, it will already be >3 weeks, hence the protocol for FUO should be followed.[9]

The clinical features, excluders, predictors, and approach to AUFI are depicted in **Figures 1A and B and Flowchart 3**.

■ CONCLUSION

Acute undifferentiated febrile illness is one of the clinically challenging scenarios which every clinician has to face. Malaria remains the most important cause of AUFI, but other causes of like dengue, leptospirosis, and typhus should also be kept in mind. An exhaustive history, extensive and thorough clinical examination, and judicious use of relevant investigations will help in diagnosing the etiology for AUFI. A presumptive treatment with doxycycline might be a reasonable approach in management of such cases when no etiology is detected despite intelligent and extensive investigations.

TAKE HOME MESSAGE

- AUFI includes a constellation of causes, with a common manifestation of unexplained fever <2 weeks.
- Causes can be varied, but most common cause in India remains malaria.
- Proper history, including travel history, and clinical examination remain the cornerstone to plan investigation and treatment.
- When the cause remains unknown, only paracetamol usage with monitoring for the red flag signs may be done for the initial 3 days of fever.
- Doxycycline may be used for fever persisting for >3 days, with the patient kept under surveillance.

■ REFERENCES

1. Joshi R, Colford JM Jr, Reingold AL, Kalantri S. Nonmalarial acute undifferentiated fever in a rural hospital in central India: diagnostic uncertainty and overtreatment with antimalarial agents. Am J Trop Med Hyg. 2008;78(3):393-9.
2. Susilawati TN, McBride WJ. Undiagnosed undifferentiated fever in Far North Queensland, Australia: a retrospective study. Int J Infect Dis. 2014;27:59-64.
3. Punjabi NH, Taylor WR, Murphy GS, Purwaningsih S, Picarima H, Sisson J, et al. Etiology of acute, non-malaria, febrile illnesses in Jayapura, north eastern Papua, Indonesia. Am J Trop Med Hyg. 2012;86(1):46-51.
4. Joshi S, Immanuel G, Arulrhaj S, Tiwaskar M, Vora A, Samavedam S. Roadmap for the management of acute undifferentiated febrile illness: An Expert Discussion and Review of Available Guidelines. J Assoc Physicians India. 2021;69(9):11-2.
5. Mueller TC, Siv S, Khim N, Kim S, Fleischmann E, Ariey F, et al. Acute undifferentiated febrile illness in rural Cambodia: a 3-year prospective observational study. PloS One. 2014;9(4):e95868.
6. Netea MG, Kullber DG, van der Meer JWM. Circulating cytokines as mediators of fever. Clin Infect Dis. 2000;31:S178-84.

7. Srikiatkhachorn A, Mathew A, Rothman AL. Immunemediated cytokine storm and its role in severe dengue. Semin Immunopathol. 2017;39(5):563-74.
8. Dalrymple NA, Mackow ER. Endothelial cells elicit immune enhancing responses to dengue virus infection. J Virol. 2012;86(12):6408-15.
9. Joshi R, Kalantri SP. Acute undifferentiated fever: management algorithm. Update on Tropical Fever. 2015:1-4.
10. Dellinger RP, Levy MM, Rhodes A, Annane D, Gerlach H, Opal SM, et al. Surviving sepsis campaign: international guidelines for management of severe sepsis and septic shock: 2012. Crit Care Med. 2013;41(2):580-637.
11. Waghdhare S, Kalantri A, Joshi R, Kalantri S. Accuracy of physical signs for detecting meningitis: a hospital based diagnostic accuracy study. Clin Neurol Neurosurg. 2010;112(9):752-7.
12. Rigau-Perez JG, Laufer MK. Dengue-related deaths in Puerto Rico, 1992-1996: Diagnosis and clinical alarm signals. Clin Infect Dis. 2006;42(9):1241-6.
13. Bhargava A, Ralph R, Chatterjee B, Bottieau E. Assessment and initial management of acute undifferentiated fever in tropical and subtropical regions. BMJ. 2018;363:k4766.
14. Chang ML, Yang CW, Chen JC, Ho YP, Pan MJ, Lin CH, et al. Disproportional exaggerated aspartate transaminase is a useful prognostic parameter in late leptospirosis. World J Gastroenterol. 2005;11(35):5553-6.
15. Abba K, Deeks JJ, Olliaro P, Naing CM, Jackson SM, Takwoingi Y, et al. Rapid diagnostic tests for diagnosing uncomplicated P. falciparum malaria in endemic countries. Cochrane Database Syst Rev. 2011;(7):CD008122.
16. Meena M, Joshi D, Joshi R, Sridhar S, Waghdhare S, Gangane N, et al. Accuracy of a multispecies rapid diagnostic test kit for detection of malarial parasite at the point of care in a low endemicity region. Trans R Soc Trop Med Hyg. 2009;103(12):1237-44.
17. Blacksell SD, Jarman RG, Bailey MS, Tanganuchitcharnchai A, Jenjaroen K, Gibbons RV, et al. Evaluation of six commercial point-of-care tests for diagnosis of acute dengue infections: the need for combining NS1 antigen and IgM/IgG antibody detection to achieve acceptable levels of accuracy. Clin Vaccine Immunol. 2011;18(12):2095-101.
18. Castro JEZ, Vado-Solis I, Perez-Osorio C, Fredeking TM. Modulation of cytokine and cytokine receptor/antagonist by treatment with doxycycline and tetracycline in patients with dengue fever. Clin Dev Immunol 2011;1-5.
19. Rothan HA, Mohamed ZA, Payder M, Rahman NA, Yusof R. Inhibitory effect of doxycycline against dengue virus replication in vitro. Arch Virol. 2014;159:711-8.
20. Holmes NE, Charles PGP. Safety and efficacy review of doxycycline. Clin Med Therapeutics. 2009;1:471-82.

Chapter 16

Fever with Rash: Approach

*Prantiki Halder, Agnibho Mondal,
Bibhuti Saha, Soumyadip Chatterjee*

■ INTRODUCTION

Fever with rash is a very common problem in tropical countries. Besides infections, there may be a host of noninfectious causes. Approach to a patient with fever and rash should be based on a meticulous history, thorough examination followed by relevant investigations.

In most situations, the chronology of fever and rash helps in pinpointing certain differential diagnoses and ordering focused investigations. **Table 1** shows the common causes of fever with rash.

■ HISTORY

A detailed and complete medical history is essential for the correct diagnosis of the underlying etiology.

Components of history should include:
- Age of patient
- Season of year
- Geographic setting
- Pattern of fever
- Nature, duration, pattern, and chronology of rash
- Previous history of rash
- Nature and pattern of joint involvement if any
- Recent medications (prescription and nonprescription including ayurvedic drugs)
- Immunizations
- Exposure to sexually transmitted disease
- Risk factors for human immunodeficiency virus (HIV) (homosexual orientation, intravenous drug abuse, and unprotected casual sex)
- Immunologic status (malignancy, chemotherapy, corticosteroid, and asplenia)
- Valvular heart disease
- Exposure to febrile or ill individuals in recent past
- Exposure to wild or rural habitats and wild animals
- Prior illnesses, including a history of drug and/or antibiotic allergies
- Travel history
- Pets.

TABLE 1: Causes of fever with rash.

Disease	Etiology	Description	Group affected/ epidemiologic factors	Clinical syndrome
Centrally distributed maculopapular eruptions				
Rubeola (measles)	Paramyxovirus	Discrete lesions that become confluent as rash spreads from hairline downward, sparing palms, and soles; lasts 3 days; Koplik's spots	Nonimmune	Cough, conjunctivitis, coryza, and severe prostration
Rubella (German measles)	Togavirus	Spreads from hairline downward, clearing as it spreads; Forchheimer spots	Nonimmune	Adenopathy, arthritis, lymphadenopathy
Erythema infectiosum	Human parvovirus B19	Bright red "slapped-cheeks" appearance followed by lacy reticular rash that waxes and wanes over 3 weeks	Most common among children 3–12 years old	Mild fever; arthritis in adults; rash following resolution of fever
Exanthem subitum (roseola)	Human herpesvirus 6	Eruption over trunk and neck; resolves within 2 days	In children <3 years old	Rash following resolution of fever; febrile seizures may occur
Primary HIV infection	HIV	Nonspecific diffuse macules and papules; less commonly, urticarial or vesicular oral or genital ulcers	Individuals recently infected with HIV	Pharyngitis, adenopathy, and arthralgias
Infectious mononucleosis	Epstein–Barr virus	Diffuse maculopapular eruption (5% of cases; 90% if ampicillin is given); urticaria, petechiae in some cases; periorbital edema (50%); palatal petechiae (25%)	Adolescent, young adults	Hepatosplenomegaly, pharyngitis, cervical lymphadenopathy, atypical lymphocytosis, and heterophile antibody

Contd...

Contd...

Disease	Etiology	Description	Group affected/epidemiologic factors	Clinical syndrome
Exanthematous drug-induced eruption	Drugs (antibiotics, anticonvulsants, diuretics, etc.)	Intensely pruritic, bright red macules and papules, symmetric on trunk and extremities; may become confluent	Occurs 2–3 days after exposure in previously sensitized individuals; otherwise, after 2–3 weeks	*Variable findings:* Fever and eosinophilia
Scrub typhus	*Orientia tsutsugamushi*	Diffuse macular rash starting on trunk; eschar at site of mite bite	Transmitted by mites	Headache, myalgias, regional adenopathy; mortality up to 30% if untreated
Leptospirosis	*Leptospira interrogans*	Maculopapular eruption; conjunctivitis; scleral hemorrhage in some cases	Exposure to water contaminated with animal urine	Myalgias; aseptic meningitis; icterohemorrhagic fever (Weil's disease)
Typhoid fever	*Salmonella typhi*	Transient, blanchable erythematous macules and papules, 2–4 mm, usually on trunk (rose spots)	Food or water born	Variable abdominal pain and diarrhea; headache, myalgias, and hepatosplenomegaly
Dengue fever	Dengue virus	Rash in 50% of cases; initially diffuse flushing; midway through illness, onset of maculopapular rash, which begins on trunk and spreads centrifugally to extremities and face; pruritus, after defervescence, petechiae on extremities in some cases	Occurs in tropics and subtropics; transmitted by mosquito	Headache, musculoskeletal pain ("breakbone fever"); leukopenia; occasionally biphasic ("saddleback") fever
Rat bite fever	*Spirillum minus*	Eschar at bite site; then blotchy violaceous or red-brown rash involving trunk and extremities	Rat bite	Regional adenopathy, recurrent fevers if untreated

Contd...

Contd...

Disease	Etiology	Description	Group affected/ epidemiologic factors	Clinical syndrome
Erythema marginatum (rheumatic fever)	Group A *Streptococcus*	Erythematous annular papules and plaques occurring as polycyclic lesions in waves over trunk, proximal extremities; evolving and resolving within hours	Patients with rheumatic fever	Pharyngitis preceding polyarthritis, carditis, subcutaneous nodules, and chorea
Systemic lupus erythematosus (SLE)	Autoimmune disease	Macular and papular erythema, often in sun-exposed areas; malar rash; vasculitis, mucosal erosions in some cases	Young to middle-aged women	Arthritis; cardiac, pulmonary, renal, hematologic, and vasculitic disease
Still's disease	Autoimmune disease	Transient 2- to 5-mm erythematous papules appearing at height of fever on trunk, proximal extremities	Children and young adults	High spiking fever, polyarthritis, and splenomegaly; erythrocyte sedimentation rate >100 mm/h
Peripheral eruptions				
Secondary syphilis	*Treponema pallidum*	Copper-colored, scaly papular eruption, diffuse but prominent on palms and soles	STI	Fever, constitutional symptoms
Chikungunya fever	Chikungunya virus	Maculopapular eruption; prominent on upper extremities and face, but can also occur on trunk and lower extremities		Arthralgia and arthritis
Hand-foot-and-mouth disease	Coxsackievirus A16	Tender vesicles, erosions in mouth; 0.25-cm papules on hands and feet with rim of erythema evolving into tender vesicles	Summer and fall; primarily children <10 years old	Transient fever

Contd...

Contd...

Disease	Etiology	Description	Group affected/ epidemiologic factors	Clinical syndrome
Erythema multiforme	Infection, drugs, idiopathic causes	Target lesions up to 2 cm; symmetric on knees, elbows, palms, soles; spreads centripetally; papular, sometimes vesicular	HSV or *Mycoplasma pneumoniae* infection; drug intake (i.e., sulfa, phenytoin, penicillin)	Variable
Bacterial endocarditis	*Streptococcus, Staphylococcus*, etc.	—	Abnormal heart valve, IDU	New heart murmur
Scarlet fever	Group A *Streptococcus*	Diffuse blanchable erythema beginning on face and spreading to trunk and extremities; circumoral pallor; "sandpaper" texture to skin; accentuation of linear erythema in skin folds (Pastia's lines); enanthem of white evolving into red "strawberry" tongue; desquamation in second week	Most common among children 2–10 years old	Fever, pharyngitis, and headache
Kawasaki disease	Idiopathic causes	Scarlatiniform rash or erythema multiforme; fissuring of lips, conjunctivitis; edema of hands, feet; desquamation later in disease	Children <8 years old	Cervical adenopathy, pharyngitis, and coronary artery vasculitis
Streptococcal toxic shock syndrome	Group A *Streptococcus*	When present, rash often scarlatiniform	Severe group A streptococcal infections	Multiorgan failure, hypotension; 30% mortality rate
Staphylococcal toxic shock syndrome	*Staphylococcus aureus*	Diffuse erythema involving palms; pronounced erythema of mucosal surfaces; conjunctivitis; desquamation 7–10 days into illness	Colonization with toxin-producing *S. aureus*	Fever >39°C (>102°F), hypotension, and multiorgan dysfunction

Contd...

Contd...

Disease	Etiology	Description	Group affected/ epidemiologic factors	Clinical syndrome
Staphylococcal scalded skin syndrome	*S. aureus*	Diffuse tender erythema, often with bullae and desquamation; Nikolsky sign	Occurs in children	Irritability; nasal or conjunctival secretions
Drug-induced hypersensitivity syndrome (DIHS)/ drug reaction with eosinophilia and systemic symptoms DRESS	Aromatic anticonvulsants; other drugs, including sulfonamides, minocycline	Maculopapular eruption (mimicking exanthematous drug rash) sometimes progressing to exfoliative erythroderma; profound edema, especially facial; pustules may occur	Individuals genetically unable to detoxify arene oxides (anticonvulsants), patients with slow N-acetylating capacity (sulfonamides)	Lymphadenopathy, multiorgan failure (especially hepatic), eosinophilia, and atypical lymphocytes; mimics sepsis
Stevens–Johnson syndrome (SJS), toxic epidermal necrolysis (TEN)	Drugs (80% of cases; often allopurinol, anticonvulsants, antibiotics), infection, idiopathic	Erythematous and purpuric macules, sometimes targetoid, or diffuse erythema progressing to bullae, with sloughing and necrosis of entire epidermis; Nikolsky sign; involves mucosal surfaces	Uncommon among children; more common among patients with HIV infection, SLE, slow acetylators	Dehydration, sepsis sometimes resulting from lack of normal skin integrity; up to 30% mortality
Varicella	Varicella-zoster virus	Macules (2–3 mm) evolving into papules, then vesicles on an erythematous base ("dewdrops on a rose petal"); pustules then forming and crusting; lesions appearing in crops; may involve scalp, mouth; intensely pruritic	Usually affects children; 10% of adults susceptible; most common in late winter and spring	Malaise; generally mild disease in healthy children; more severe disease with complications in adults and immunocompromised children

Contd...

Contd...

Disease	Etiology	Description	Group affected/ epidemiologic factors	Clinical syndrome
Primary herpes simplex virus (HSV) infection	HSV	Erythema rapidly followed by hallmark painful *grouped vesicles* that may evolve into pustules that ulcerate, especially on mucosal surfaces	Primary infection most common among children and young adults for HSV-1 and among sexually active young adults for HSV-2	Regional lymphadenopathy
Ecthyma gangrenosum	*P. aeruginosa*, other Gram-negative rods, fungi	Indurated plaque evolving into hemorrhagic bulla or pustule that sloughs, resulting in eschar formation; erythematous halo; most common in axillary, groin, perianal regions	Usually affects neutropenic patients; occurs in up to 28% of individuals with *Pseudomonas* bacteremia	Clinical signs of sepsis
Urticarial vasculitis	Serum sickness, often due to infection (including hepatitis B, enteroviral, parasitic), drugs; connective tissue disease	Erythematous, edematous "urticaria-like" plaques, pruritic or burning; unlike urticaria	Patients with serum sickness, connective tissue disease	Fever variable; arthralgias/ arthritis
Disseminated infection	Fungi, mycobacteria	Subcutaneous nodules (up to 3 cm); fluctuance, draining common with mycobacteria; necrotic nodules (extremities, periorbital or nasal regions) common with *Aspergillus, Mucor*	Immunocompromised hosts	Features vary with organism

Contd...

Contd...

Disease	Etiology	Description	Group affected/ epidemiologic factors	Clinical syndrome
Erythema nodosum	Infections (e.g., streptococcal, fungal, mycobacterial, yersinial); drugs (e.g., sulfas, penicillin, and oral contraceptives); sarcoidosis; idiopathic causes	Large, violaceous, nonulcerative, subcutaneous nodules; exquisitely tender; usually on lower legs but also on upper extremities	More common among girls and women 15–30 years old	Arthralgias (50%); features vary with associated condition
Acute meningococcemia	*Neisseria meningitidis*	Initially pink maculopapular lesions evolving into petechiae; petechiae rapidly becoming numerous; trunk, extremities most commonly involved; may appear on face, hands, and feet	Most common among children, individuals with asplenia or terminal complement component deficiency (C5–C8)	Hypotension and meningitis
Disseminated gonococcal infection	*Neisseria gonorrhoeae*	Papules evolving over 1–2 days into hemorrhagic pustules with grey necrotic centers; hemorrhagic bullae occurring rarely; lesions distributed peripherally near joints	Sexually active individuals	Low-grade fever, tenosynovitis, and arthritis
Viral hemorrhagic fever	Arboviruses (including dengue) and arenaviruses	Petechial rash	Residence in or travel to endemic areas	Triad of fever, shock, hemorrhage from mucosa or gastrointestinal tract
Thrombotic thrombocytopenic purpura (TTP)/ hemolytic-uremic syndrome (HUS)	Idiopathic, *Escherichia coli* O157:H7 (Shiga toxin), drugs	Petechiae	Individuals with *E. coli* O157:H7 gastroenteritis	Fever (not always present), hemolytic anemia, thrombocytopenia, renal dysfunction, and neurologic dysfunction

(HIV: human immunodeficiency virus; IDU: intravenous drug use; STI: sexually transmitted infection)

Age

Primarily viral exanthems are seen in children but due to immunization changing pattern has been seen.[1] Acute maculopapular rashes in children are usually caused by viral infections but in adults, it is often due to drug reactions.[2]

Season of the Year

Parvovirus B-19 infections are often seen in the winter or spring. Rubella infections appear most commonly in the springtime but can be seen in any month of the year. Dengue fever (DF) is seen more commonly when the monsoon arrives. DF outbreaks are often influenced by rainfall, temperature, and humidity.[3] Enteroviruses such as *Echovirus* and *Coxsackie* cause infections primarily in the summer and autumn months. In endemic areas, particularly the hilly area of north-eastern states, Scrub typhus is seen in rainy season but in South India, it is seen in winter period.[4]

Geographical Settings

Historically DF is considered a disease of urban population due to high density of population and short flying distance of *Aedes aegypti*. But rural outbreak has also been reported in Asia and Latin America.[5] Scrub typhus outbreak had been reported from sub-Himalayan belt, from Jammu to Nagaland. Foci of outbreak have also been reported from South India in recent past.[6] Current outbreak of Chikungunya started in Southern and spread to Western and Eastern states.

Travel History

Diagnosing the cause of fever with rash in travelers is challenge. A few examples are presented in **Table 2**.

Morphology of rash in different diseases is shown in **Table 3**. Presence or absence of pruritus may also help in narrowing the differential diagnosis as shown in **Table 4**.

The concomitant clinical features present in a case of fever and rash also helps in pinpointing the diagnosis **(Table 5)**.

Although generalized rashes are often painless, they may be painful in patients with Stevens–Johnson syndrome, Sweet syndrome, and Kawasaki disease. In some disease conditions, the rashes tend to avoid or favor certain parts of the body **(Table 6)**.

Patients should be asked where the rash first appeared and how it progressed in due course of disease. Vasculitic rashes usually spread from periphery to centrally, whereas viral rashes (e.g., varicella) start centrally and spread peripherally.[7]

TABLE 2: Infectious agents causing fever with rash in travelers.

Infectious agent	Geographical location
Ancylostoma braziliense	Southeast United States, Caribbean, Asia, Africa, and South America
Dengue virus	Tropical countries
Leishmania spp.	Central and South America, Africa, Asia, Mexico, and Southern Europe
Onchocerca volvulus	Africa, Central America, and South America
Rickettsia akari	United States, Russia, and South Africa
Rickettsia conorii	Mediterranean, Russia, and African bush country
Rickettsia tsutsugamushi	Southeast Asia, Nepal, India, Korea, Australia, China, and Southern-Western Pacific
Schistosoma mansoni	Africa, South America, Middle East, and Caribbean Islands
Schistosoma japonicum	Eastern Asia and Philippines
Schistosoma haematobium	Middle East and Africa
Strongyloides stercoralis	United States, Asia, Africa, Central America, and Eastern Europe
Trypanosoma cruzi	Mexico, South America, and Central America

TABLE 3: Morphology of rash in different diseases.

Morphology of rash	Causes
Maculopapular	Measles, rubella, roseola infantum, Kawasaki disease, Scarlet fever, erythema infectiosum, HIV seroconversion, and acute HBV or HCV infection
Vesicular	Varicella
Vesiculobullous	SJS/TEN, drugs
Hemorrhagic	Meningococcal septicemia, ITP, HSP, Acute leukemia, and bleeding disorders
Erythematous	Urticaria due to hypersensitivity, Scarlet fever, staphylococcal scalded skin syndrome (SSSS), toxic shock syndrome (TSS), early stages of Stevens–Johnson syndrome (SJS), rheumatic fever, juvenile arthritis, systemic lupus erythematosus (SLE), sarcoidosis, and Lyme disease.
Eschar	Scrub typhus
Annular	Erythema chronicum migrans

(HBV: hepatitis B virus; HCV: hepatitis C virus; HIV: human immunodeficiency virus; HSP: Henoch–Schönlein purpura; ITP: idiopathic thrombocytopenic purpura; TEN: toxic epidermal necrolysis)

TABLE 4: Differential diagnosis of fever with rash based on presence of pruritus.

Common	Variable	Absent or rare
• Scabies with secondary infection • Varicella • Urticarial	• Drug eruption • Erythema multiforme • Kawasaki disease • TEN • Toxic shock syndrome	• HIV seroconversion • Erythema infectiosum • Meningococcemia • Roseola • Rubella • Scarlet fever • Secondary syphilis • Staphylococcal scalded skin syndrome • SJS

(HIV: human immunodeficiency virus; SJS: Stevens–Johnson syndrome; TEN: toxic epidermal necrolysis)

TABLE 5: Different clinical features associated with fever and rash.

Rashes and concomitant clinical features	Suspected diseases
Rash and shock	Dengue, MIS-A (multisystem inflammatory syndrome in adults), TSS (toxic shock syndrome), meningococcemia, pneumococcal sepsis, *Staphylococcus aureus* sepsis, and viral hemorrhagic fever
Rash and arthralgia	Dengue, chikungunya, Zika virus infection, primary HIV infection, and erythema nodosum
Rash and arthritis	SLE and Still's disease
Rash and conjunctivitis	MIS-A, Kawasaki diseases, measles, TSS
Rash and abdominal pain	MIS-A, typhoid fever, scarlet fever, *Vibrio vulnificus*, and SLE
Rash and diarrhea	MIS-A, *V. vulnificus*, gas gangrene, and TSS
Rash and mental changes	SLE, meningococcemia, and typhoid fever
Rash and pulmonary infiltrates	SLE and atypical measles
Rash and relative bradycardia	Typhus, typhoid fever, and drug fever
Rash and purpura	Cutaneous small vessel vasculitis (leukocytoclastic vasculitis), viral hemorrhagic fever, and meningococcemia
Rash and adenopathy	Infectious mononucleosis, rubella, primary HIV infection, scrub typhus, Kawasaki diseases
Rash and splenomegaly	Typhoid fever and Still's disease

(HIV: human immunodeficiency virus; SLE: systemic lupus erythematosus)

TABLE 6: Fever with rash involving palm and sole.	
Common	**Absent**
• Rubella • Erythema multiforme • SSSS • SJS/TEN • TSS • Kawasaki disease	• Scarlet fever • Roseola • Varicella • Erythema infectiosum

(SJS: Stevens–Johnson syndrome; SSSS: staphylococcal scalded skin syndrome; TEN: toxic epidermal necrolysis; TSS: toxic shock syndrome)

Time interval between fever and appearance of rash also provides important diagnostic clues. As for example rash of varicella appears on the same day of fever, in scarlet fever, it appears on the 2nd day of fever, in measles on 4th to 5th day of fever, in dengue and typhoid on 6th to 7th day of fever.

Prodromal symptoms are present in many cases of fever with rash. Prodromal symptoms are absent in cases of varicella in children.

Past history may also lead to important diagnostic clues. For example, patients with an intravenous (IV) drug use, artificial heart valve, or cardiac valvular lesions may have endocarditis. Certain cutaneous conditions tend to recur in the same patient, such as herpes zoster associated with HIV or recurrent erythema multiforme following herpes simplex or mycoplasma infections.

Exposure to Sexually Transmitted Diseases

Risk factors for HIV infection should be reviewed when evaluating the patient with unexplained fever and rash. Exposure to other sexually transmitted diseases (STDs) may be elicited at the same time. Rash, tenosynovitis, fever, and malaise with or without arthritis characterize disseminated gonococcal infections (DGIs), skin lesions are in different stages of development.[8] The constellation of urethritis, conjunctivitis, arthritis, and mucocutaneous lesions, particularly in a young, HLA-B27 antigen positive should invoke a differential diagnosis that includes Reiter syndrome.

Immune Status of the Patient

Patients with neutropenia or neutrophil dysfunction are at increased risk for developing infections with *Staphylococcus spp.*, *Streptococci viridians*, *Enterococcus spp.*, *Enterobacteriaceae*, *Pseudomonas aeruginosa*, *Stenotrophomonas maltophilia*, anaerobic bacteria, *Candida spp.*, *Fusarium spp.*, *Trichosporon spp.*, and *Aspergillus spp.* Patients with humoral immune dysfunction including hypogammaglobulinemia or complement deficiencies are at risk for infection with *Streptococcus pneumoniae*,

Haemophilus influenzae, Salmonella, Mycoplasma, Neisseria meningitidis, and *Enteroviruses,* to name a few. Cell-mediated immune dysfunction (CMI) increases the risk of infection with *Mycobacteria spp., Nocardia spp., Listeria spp., Salmonella spp.,* herpes viruses, *Coccidioides immitis, Blastomyces dermatitidis, Histoplasma capsulatum, Cryptococcus neoformans, Leishmania spp., Strongyloides spp.,* and *Toxoplasma spp.*

Immunization history is of great importance but it is difficult to reveal in our country due to lack of records and awareness.

Physical Examination

Characteristic clinical associations are helpful when evaluating patients with fever and rash syndromes and should include a search for associated lymphadenopathy, arthritis, lung involvement, cardiac involvement, and meningeal signs[9] **(Table 7)**.

The common appearance of rash caused by different etiologies are shown in **Table 8**.

The differential for fever and rash with associated joint pains includes connective tissue diseases such as systemic lupus erythematosus and infections such as Chikungunya, dengue, Lyme disease, DGI, acute rheumatic fever, parvovirus B19, rubella, and roseola.[9]

TABLE 7: Fever and rash: Physical examination.

Vital signs	• Temperature? • Pulse? • Respiration? • Blood pressure?
General appearance	• Alert? • Acutely ill? • Chronically ill? • Toxic?
Lymphadenopathy	Location/size/tenderness/whether matted
Features of rash	• Type? • Discrete or uniform? • Desquamation? • Configuration of individual lesion? • Arrangement of lesion? • Distribution pattern: Exposed area? • Centripetal or centrifugal?
Other features	• Conjunctival, mucosal, or genital lesion? • Hepatosplenomegaly? • Arthritis or arthralgia? • Neurological dysfunction or neck rigidity?

CHAPTER 16: Fever with Rash: Approach 169

TABLE 8: Morphology of rash in different diseases.

Morphology of rashes	Causes
Maculopapular 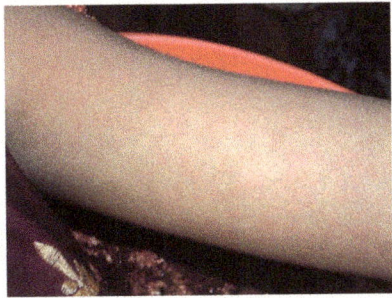	Measles, rubella, roseola infantum, Kawasaki disease, Scarlet fever, erythema infectiosum, HIV seroconversion, coxsackie, Echo, CMV, acute HBV or HCV infection
Erythematous 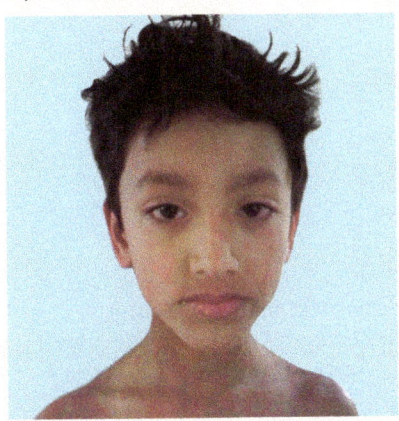	Urticaria due to hypersensitivity, Scarlet fever, staphylococcal scalded skin syndrome (SSSS), toxic shock syndrome (TSS), early stages of Stevens–Johnson syndrome (SJS), rheumatic fever, juvenile arthritis, systemic lupus erythematosus (SLE), and sarcoidosis
Vesicular 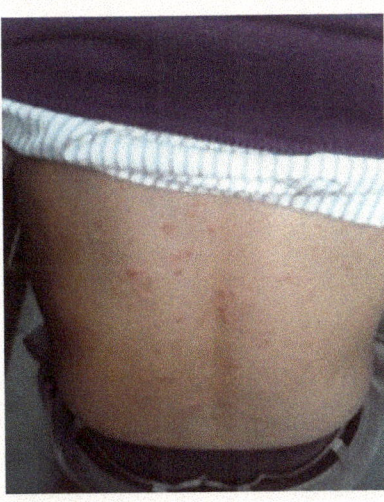	Varicella, herpes simplex, echo, coxsackie including coxsackie A16 causing hand-foot-and-mouth disease)

Contd...

Contd...

Morphology of rashes	Causes
Bullous 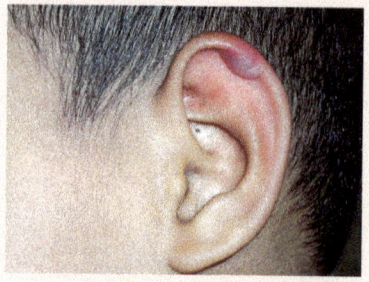	Gr A streptococcal erysipelas with necrotizing fasciitis, ecthyma gangrenosum, *Vibrio vulnificus*, *Staphylococcus/Streptococcus* cellulitis
Vesiculobullous 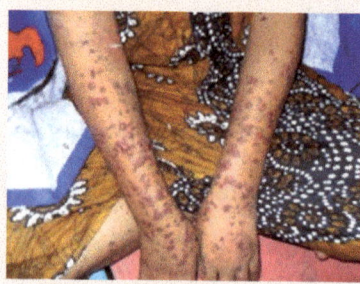	SJS/TEN and drugs
Petechiae 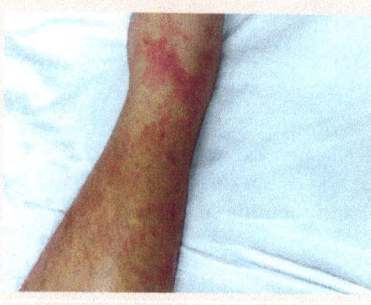	Gram-negative sepsis, invasive *Neisseria meningitidis* infection, rickettsial infections, and viral hemorrhagic fever
Eschar 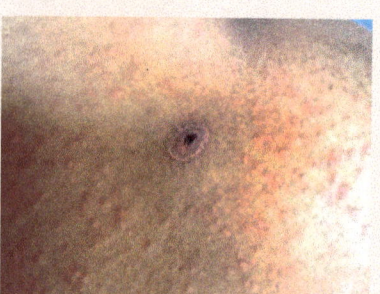	Rickettsial infections

(HBV: hepatitis B virus; HCV: hepatitis C virus; HIV: human immunodeficiency virus; CMV: cytomegalovirus; TEN: toxic epidermal necrolysis)

Generalized lymphadenopathy can be associated with Epstein–Barr virus (EBV)-associated mononucleosis, secondary syphilis, HIV, and sarcoidosis. Local lymphadenopathy is seen in cat-scratch disease, tularemia, primary syphilis, and rubella. Retroauricular and suboccipital lymphadenopathy are characteristic of rubella in children.[10]

The physician should consider mycobacteria, endemic fungal infections, varicella zoster, and sarcoidosis in patients with pulmonary abnormalities.[9]

■ INVESTIGATIONS

Laboratory testing should be guided by salient clinical data. Unfortunately, diagnostic test results are often not available quickly enough to have impact upon initial therapeutic decisions.

In general, initially nonspecific tests such as the complete blood count, serum chemistry studies, and urinalysis should be done. Blood cultures can be particularly helpful when bacteremia and certain systemic fungal infections are being considered.

Cultures of other body sites may be helpful including cerebrospinal fluid in the setting of meningococcemia or the oropharynx, throat, and rectum in cases of suspected DGI. Microscopic examination of the buffy coat smear may identify patients with *N. meningitidis* or *S. pneumoniae* bacteremia. Gram stain and culture of aspirates from pustules or petechiae may reveal *N. meningitidis* in as many as 50–70% of cases of acute meningococcemia.[11] Vesicular lesions due to herpes simplex or varicella-zoster should be unroofed so that Wright-Giemsa-stained exudate from the base of these lesions can be examined for the presence of multinucleated giant cells. Dark-field microscopy can demonstrates *spirochaetes* in exudative material from the lesions of early syphilis.

Serologic tests may be helpful when evaluating the patient with suspected DF, chikungunya, syphilis, leptospirosis, Lyme disease, cryptococcosis, coccidioidomycosis, toxoplasmosis, hepatitis B and C, HIV, typhoid, though diagnosis in many cases requires both acute and convalescent titers. Biopsy material from skin lesions can be appropriately stained and cultured to detect bacterial, fungal, mycobacterial and viral organisms. Immunofluorescent studies in skin biopsy specimens can assist in the diagnosis of systemic lupus erythematosus, Henoch–Schöenlein purpura, and pemphigoid.

■ CONCLUSION

The differential diagnosis of fever with rash is broad and diagnosis is often confusing due to variable presentation. Careful history, epidemiological details including immunization profile, meticulous systemic examination, and relevant laboratory reports are the essential component to make a correct diagnosis.

REFERENCES

1. Cherry JD. Contemporary infectious exanthems. Clin Infect Dis. 1993;16(2): 199-207.
2. Drago F, Rampini P, Rampini E, Rebora A. Atypical exanthems: morphology and laboratory investigations may lead to an aetiological diagnosis in about 70% of cases. Br J Dermatol. 2002;147(2):255-60.
3. Raheel U, Faheem M, Riaz MN, Kanwal N, Javed F, Zaidi N us SS, et al. Dengue fever in the Indian subcontinent: an overview. J Infect Dev Ctries. 2010;5(04):239-47.
4. Kumar D, Raina DJ, Gupta S, Angurana A. Epidemiology of scrub typhus. JK Sci. 2010;12(2):60-2.
5. Guha-Sapir D, Schimmer B. Dengue fever: new paradigms for a changing epidemiology. Emerg Themes Epidemiol. 2005;2(1):1.
6. Vivekanandan M, Mani A, Priya YS, Singh AP, Jayakumar S, Purty S. Outbreak of scrub typhus in Pondicherry. J Assoc Physicians India. 2010;58:24-8.
7. Cherry JD, Demmler-Harrison GJ, Feigin RD. Measles virus. In: Textbook of Pediatric Infectious Diseases, 6th edition. Philadelphia: Saunders; 2009. p. 2427.
8. Martin DH, Mroczkowski TF. Dermatologic manifestations of sexually transmitted diseases other than HIV. Infect Dis Clin North Am. 1994;8(3):533-82.
9. Hurst J, Butterworth-Heinemann. Fever and rash. In: Medicine for the Practicing Physician, 3rd edition. Massachusetts: Stoneham; 1992. p. 273-81.
10. Garcia JJG. Differential diagnosis of viral exanthemas. Open Vaccine J. 2010;3:65-8.
11. Salzman MB, Rubin LG. Meningococcemia. Infect Dis Clin North Am. 1996;10(4):709-25.

Chapter 17

Hemorrhagic Fever

Ketan K Patel, Atul K Patel

■ INTRODUCTION

The term hemorrhagic fever (HF) describes a life-threatening clinical syndrome characterized by fever with musculoskeletal and gastrointestinal symptoms progresses to organ dysfunction and failure (liver and kidney) followed by bleeding manifestations and shock. Common pathological features of HF are thrombocytopenia, abnormal markers of coagulations, and capillary leak syndrome leading to bleeding diathesis.

Several reports describes an emergence and re-emergence HF with changes in epidemiology in last two decades. Most notably, outbreak of Crimean-Congo hemorrhagic fever (CCHF) in Gujarat, India, in 2011,[1] and Ebola in western part of Africa in 2014–2016.[2] Apart from these two dengue HFs, leptospirosis and rickettsial fevers are also increasingly reported from different parts of the world (especially tropical countries) and India. Other pathogens implicated in the HF are mainly viral infections, e.g., yellow fever virus, Saint Louise virus, hantavirus, Arena virus, bacterial pathogens (leptospirosis, rickettsia), and parasitic infections, e.g., malaria. Infections causing hemorrhagic manifestations relevant to India are included in this chapter, several other viruses are also implicated in causing viral infections across the world.

Hemorrhagic fever is usually arthropod borne disease transmitted by tick or mosquitoes bites. Person-to-person transmission can occur with CCHF and Ebola viruses via direct contact with infected blood or body secretions. Leptospirosis is generally acquired by exposure to contaminated water and soil, infected rodents urine, or infected animal tissues. Portals of entry are cuts or abraded skin, mucous membrane, or conjunctiva. Animal reservoirs for HFs pathogens are wild rodents, domestic livestock, monkeys, and other primates. Treatment options as well as prophylaxis are limited, so early detection and strict adherence to infection control measures are most essential.

■ ETIOLOGY AND EPIDEMIOLOGY

Table 1 described the common viral, bacterial, and parasitic causes for HF with important clinical, laboratory features, diagnosis, and treatment.

TABLE 1: Clinical and Laboratory parameters of common hemorrhagic fevers.

Diseases	Viral infections					Bacterial infections		Parasitic
	Dengue fever	CCHF	Ebola viral disease	Yellow fever	Hantavirus	Leptospirosis	Rickettsia	Malaria
Distribution	Worldwide especially in tropical and subtropical countries	Africa, Balkans, Middle East, Asia	West Africa	Sub-Saharan Africa and tropical South America	Europe, Asia and America	Tropical and subtropical countries	Worldwide	Sub Saharan Africa, South East Asia, Eastern Mediterranean, Western Pacific Americas
Reservoir	Human/*Ades aegypti*	Ixodid tick	Bats, nonhuman primates	Monkeys	Rodent	Rodent	Tick, mite, lice	Humans
Transmission	Mosquito bite	Tick bite, person-person	Direct contact with the blood, secretions, body fluid	Mosquitoes	Urine/feces contaminate water/soil contact with cut/abraded skin	Urine/feces contaminate water/soil contact with cut/abraded skin	Tick bite	Mosquito bite

Contd...

Contd...

Diseases	Viral infections					Bacterial infections		Parasitic
	Dengue fever	CCHF	Ebola viral disease	Yellow fever	Hantavirus	Leptospirosis	Rickettsia	Malaria
Clinical features:								
• Fever	+++	++	++	++	+++	+++	+++	+++
• Headache	+++	++	+++	++	++	++	++	+++
• Musculoskeletal	++++	++	+++		+++	++++		+
• GI symptoms	+	+	++	++	++		++	
• Rashes	++	+			–	+	+++	
Laboratory features								
• WBC	N to Low	N to Low	Low	Low	High	N to high	N to Low	Normal
• Platelets	Low	Low	Low	Low	Low	N to Low	Low	N to Low
Liver/renal involvement	Uncommon	Common	Common	Common	Common	Common	Common	Uncommon
Diagnosis	PCR, NS1 antigen, serology	PCR	PCR, serology	PCR, serology	Serology, PCR only during early stage	Serology, PCR, MAT	Serology	Blood smear
Treatment	Supportive	Supportive	Supportive, monoclonal antibodies	Supportive	Supportive	Penicillin, ceftriaxone doxycycline	Doxycycline, chloramphenicol, azithromycin	Artemisinin-based combination therapy (ACT)
Case fatality	<1%	10–40%	25–90%	15–50%	35%	0–15%	20–60% in untreated, 4% with treatment	

(GI: gastrointestinal; PCR: polymerase chain reaction; MAT: microscopic agglutination test; WBC: white blood cell)

Kyasanur Forest disease (KFD) is described separately in viral HF section below.

Viral Hemorrhagic Fever

Viral hemorrhagic fever is caused by single-stranded RNA viruses with lipid envelope and belong to four families which includes *Filoviridae* (Marburg and Ebola virus), *Arenaviridae* (Lassa fever, Argentine HF, Brazilian HF, Bolivian HF, and Venezuelan HF), *Bunyaviridae* (Crimean Congo HF, hantavirus rift valley fever), and *Flaviviridae* (Dengue Fever). All of the VHF agents cause sporadic disease or epidemics in the areas of endemicity. The routes of transmission are variable, but most are zoonotic with spread via arthropod bites or contact with infected animals. Person-to-person spread is a major form of transmission for the Ebola and CCHF. HF has restricted geographical location according to their vectors/animal reservoirs lives.[3,4] Many reports have demonstrated the changing and expanding global epidemiology. The population growth, urbanization, climate changes, and extensive global air travelling facilitated the changes in the global epidemiology of HF. The classical example is spread of Ebola to seven more countries: Italy, Mali, Nigeria, Senegal, Spain, the United Kingdom, and the United States mainly infecting healthcare settings.

Most of the VHF share the common pathological pathways to produce symptoms and hemorrhagic manifestations. Fever and myalgia are frequently associated with flushing, conjunctival injection, petechiae are common due to endothelial infection. These can progress to frank mucocutaneous hemorrhages from natural orifices or in the organs (pulmonary hemorrhages) with other features such as hypotension and shock. Initial illness is characterized by viremic phase in which the replicating viruses can triggering cytokine activations leading to increased vascular permeability and shock. Hemorrhagic manifestations are usually multifactorial. Increase vascular permeability, thrombocytopenia, acute liver injury resulting into impaired coagulation, and this can progress to disseminated intravascular coagulations (DICs) and multiorgan involvement and failure. Kidney involvement is also multifactorial in HF; rhabdomyolysis with myoglobinuria blocking the renal tubules, DIC, microvascular thrombosis, and hypotension contributes to renal injury.

Kyasanur Forest disease is tick-borne VHF endemic to Karnataka state of India characterized by biphasic illness: Phase I is characterized by acute onset of fever, myalgias, headache, skin flushing, conjunctival involvement, lymphadenopathy, GI symptoms, and hemorrhagic manifestations, lasting for 6–11 days. Important laboratory parameters are leukopenia, thrombocytosis, and transaminitis. Half of the patients may go on to develop the second phase with meningoencephalitis. Case fatality with KFD ranges from 3 to 10%.

Reverse transcription polymerase chain reaction (RT-PCR) and serological tests are used to make diagnosis of KFD. A killed vaccine for KFD prevention is available and is used in endemic areas. Treatment is mainly symptomatic and supportive.

Bacterial Hemorrhagic Fever

Leptospira and rickettsia are two bacterial agents that can have hemorrhagic manifestations. Many rickettsia species cause diseases in humans and animals. In India and Asia Pacific, scrub typhus, caused by *Orientia tsutsugamushi*, transmitted by mite is common while rocky mountain spotted fever (RMSF), caused by *Rickettsia rickettsii*, transmitted by tick is prevalent in United States, Canada, Mexico, Central America, and in parts of South America.

Parasitic Hemorrhagic Fever

Malaria, caused by *Plasmodium vivax/falciparum*, is transmitted by bites of infected *Anopheles* mosquitoes. Hemorrhagic manifestations can occur in small numbers of patients with complicated malaria. Malarial infections are predominantly distributed in tropical countries. African countries contribute to high share (95%) of the global malaria burden and 96% of malaria deaths. Though hemorrhagic manifestations are not common but due to widespread of disease in tropical countries, it is an important differential diagnosis of HF.

■ CLINICAL FEATURES

Table 1 describes general features of HF. Most of the presenting clinical features are overlapping for viral, bacterial, and parasitic HF.

■ DIAGNOSIS OF HEMORRHAGIC FEVER

The diagnosis of HF is suspected in a febrile patient with thrombocytopenia with or without transaminitis, renal involvement, and relevant epidemiological risk factor. Clinicians should be aware about geographical mapping of HF to suspect and send appropriate diagnostic tests for HF. In general, molecular diagnostic tests (RT-PCR) are sensitive and specific for most of the VHFs during first week of their illness. CCHF, Ebola viral disease, hantavirus, yellow fever, dengue fever, and other viral infections are diagnosed with RT-PCR testing from serum, whole blood, or plasma.[4] RT-PCR is also useful to reach the diagnosis of leptospirosis. Drawbacks of RTPCR are narrow window for testing opportunity and may become negative after 1 week of onset of illness or resolution of fever, expensive, not readily available at many places, and turnaround time is generally 24 hours and for referral centers, it may take even longer.

Serological tests are useful to reach diagnosis of VHF, bacterial pathogens such as leptospirosis and scrub typhus. Patients generally start mounting IgM antibodies response after 5th day of symptom onset and majority of patients will have detectable IgM antibodies by the end of first week of illness. Window of testing opportunity is longer with serological testing and IgM antibody testing can be used for diagnosis in a patient who is recovering from illness, as positive IgM antibodies may last for first 3–6 months after symptom onset. The major disadvantage of serological testing is cross reactivity with infection with members from the same virus family and false positive results.

Microscopic agglutinin tests are useful to make diagnosis of leptospirosis as apart from antibodies level, it also provides an additional information about serovar.

Malaria diagnosis is arrived by peripheral smear examination.

■ TREATMENT

Supportive treatment is the mainstay in the management of VHF. Supportive care includes maintenance of fluid and electrolyte balance, maintenance of adequate circulating volume, and organ perfusions. Supportive care for organ dysfunction, replacement of coagulation factors, plasma, platelets in patients with bleeding. Control of fever with paracetamol. Specific antiviral agents are not available for the treatment of most of the VHF. Ribavirin and remdesivir have been tried in the treatment of CCHF, hantavirus, and Ebola viral diseases. Ribavirin has been used in the treatment of CCHF with variable success and in one study it has shown mortality benefit.[5]

The triple-monoclonal antibody (mAb) product atoltivimab, maftivimab, and odesivimab (REGN-EB3) was approved by the US Food and Drug Administration (FDA) for the treatment of Ebola virus diseases and provides a potent virus neutralization.[6] Another mAb, ansuvimab (mAb114), isolated from a survivor of Ebola virus disease and neutralizes the virus is also approved by US FDA. Routine antimicrobials are generally not recommended in the treatment of VHF except patients with shock and organ dysfunction requiring intensive care unit (ICU) care and invasive supports. Treatment is mainly supportive for yellow fever and dengue fever.

Bacterial HF: Penicillin, third-generation cephalosporin (Ceftriaxone) and doxycycline are effective antibiotics for the treatment of leptospirosis. Doxycycline is also a drug of choice for scrub typhus. Other useful antimicrobials are rifampicin and azithromycin.

■ PREVENTION AND INFECTION CONTROL

General Measures

General measures such as vector control, reduction in exposure, use of mosquitoes nets, and repellent are effective in preventing HF.[3]

Infection control measures should be instituted immediately following diagnosis. Restrict staff and visitors from entering the room. All the staff entering the room should wear gloves and gowns and persons coming within 3 feet of the patient should wear face shields or surgical masks with eye protection (including side shields). If large amounts of blood or other body fluids are present in the environment, use leg and shoe coverings. Before exiting the room, discard all used protective barriers and clean shoes with a hospital disinfectant or solution of household bleach.

Vaccine

Vaccination for yellow fever is the main tool for prevention. Two vaccines are also available for prevention of Ebola during outbreak while malarial vaccine is under development. Several human vaccine has been developed for leptospirosis, all are specific to serovar and none is available for clinical use.

Chemoprophylaxis

Doxycycline is used for prophylaxis of leptospirosis.

> **TAKE HOME MESSAGE**
>
> Transaminitis with renal involvement in a febrile patient with thrombocytopenia and relevant epidemiological risk factor should raise possibility of HF. Clinicians should be aware about geographical mapping of HF to suspect and send appropriate diagnostic tests for HF. Treatment is mainly supportive for VHF while specific antibacterial are highly effective for the treatment of bacterial HF.

■ REFERENCES

1. Patel AK, Patel KK, Mehta M, Parikh TM, Toshniwal H, Patel K. First Crimean-Congo hemorrhagic fever outbreak in India. J Assoc Physicians India. 2011;59: 585-9.
2. Coltart CE, Lindsey B, Ghinai I, Johnson AM, Heymann DL. The Ebola outbreak, 2013-2016: old lessons for new epidemics. Philos Trans R Soc Lond B Biol Sci. 2017;372(1721):20160297.
3. Pigott DC. Hemorrhagic fever viruses. Crit Care Clin. 2005;21(4):765-83.
4. Racsa LD, Kraft CS, Olinger GG, Hensley LE. Viral hemorrhagic fever diagnostics. Clin Infect Dis. 2016;62(2):214-9.
5. Fabara SP, Ortiz JF, Smith DW, Parwani J, Srikanth S, Varghese T, et al. Crimean-Congo hemorrhagic fever beyond ribavirin: a systematic review. Cureus. 2021; 13(9):e17842.
6. Markham A. REGN-EB3: first approval. Drugs. 2021;81(1):175-8.

Fever with Hepatorenal Dysfunction

Chapter 18

D Suresh Kumar, N Naveen Kumar

INTRODUCTION

India is endemic for many tropical diseases that present with fever and liver involvement and renal dysfunction, commonly labeled as tropical fever with hepatorenal syndrome. In the recent past, many infections are emerging and re-emerging (such as dengue, melioidosis, zika, COVID-19) and the clinical spectrum is also changing.[1] However, the epidemiology and the diagnostic and treatment approaches were not periodically updated, hence in this review, the epidemiology, the etiology, pathophysiology, and diagnostic and treatment approaches were reviewed.

EPIDEMIOLOGY

Most of the diseases under fever with hepatorenal dysfunction syndrome were neglected and the true incidence and prevalence is underestimated and reported in the literature. According to the World Health Organization (WHO) reports, incidences of leptospirosis range from approximately 0.1–10 per 100,000 per year globally and periodic outbreaks have been reported in different parts of India. Incidence of scrub typhus varies widely from most common cause of fever in Vellore to 2–20/100,000 population. Hantavirus has been reported from Tamil Nadu. The seroprevalence of hantavirus infections in the general population is about 4% in India. Estimated 33 million clinically apparent dengue cases occur in India each year, contributing to a third of the total global dengue burden. The number of malaria cases in India dropped from approximately 20 million cases to about 6 million cases, but still it causes multiorgan dysfunction and it should be still considered in the differential diagnosis.

ETIOLOGY

The common causes of fever with hepatorenal syndrome are classified on the basis of incubation period and mode of presentation **(Table 1)**.

PATHOPHYSIOLOGY

Generally, the organism enters the susceptible host and multiples, enters multiple organs including liver and kidney, and causes injury either

CHAPTER 18: Fever with Hepatorenal Dysfunction

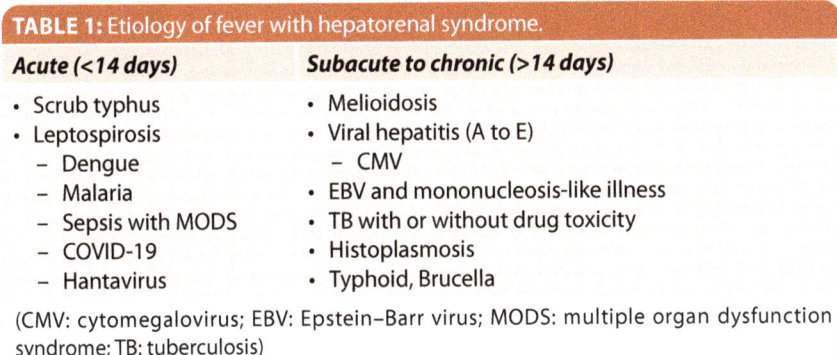

TABLE 1: Etiology of fever with hepatorenal syndrome.

(CMV: cytomegalovirus; EBV: Epstein–Barr virus; MODS: multiple organ dysfunction syndrome; TB: tuberculosis)

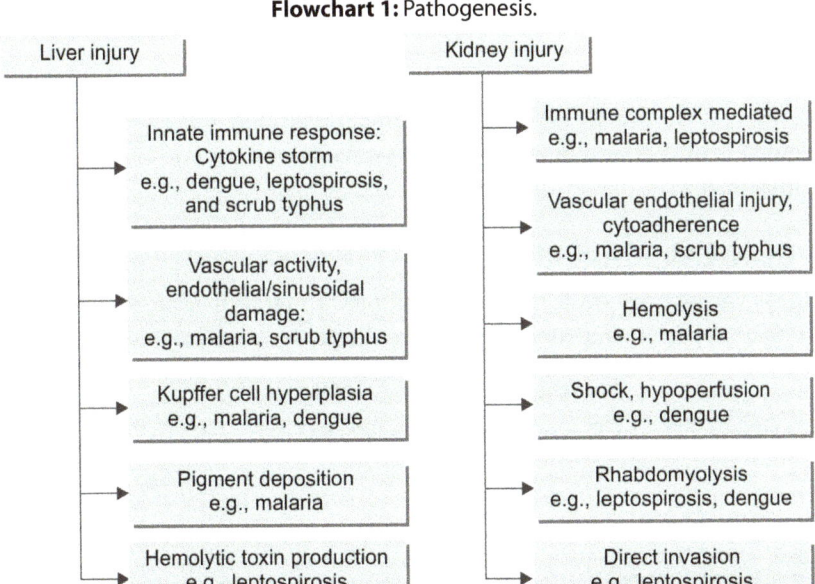

Flowchart 1: Pathogenesis.

directly or indirectly. There are several mechanisms of pathogenesis of liver injury and kidney injury in different etiologies causing the syndrome **(Flowchart 1)**.[2,3]

Leptospirosis

Leptospira enters our body through a broken skin and binds to factor H, escapes the immune system and multiples, infiltrates the solid organs. In liver, it enters the space of Disse and disrupts intercellular junction leading to bile leakage. In kidney, it causes tubular damage and interstitial damage leading to nephritis.

Scrub Typhus

Scrub typhus is caused by *Orientia tsutsugamushi*, through cutaneous entry by mite bite. It causes liver damage either by direct injury or microvascular injury by disseminated intravascular coagulation (DIC) transaminitis (63%). Renal involvement includes acute kidney injury (AKI) (53%) and proteinuria (60%). Oliguric AKI is a predictor of poor outcome.

Hantavirus

Hantaviruses are carried and transmitted by rodents (striped field mouse). People acquire this virus after exposure to aerosolized urine, droppings, saliva, or after exposure to dust from their nest. Functional impairment of vascular endothelium is the main pathology involved.

Dengue

Dengue is caused by dengue virus (*Flavivirus*). There are four serotypes DENV-1, 2, 3, and 4. They are antigenically similar but they elicit cross protection only for few months following infection by any one of the serotypes **(Flowchart 2)**.

■ CLINICAL FEATURES

Illness varies from mild self-limiting illness to fatal disease. Based on the incubation period, infection can manifest in days or weeks after the entry. The

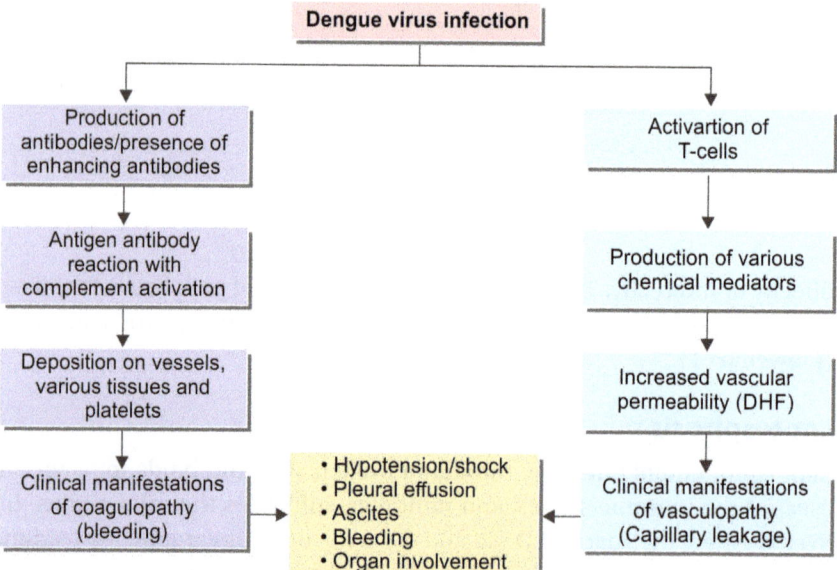

Flowchart 2: Pathogenesis of Dengue fever.

(DHF: dengue hemorrhagic fever)

CHAPTER 18: Fever with Hepatorenal Dysfunction

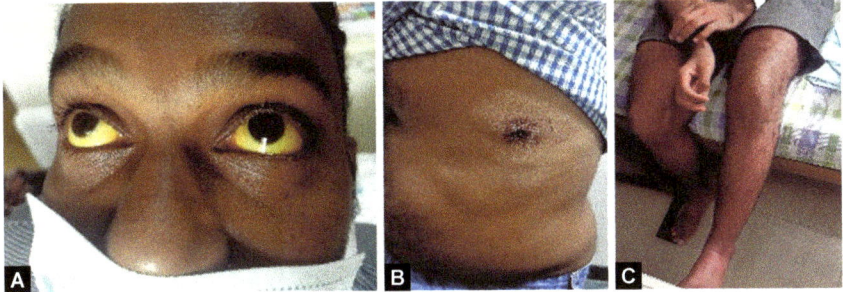

Figs. 1A to C: Common clinical features of fever with hepatorenal manifestations: (A) Jaundice; (B) eschar; and (C) diffuse erythema.

symptoms commonly noted are fever, myalgia, abdominal pain, vomiting, yellowish discoloration of eyes and urine, skin rash [eschar, diffuse erythema, **(Fig. 1C)**], decreased urine output, and hematuria. The specific symptoms in each disease are as follows:
- *Leptospirosis:* Conjunctival congestion, jaundice **(Fig. 1A)**, oliguria, hepatorenal dysfunction (Weil's disease), retro-orbital pain, and muscular pain
- *Scrub typhus:* Eschar **(Fig. 1B)** at site of mite bite, fever, headache and regional lymphadenopathy
- *Malaria:* Fever with chills and rigors, pallor, and splenomegaly.

■ INVESTIGATIONS (TABLE 2)
Basic Investigation
- Complete hemogram
- Renal function test
- Liver function test
- Peripheral smear/Quantitative buffy coat/rapid card-based test for malaria
- Urine routine examination
- Blood cultures
- Ultrasonography (USG) of the abdomen, Computed tomography (CT) of the abdomen/chest.

■ TREATMENT
Treatment involves supportive therapy and specific therapy with appropriate antibiotics.[4]

Supportive Therapy
It is given irrespective of any culture or serological testing.
- Intravenous fluids
- Antipyretics (acetaminophen)

TABLE 2: Infection and their specific investigations.

Infection suspected based on clinical history	Specific investigation
Leptospirosis	• IgM for leptospirosis • Microscopic slide agglutination • PCR
Scrub typhus	• IgM scrub • PCR
Dengue	• NS1Ag • IgM, IgG dengue antibodies
Malaria	Peripheral smear/MP QBC/rapid card test
Blood cultures	Minimum 20 mL of blood, ideal 40 mL of blood
Hantavirus	• Anti-Hantavirus IgM • PCR
Viral hepatitis	• Hepatitis A and E IgM • HBsAg, anti-HCV antibody
Others (second line tests)	• COVID-19 PCR, EBV VCA IgM, CMV IgM, urine for histoplasma antigen, sputum/tissue for gene Xpert for MTB and tissue/node biopsy for histopathological examination • ANA, DS DNA, C and P ANCA

(ANCA: antineutrophil cytoplasmic antibody; ANA: antinuclear antibody; CMV: cytomegalovirus; EBV: Epstein–Barr virus; HBsAg: hepatitis B surface antigen; HCV: hepatitis C virus; IgE: immunoglobulin E; IgM: immunoglobulin M; MTB: mycobacterium tuberculosis; PCR: polymerase chain reaction; VCA: viral capsid antigen)

- Blood supports:
    - Platelets—thrombocytopenia
    - Fresh frozen plasma—coagulopathy
    - Packed red cells—anemia
- Renal replacement therapy for AKI
- Encephalopathy measures.

Specific Therapy

Empirical therapy for suspected fever with hepatorenal syndrome is ceftriaxone 2 g intravenous (IV) OD and doxycycline 100 mg PO BD for patients in intensive care units and oral azithromycin for patients in OP/wards with >5–7 days of fever till initial investigations results **(Table 3 and 4)**.

Definite Therapy

Leptospirosis

Scrub Typhus

Standard regimen: Doxycycline 100 mg BD—7 days

TABLE 3: Leptospirosis treatment.

Indication	Treatment
Mild leptospirosis	- Doxycycline mg PO BD - Azithromycin 500 mg OD - *Duration:* 7 days
Moderate/severe leptospirosis	- Ceftriaxone 2 g IV/OD - Doxycycline 100 mg IV q 12h - *Duration:* 7 days - Crystalline penicillin is not preferred (due to administrative difficulties)

(IV: intravenous)

TABLE 4: Malaria treatment.

Uncomplicated malaria (Non-*Falciparum*)	*Chloroquine sensitive:* Chloroquine of 10 mg/kg base stat followed by 10 mg/kg at 24 hours and 5 mg/kg at 48 hours
Uncomplicated malaria (*Falciparum*)	Artemether + lumefantrine (AM + L) (weight based)
Complicated falciparum malaria	- Artesunate (2.4 mg/kg IV followed by 2.4 mg/kg at 12 and 24 hours and then daily if necessary; children <20 kg given 3 mg/kg/dose plus doxycycline after clinical improvement change it to oral (AM+L) - Artemether 3.2 mg/kg IM followed by 1.6 mg/kf qd

TABLE 5: Implication of hematocrit in dengue fever.

Hematocrit ↑	Fluid leakage	Replace with crystalloids
Hematocrit ↓	Hemorrhage/blood loss	Replace with blood

Azithromycin 1000 mg loading dose on day 1 followed by 500 mg for next 2 days. In children and pregnancy, azithromycin is preferred.

Hantavirus

The treatment is supportive with hydration and ribavirin is not indicated for hepatorenal involvement.

Dengue (Table 5)

- Symptomatic management
- *Platelet transfusion:* <10,000 counts
- IV fluids/blood support based on hematocrit.

Malaria

See **Table 4**

DIAGNOSTIC AND TREATMENT APPROACH

The simplified approach to common tropical infections with hepatorenal syndrome is detailed history and head-to-toe physical examination along with basic investigations **(Table 6)**.[5]

	Scrub	*Leptospirosis*	*Dengue*	*Malaria*	*Melioidosis*
History	Rural back ground, exposure to bushy areas	Exposure to rain water/ floods, agriculture field, swimming	Sudden onset of fever, back pain, headache. Mosquito bite	Fever with chills and rigors, mosquito bite	Rural back ground, agriculture field /flood exposure poorly controlled diabetes, alcohol intake
Physical examination	Eschar Regional lymphadenopathy	Conjunctival congestion, jaundice	Blanching skin rash, conjunctival congestion	Pallor, splenomegaly	Parotid and abscess in internal organs
CBC	Elevated WBC, low platelets	Elevated WBC, low platelets	Elevated HB, low WBC counts, reactive lymphocytes, very low platelets	Low HB, low platelets	Elevated WBC and low platelets
LFT	Mixed pattern - both ALT/AST and Alk, GGTP elevation	Cholestatic picture (elevated bilirubin, Alk, GGTP)	Hepatocellular pattern- AST >ALT and normal Alk and GGTP	Indirect bilirubin may be elevated	Cholestatic picture
Therapeutic trial	Allowed	Allowed	Supportive care	Tried to confirm all means	After cultures allowed
Treatment options	Doxycycline Azithromycin Rifampicin	Doxycycline Azithromycin Ceftriaxone Crystalline penicillin	Symptomatic care	*P. vivax*: Chloroquine *P. falciparum*: Artemisinin based therapy	Intensive phase: Ceftazidime/ meropenem maintenance phase: doxycycline/ co-trimoxazole

(ALT: alanine aminotransferase; AST: aspartate aminotransferase; CBC: complete blood count; HB: hemoglobin; LFT: liver function test; GGTP: gamma-glutamyl transpeptidase; WBC: white blood cell)

PREVENTION (TABLE 7)

TABLE 7: Preventive strategies for tropical infections.

Organism	Preventive measures
Leptospirosis	• Avoidance of exposure to urine and tissues from infected animals through proper footwear • Animal vaccination
Scrub typhus	• Insect repellents—DEET • No licensed vaccines
Dengue and malaria	Personal protection against mosquito bite sleeping in bed nets, insect repellents such as DEET

(DEET: N,N-diethyl-meta-toluamide)

TAKE HOME MESSAGE

- Tropical infection has varied presentation and nonspecific manifestation and it should be considered as differential diagnosis in any patient presenting with fever in India.
- Early diagnosis by timely clinical decision and treatment can prevent complications.
- Detailed history, head-to-toe physical examination, and basic laboratory tests will give clues to identify fever with hepatorenal syndrome.
- Scrub typhus and leptospirosis clinical diagnosis is allowed, but for malaria, all efforts to be taken to make definite diagnosis.
- Oral azithromycin or doxycycline will be sufficient for most of the fever with hepatorenal syndrome.

REFERENCES

1. Gopalakrishnan R, Sureshkumar D, Thirunarayan MA, Ramasubramanian V. Melioidosis: an emerging infection in India. J Assoc Physicians India. 2013;61(9):612-4.
2. Samanta J, Sharma V. Dengue and its effects on liver. World J Clin Cases. 2015;3(2):125-31.
3. Basu G, Chrispal A, Boorugu H, Gopinath KG, Chandy S, Prakash JA, et al. Acute kidney injury in tropical acute febrile illness in a tertiary care centre – RIFLE criteria validation. Nephrol Dial Transplant. 2011;26(2):524-31.
4. Singhi S, Chaudhary D, Varghese GM, Bhalla A, Karthi N, Kalantri S, et al. Tropical fevers: management guidelines. Indian J Crit Care Med. 2014;18:62-9.
5. Bhargava A, Ralph R, Chatterjee B, Bottieau E. Assessment and initial management of acute undifferentiated fever in tropical and subtropical regions. BMJ. 2018;363:k4766.

Chapter 19

Fever with Central Nervous System Dysfunction

Suba Guruprasad, Ramasubramanian, Prasun Chatterjee

■ INTRODUCTION

The central nervous system (CNS) may be impacted by an infectious process in several ways. From encephalopathy during a sepsis event to direct invasion by a neurotropic pathogen, the involvement of the CNS can have devastating consequences. In recent years, neglected tropical infections are being increasingly identified as a cause of acute febrile encephalopathy.[1,2] In this article, we discuss the prevalent infectious causes associated with CNS dysfunction.

Neurological involvement during an infection can occur due to direct affection of the neurons as in rabies, by causing local inflammatory reaction or mass effect (neurocysticercosis), due to the systemic inflammatory response at the time of infection (sepsis) or at the time of treatment (filariasis), by predisposing to cerebral vascular disease such as in Chaka's disease or by immune-mediated nerve injury as seen in leprosy.[3]

■ VIRUSES AND CENTRAL NERVOUS SYSTEM DYSFUNCTION

Dengue

Dengue is an important arboviral disease in tropical countries such as India. The virus belongs to the *Flavivirus* family and is transmitted by *Aedes aegypti* mosquito. CNS involvement may be seen in up to 21% of the patients and has been mainly seen with DEN-2 and DENV-3 stereotypes of the virus.[4,5]

The involvement of CNS in dengue can take many forms including encephalitis, meningitis, meningoencephalitis, or myelitis. Headache, fever, irritability vomiting seizures, and coma were reported manifestations. Rarer complications include hemorrhagic stroke, lumbosacral plexopathy, and mononeuropathy as well as postinfectious Guillain–Barré syndrome, acute disseminated encephalomyelitis, and Parkinsonism.[6,7]

Clinical presentation includes fever, headache, altered sensorium, behavioral changes, seizures, and focal deficits. Magnetic resonance imaging (MRI) of the brain may show cerebral edema or nonspecific changes. The diagnosis is supported by presence of lymphocyte predominant cells in the cerebrospinal fluid (CSF), detection of dengue immunoglobulin M (IgM), NS1 antigen in serum, a positive polymerase chain reaction (PCR), or isolation of virus in CSF.

Nipah Virus Encephalitis

Nipah virus belongs to the family of *Paramyxoviridae* and is found in fruit bats or flying foxes. Humans acquire infection when they come in contact with pigs, which are intermediate host, through consumption of fruits contaminated with bat urine or bat saliva or direct human-to-human transmission.

The patient typically experiences a viral prodrome followed by altered sensorium that can rapidly progress to coma, seizures, myoclonus, areflexic weakness, meningism, cerebellar ataxia, and brain stem involvement with autonomic dysfunction. Neurological symptoms may also occur after several months or years usually due to reactivation of latent CNS infection. CSF examination shows lymphocytic pleocytosis and electroencephalogram (EEG) shows diffuse slowing or periodic complexes. Nipah IgG and IgM antibodies can be detected in the serum. Case fatality is over 70%.

Rabies

Dogs are the primary reservoir for the virus. Following the bite of an infected animal, the virus propagates from the muscle and the nerves to the dorsal root ganglion and the CNS. The encephalitic form manifests as fever, encephalopathy, hydrophobia or acrophobia, inspiration spasm, autonomic signs, and the paralytic form has features of neuropathic pain, progressive ascending weakness, and areflexia. Further anterograde propagation of the virus to extraneural tissues including, skin, heart, and blood vessels can lead to multiorgan dysfunction. The infection is invariably fatal.

Chikungunya

Belonging to the *Togavirus* family, the chikungunya virus is transmitted by *Aedes* mosquito. Clinically presents with symmetrical peripheral arthropathy. CNS maybe involved in up to 25% of the patients and generally manifests as meningitis, encephalitis, encephalopathy neuropathy, and myopathy. Diagnosis is made, based on the detection of serum IgM and IGG antibodies and viral RNA by PCR in CSF or serum.

Zika

Zika belongs to the *Flaviviridae* family. Neurological complications include Guillain-Barré syndrome, which is the most common manifestation, encephalopathy, acute demyelination, encephalomyelitis, and stroke. MRI may show alterations in the subcortical areas and CSF may show leukocytosis with neutrophilic predominance. Detection of the RNA by PCR and IgM in CSF helps establish the diagnosis.

Intrauterine exposure to the virus may cause congenital Zika syndrome, which is associated with microcephaly, cerebral atrophy, intracranial calcification, neural tube defects, optic nerve abnormalities, and hearing loss.

Chandipura Virus

Belonging to the genus vesiculovirus of the *Rhabdoviridae* family, this virus has caused several outbreaks of acute encephalitis syndrome, particularly in children, in parts of India. The disease manifests as sudden high fever followed by seizures, altered sensorium, diarrhea, and vomiting. It is rapidly progressive and is fatal in most cases.[8,9] No definitive treatment is currently available.

Japanese Encephalitis

This is caused by a *Flavivirus* and transmitted by the *Culex* mosquito. Japanese encephalitis begins as a nonspecific febrile illness followed by headache, vomiting, and altered sensorium.[10] Seizures generally follow. Extrapyramidal symptoms such as head nodding and opsoclonus-myoclonus have also been reported. The treatment is supportive and mortality associated with it is in the range of 30%.

BACTERIAL INFECTIONS ASSOCIATED WITH CENTRAL NERVOUS SYSTEM DYSFUNCTION

Tuberculosis and the Central Nervous System

Tubercular meningitis, one of the most disabling forms of tuberculosis, is a common cause of cerebral dysfunction particularly in children. Inflammatory reaction triggered by the bacteria may lead to meningitis, tuberculous, arteritis, obstruction of the CSF (**Fig. 1**), and vascular complications including stroke.[11] With the advent of molecular and PCR-based technologies, the diagnosis of tubercular meningitis is more reliable. Treatment for drug-sensitive TB is a four drug antitubercular regimen including rifampicin, ethambutol, isoniazid, and pyrazinamide, with or without steroids.

Melioidosis

Caused by *Burkholderia pseudomallei*, a facultative intracellular bacterium, it can cause CNS syndromes such as cerebral and epidural abscess, brain stem encephalitis, aseptic meningitis, and transverse myelitis.[12] The CSF profile may show normal glucose and mononuclear pleocytosis. MRI changes reported in literature include rim-enhancing lesions, nodular leptomeningeal, and linear enhancements. The mortality associated with neuromelioidosis is reported to be approximately 20%.

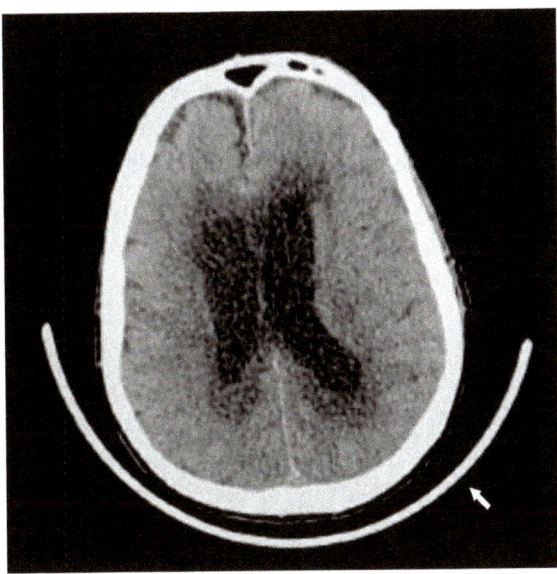

Fig. 1: Computed tomography (CT) image showing hydrocephalus with periventricular ooze in tuberculosis (TB) meningitis.
(*Courtsey:* Dr V Ramasubramanian)

Brucellosis

Brucellosis is a zoonotic disease transmitted to humans by direct or indirect contact with infected animals such as cattle and sheep camels. Most cases are caused by *Brucella melitensis*. The condition begins insidiously with fever, malaise, and night sweats. Neurological involvement may occur in up to 10% of the patients and may present as meningitis, encephalitis, brain abscess, myelitis, or cranial or peripheral neuritis.[12-14] Diagnosis is made by culturing the organism in blood or CSF. Prolonged therapy generally needed with gentamicin is given along with rifampicin or doxycycline for at least 6–12 weeks. In children and pregnant women, doxycycline is replaced with trimethoprim-sulfamethoxazole.

Lyme Disease

This is a tick borne illness caused by the spirochete, *Borreliella*. The clinical course is divided into three phases:
1. *The early-localized disease:* Characterized by appearance of characteristic skin lesions, erythema migrans.
2. *The early-disseminated disease:* Neurological involvement is typically seen in this phase and may present as lymphocytic meningitis, cranial nerve palsies, radiculopathy, mononeuritis multiplex, and rarely cerebellar ataxia. Other manifestations of disseminated phase include carditis and ocular manifestations such as iridocyclitis.

3. *Late disease:* Neurological involvement may rarely be seen in this phase in the form of mononeuropathy multiplex and encephalomyelitis.[15] Diagnosis in the early-disseminated phase is made by testing for antibodies but is usually interpreted in conjunction with the clinical scenario. In cases with CSF pleocytosis, a simultaneous CSF/serum antibody index may help in establishing the diagnosis.[16] Treatment is generally with doxycycline or ceftriaxone for 14–21 days.

Rickettsia

This is a mite-borne infection caused by *Orientia tsutsugamushi* and transmitted by trombiculid mites. Generally, this begins as a febrile illness with headache, anorexia, and malaise. Diffuse rashes may also be present and often the site of the bite from the mite may form an eschar. CNS involvement generally occurs due to vasculitis of the cerebral vessels and may produce mononuclear pleocytosis and encephalitis. Diagnosis is usually made by indirect fluorescent antibody testing in concurrence with clinical and other laboratory parameters such as leukocytosis and thrombocytopenia. Doxycycline is the drug of choice and clinical improvement is seen rapidly once treatment is initiated.

Tetanus

Caused by *Clostridium tetani*, the infection typically follows a deep penetrating wound. Neurological involvement occurs due to the toxin-mediated inhibition of the neurotransmitter gamma-amino butyric acid in the neurons.[17] Lock jaw, caused by the spasm of the masseter, is usually the most common feature. Generalized tetanus may present with pain, headache, stiffness, rigidity, opisthotonus, and spasms. Death usually occurs due to respiratory arrest. The diagnosis is clinical and penicillin remains the treatment of choice.

Enteric Fever

Caused by *Salmonella enterica serovar typhi*, typhoid fever is a common cause of fever without a focus in tropical countries.[18] Most cases present with fever and a diarrheal illness and the CNS involvement occur late in the disease, generally in the second week. The most common manifestation includes delirium and altered sensorium. Hallucinations and other psychotic symptoms have also been described. Less commonly, stroke, cerebellar involvement and extrapyramidal signs may be seen. Blood cultures give the definitive diagnosis and treatment varies based on the local resistance pattern and generally involves combination therapy with a third-generation cephalosporin and azithromycin.

PROTOZOAL AND HELMINTHIC INFECTIONS AND CENTRAL NERVOUS SYSTEM DYSFUNCTION

Cerebral Malaria

Malaria is reported to be the most common cause of encephalopathy in the world.[19] It is caused by *Plasmodium falciparum* and is transmitted by the female anopheles mosquito.

Nervous system involvement typically occurs due to the sequestration of the parasite in the brain. It presents with diffuse encephalopathy and focal signs are rare. Most adults have generalized seizures although partial motor seizures have also been reported. Neurological involvement is accompanied by multiorgan dysfunction. Mortality of cerebral malaria is reported to be around 52% particularly if other systems are involved and most deaths occur within the first 48 hours of admission. Prompt administration of intravenous antimalarial agents has a dramatic impact on the outcome. Intravenous quinine is the drug of choice, followed by oral antimalarials once the patient is able to swallow.

Schistosomiasis

Schistosomiasis is a helminthic fluke infection caused by the genus Schistosoma.[20] Human beings are the definitive hosts, while snails are the intermediate host of the parasite. Neurological involvement occurs in different forms. Acute schistosomal encephalopathy, caused mainly by *Schistosoma japonicum* is seen 3 weeks after the onset of systemic symptoms. It presents with headache, altered mental status, seizures, and sensory disturbances. Many of the findings are transient and resolve in a few days to weeks. Diagnosis is generally based on history of exposure to schistosomes and positive serological tests. Pseudotumor encephalic schistosomiasis is seen in about 3.5% of infections with *S. japonicum*. They present as a tumor-like slowly expanding lesion that causes increased intracranial pressure resulting in headache, vomiting, focal deficits, and visual disturbances. The disease may also involve the spinal cord. Treatment options include antischistosomal drugs such as praziquantel, corticosteroids, and surgery.

Leishmaniasis

Central nervous system involvement in leishmaniasis is less common and may present as meningoencephalitic involvement such as mental changes and altered behavior. Generalized seizures are also a common manifestation. Treatment is usually with sodium stibogluconate and amphotericin B and outcomes are good.

Neurocysticercosis

Cysticercosis develops following the ingestion of *Taenia solium* eggs and the migration of the larvae into the host tissue. Infiltration of the brain causes neurocysticercosis. It is one of the leading causes of preventable seizures. The larvae may be found in the parenchyma, in the intraventricular spaces, or the spinal cord. Headache and seizures are the most common manifestations and psychiatric symptoms are rare. Imaging of the brain **(Fig. 2)** is the

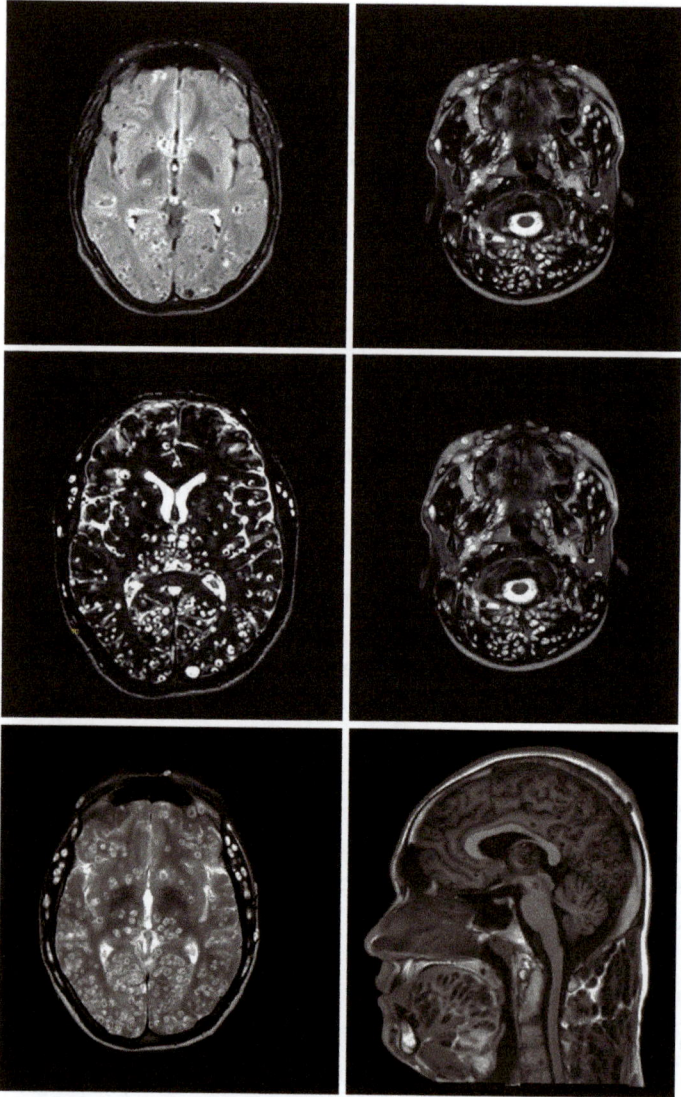

Fig. 2: Magnetic resonance imaging (MRI) features of a case with miliary neurocysticercosis.
(*Courtsey:* Dr V Ramasubramanian)

gold standard in making a diagnosis. Treatment with antihelminthic drugs such as albendazole and praziquantel along with steroids has good outcomes.

APPROACH TO A PATIENT WITH FEVER AND CENTRAL NERVOUS SYSTEM DYSFUNCTION

A detailed history is essential to narrow down the cause of a tropical fever causing encephalopathy **(Table 1)**. Exposure to mites, mosquitoes, consumption of unpasteurized milk, untreated water, or undercooked meat can give an idea of a likely etiology. Presence of eschars, lymphadenopathy, and rashes on examination can also be useful pointers to likely diagnosis. Initial tests should include a complete blood picture with peripheral smear to look for parasites such as *Falciparum* or *Leishmania*. A high count with low platelet count may be seen in scrub typhus, while leukopenia and thrombocytopenia are more characteristic of dengue or enteric fever. For any febrile patients presenting with encephalopathy, it is important to rule out raised intracranial pressure and meningitis with imaging studies followed by a lumbar puncture. Imaging and CSF examination are also essential in encephalopathy syndrome. Rapid tests for dengue and malaria can be helpful in establishing the diagnosis early and help make treatment decisions. Empiric treatment at presentation must include a third-generation cephalosporin, acyclovir, and doxycycline.

TABLE 1: Key points in history for a suspected case of tropical fever.[21]

History	Implications or Associated Diseases
• Day-by-day itinerary	• Provides geographic disease associations
• Vaccinations and malaria prophylaxis	• Narrow the differential diagnosis but do not rule out vaccine-preventable diseases or malaria
• Other drugs taken while or since traveling	• Partial treatment of infection may delay or alter disease presentation (e.g., malaria)
• Immune status (diabetes, glucocorticoid treatment, renal failure, splenectomy, diseases associated with immune deficit)	• Melioidosis, listeriosis, tuberculosis, fungal infections, CMV infection
• Consumption of unclean water, unpasteurized milk, or improperly cooked or raw food	• Travelers' diarrhea, giardiasis, nontyphoidal salmonellosis, enteric fever, shigellosis, campylobacter infection, hepatitis A and E, amebic dysentery, brucellosis, listeriosis

Contd...

Contd...

History	Implications or Associated Diseases
• Exposure to fresh water (rafting, kayaking, swimming in rivers or lakes, floods)	• Leptospirosis, acute schistosomiasis
• Skin contact with soil (e.g., walking barefoot)	• Strongyloidiasis, melioidosis
• Tattoos, piercings, intravenous drug use, or medical procedures (e.g., injections and blood-product transfusions)	• Hepatitis B or C virus infection, acute HIV infection, CMV infection, malaria, babesiosis
• Sexual contact, specifically unprotected sex with a new partner, commercial sex workers, or multiple partners	• Primary herpesvirus infection; acute HIV infection; hepatitis A, B, or C virus infection; syphilis; gonorrhea; Zika virus infection; viral hemorrhagic fevers
• Visits with relatives or friends while abroad (Was anyone ill?)	• Tuberculosis, other infections transmitted by exposure to ill persons
• Insect bites	
– Mosquitoes	• Malaria, dengue fever, chikungunya, Zika virus infection, Japanese encephalitis, yellow fever, Rift Valley fever, West Nile virus infection, filarial fever
– Ticks	• Rickettsioses, Q fever, tickborne relapsing fever, Lyme disease, tickborne encephalitis, babesiosis, Crimean-Congo hemorrhagic fever, tularemia
– Mites	• Scrub typhus, rickettsialpox *(R. akari)*
– Fleas	• Murine typhus, plague
– Lice	• Louseborne relapsing fever *(B. recurrentis)*, epidemic typhus *(R. prowazekii)*, trench fever *(Bartonella quintana)*
– Flies	• Leishmaniasis, African sleeping sickness, bartonellosis, phlebotomus (sandfly) fever
– Triatomine bugs	• Chagas' disease
• Animal bites	• Rabies, cat-scratch fever *(B. henselae)*, rat-bite fever *(Spirillum minus or Streptobacillus moniliformis infection)*, simian herpesvirus B infection
• Close contact with animals	• Toxoplasmosis, anthrax, Q fever, hantavirus infection, Nipah virus, Hendra virus, plague, psittacosis, diseases from animal ectoparasites
• Close contact with wild or pet birds	• Psittacosis, avian influenza

(CMV: cytomegalovirus; HIV: human immunodeficiency virus)

CHAPTER 19: Fever with Central Nervous System Dysfunction

> **TAKE HOME MESSAGE**
> - The CNS involvement in tropical infections can take various forms, from encephalopathy due to edema to demyelination.
> - A detailed history including dietary and travel history is essential in arriving at a probable etiology. Thorough physical examination (to look for clues like an eschar) can aid in clinching the diagnosis.
> - PCR and serology on the CSF are often helpful in establishing the diagnosis.
> - Most conditions are self-limiting or have an effective treatment and hence early identification, good supportive care, and prompt initiation of appropriate therapy is important to ensure good clinical outcomes.

■ REFERENCES

1. Joshi R, Kalantri SP, Reingold A, Colford JM Jr. Changing landscape of acute encephalitis syndrome in India: a systematic review. Natl Med J India. 2012; 25(4):212-20.
2. Ranawaka UK. The challenge of treating central nervous system infections in the developing world. J Ceylon Coll Physicians. 2018;49:2-15.
3. Berkowitz AL, Raibagkar P, Pritt BS, Mateen FJ. Neurologic manifestations of the neglected tropical diseases. J Neurol Sci. 2015;349(1):20-32.
4. Carod-Artal FJ, Wichmann O, Farrar J, Gascón J. Neurological complications of dengue virus infection. Lancet Neurol. 2013;12(9):906-19.
5. Puccioni-Sohler M, Rosadas C, Cabral-Castro MJ. Neurological complications in dengue infection: a review for clinical practice. Arq Neuropsiquiatr. 2013; 71(9B):667-71.
6. Azmin S, Sahathevan R, Suehazlyn Z, Law ZK, Rabani R, Nafisah WY, et al. Post-dengue parkinsonism. BMC Infect Dis. 2013;13(1).
7. Fong CY, Hlaing CS, Tay CG, Ong LC. Post-dengue encephalopathy and Parkinsonism. Pediatr Infect Dis J. 2014;33(10):1092-4.
8. Rao BL, Basu A, Wairagkar NS, Gore MM, Arankalle VA, Thakare JP, et al. A large outbreak of acute encephalitis with high fatality rate in children in Andhra Pradesh, India, in 2003, associated with Chandipura virus. Lancet (London, England). 2004;364(9437):869-74.
9. Chadha MS, Arankalle VA, Jadi RS, Joshi MV, Thakare JP, Mahadev PV, et al. An outbreak of Chandipura virus encephalitis in the eastern districts of Gujarat state, India. Am J Trop Med Hyg. 2005;73(3):566-70.
10. Solomon T, Dung NM, Kneen R, Gainsborough M, Vaughn DW, Khanh VT. Japanese encephalitis. J Neurol Neurosurg Psychiatry. 2000;68(4):405-15.
11. Wilkinson RJ, Rohlwink U, Misra UK, Van Crevel R, Mai NTH, Dooley KE, et al. Tuberculous meningitis. Nat Rev Neurol. 2017;13(10):581-98.
12. Zamzuri M 'Ammar IA, Jamhari MN, Nawi HM, Hassan MR, Pang NTP, Kassim MAM, et al. Epidemiology of Neuromelioidosis in Asia-Pacific: a systematic review. Open Access Maced J Med Sci. 2021;9(F):318-26.
13. Araj GF. Update on laboratory diagnosis of human brucellosis. Int J Antimicrob Agents. 2010;36 Suppl 1.
14. Doganay M, Aygen B. Human brucellosis: an overview. Int J Infect Dis. 2003;7(3): 173-82.

15. Balmelli T, Piffaretti JC. Association between different clinical manifestations of Lyme disease and different species of Borrelia burgdorferi sensu lato. Res Microbiol. 1995;146(4):329-40.
16. Lantos PM, Rumbaugh J, Bockenstedt LK, Falck-Ytter YT, Aguero-Rosenfeld ME, Auwaerter PG, et al. Clinical Practice Guidelines by the Infectious Diseases Society of America (IDSA), American Academy of Neurology (AAN), and American College of Rheumatology (ACR): 2020 Guidelines for the Prevention, Diagnosis and Treatment of Lyme Disease. Clin Infect Dis. 2021;72(1):1-8.
17. Farrar JJ, Yen LM, Cook T, Fairweather N, Binh N, Parry J, et al. Tetanus. J Neurol Neurosurg Psychiatry. 2000;69(3):292-301.
18. Ahmed AIA, Prabhakar AT. Typhoid fever and its nervous system involvement. In: Saxena SK, Hridayesh P, (eds). Innate Immunity in Health and Disease. Germany: Books on Demand; 2021.
19. Newton CRJC, Hien TT, White N. Cerebral malaria. J Neurol Neurosurg Psychiatry. 2000;69:433-41.
20. ClinicalKey. Neuroschistosomiasis: clinical symptoms and pathogenesis. [online] Available from: https://www.clinicalkey.com/#!/content/playContent/1-s2.0-S1474442211701703?scrollTo=%23hl0000422. [Last accessed May 2022].
21. Thwaites GE, Day NP. Approach to fever in the returning traveler. N Engl J Med. 2017;376(6):548-60.

Chapter 20

Fever with Acute Respiratory Distress Syndrome

Chandrasekhar Valupadas

■ INTRODUCTION

Fever is a common clinical problem, particularly during rainy season. Many fevers in India, during the season from July to September, increase the incidence of acute febrile illness (AFI), which may lead to increase in morbidity and mortality. Most common complications in the seasonal fevers in tropics include multiorgan failure, and most common cause of death is acute respiratory distress syndrome (ARDS).[1]

Most often, these fevers are likely to be vector-borne diseases transmitted by mosquitoes and other insect bites. It is imperative from the fact that there exists vast geographical and seasonal variations in the Indian subcontinent;[2] wide variations exist in prevalence, incidence, clinical presentations, and outcomes. The differential diagnosis of AFI by infectious agent is critical when patient getting admitted into emergency department and intensive care unit (ICU). Most fevers may have overlapping clinical syndromes with complications such as shock, cytopenias, hypoxia, respiratory distress, and renal failure requiring vasopressor support, blood component transfusions, renal replacement therapy, and ventilator support. Examples include malaria, scrub typhus, leptospirosis, dengue fever, and enteric fever. High index of suspicion and prompt intervention are often life-saving as time available for clinical judgment and decision-making is very minimal.

■ ACUTE RESPIRATORY DISTRESS SYNDROME

Acute respiratory distress syndrome is an acute, diffuse, and inflammatory lung injury **(Fig. 1)** that leads to increased pulmonary vascular permeability, loss of aerated tissue, and increased lung weight resulting acute respiratory failure with hypoxia and/or hypercarbia. Clinically, ARDS manifests with hypoxia and diffuse alveolar opacities. It is also based on Berlin Criteria[3] **(Box 1)** and severity is expressed as PaO_2 (partial pressure of oxygen in arteries)/FiO_2 (fractional inspired oxygen) ratio. It is also called as Horowitz index and Carrico index. Based on this ratio, ARDS is classified into three categories: Mild (200–300), moderate (100–200), and severe (<100).

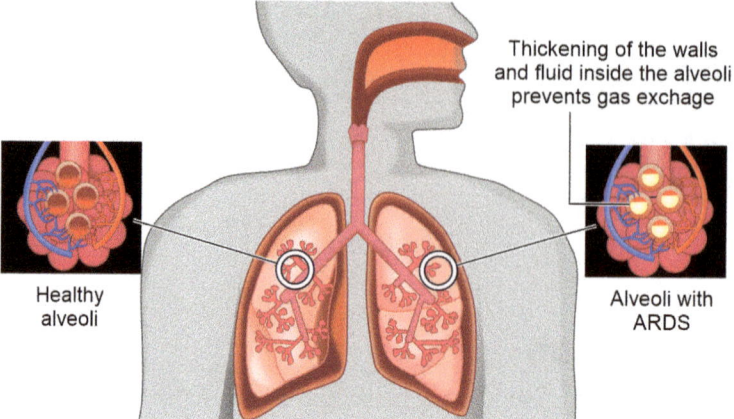

Fig. 1: Acute respiratory distress syndrome.

> **BOX 1:** Definition of Berlin criteria for the diagnosis of ARDS.
> - Onset within 1 week of respiratory insult
> - Bilateral opacities in the chest radiograph (excluding atelectasis, consolidation, and pleural effusions)
> - Pulmonary edema (not explained by cardiac origin)
> - Abnormal PaO_2/FiO_2 ratio on continuous positive airway pressure (CPAP)

■ CLINICAL FEATURES

Clinical features depend on time of onset of cause, severity pathogenesis, underlying comorbidities, and number of precipitating factors present. In the due course of time, there may be signs and symptoms of complications of ARDS add-on such as cyanosis due to intrapulmonary shunting and right heart failure due to development of pulmonary arterial hypertension **(Table 1)**.

■ ETIOLOGY

The causes of ARDS may broadly classify based on direct and indirect lung injury. Nevertheless, isolation of infectious agent is paramount important to initiate specific treatment at the earliest. In the setting of fever with ARDS, the direct and indirect lung injury causes need to be identified at the earliest as these factors may precipitate, prolong the course of illness, and may be responsible for adverse outcomes.
- *Indirect lung injury* may be due to sepsis, trauma, pancreatitis, shock, intracranial hemorrhage, blood transfusion-related lung injury, drug overdose, amniotic embolism, and long bone fracture (i.e., fat embolism).
- *Direct lung injury* may due to pneumonia, gastric contents aspiration, toxic inhalational, pulmonary bruise, embolism, and near-drowning.

TABLE 1: Clinical features of ARDS.

Symptoms	Signs
• Tachycardia	• Crackles (bilateral, mostly asymmetrical)
• Tachypnea	• Wheezes (bilateral, mono/polyphonic)
• Dyspnea	• Cyanosis
• Cough with/without sputum, hemoptysis	• Hypercarbia
• Chest pain	• P2 loud (pulmonary arterial hypertension)
• Diaphoresis	• Parasternal heave (right-sided heart failure)
• Accessory muscle use	• Right-sided murmurs

(ARDS: acute respiratory distress syndrome)

■ PATHOPHYSIOLOGY

Acute respiratory distress syndrome is a secondary disease process and its severity is based upon hypoxemia (PaO_2/FiO_2). Primary triggers for ARDS are sepsis, trauma, multiorgan failure, pulmonary insult, pancreatitis, drug overdose, blood transfusion, etc. Any triggering insult results in release of inflammatory mediators promoting neutrophil accumulation in microcirculation of the lung. Neutrophils damage vascular endothelium and alveolar epithelium leading to pulmonary edema, hyaline membrane formation, and difficult in gaseous exchange. The pathophysiological events are illustrated in **Flowchart 1**.

■ COURSE OF ACUTE RESPIRATORY DISTRESS SYNDROME

Acute respiratory distress syndrome is developed through three phases.
1. *Early phase:* This is period usually spreads across first 3 days and marked with uncontrolled inflammation by neutrophils, macrophages, platelets, and activated cytokines (cytokine storm) associated with cell injury. Damage to type 2 alveolar cells leads to acute deficiency of surfactant causing decreases compliance and increases mechanical work of lung. Alveolar edema and respiratory membrane dysfunction because of increased permeability in turn affects gas exchange causing hypoxia and/or hypercarbia.
2. *Proliferative phase:* This period may be lasting as long as 3 weeks, during which reparative work is initiated like proliferation of type 2 cells and lymphatic drainage of edema fluid.
3. *Fibrotic phase:* This is extended period, which is associated with complications of ARDS-like fibrosis of lung parenchyma causing reduced functional reserve capacity of lungs, which may cause persistent respiratory failure leading to permanent dependence on oxygen at home. Decreased forced vital capacity (FVC) and fibrosis result in increased load on right ventricle to cause right heart failure ultimately.

Flowchart 1: Pathophysiological events related with the development of ARDS.

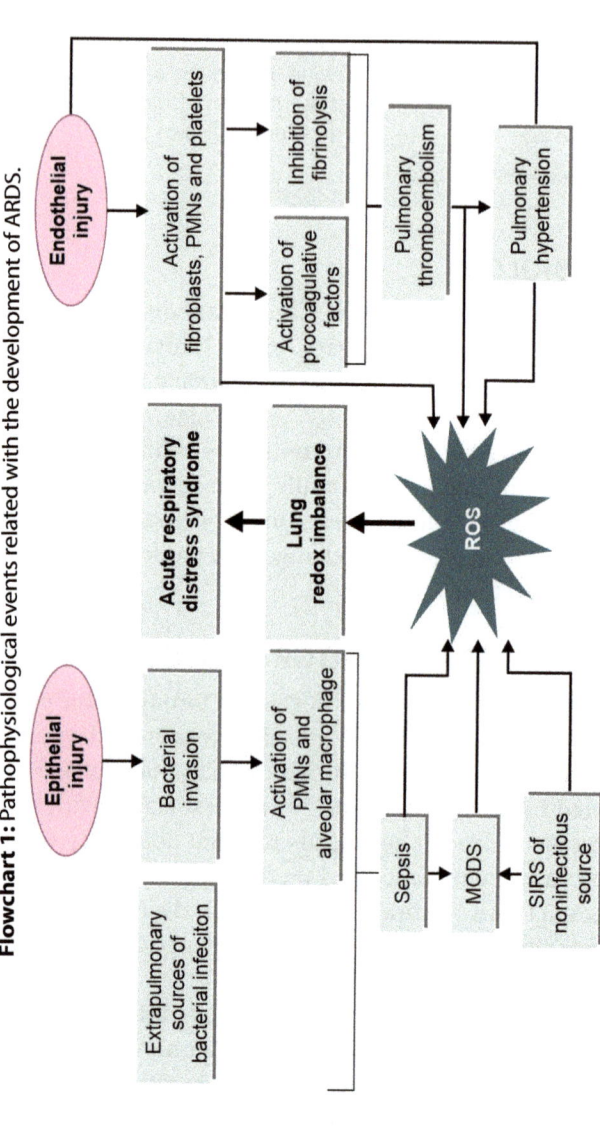

(ARDS: acute respiratory distress syndrome; MODS: multiorgan dysfunction syndrome; PMNs: polymorphonuclear neutrophils; SIRS: systemic inflammatory response syndrome; ROS: reactive oxygen species)

DIAGNOSIS

The diagnosis of ADRS is based on clinical features alone, but some of the investigations may be required to identify infective agent and precipitating factors, and to rule out alternative diagnosis. Clinical features are given in **Table 1** and standard definition of ARDS based on Berlin Criteria is given in **Box 1**. Useful investigations could be chest radiograph, computed tomography (CT) scan chest, arterial blood gas (ABG) analysis, 2D echocardiography, DLCO (diffusing capacity of the lung for carbon monoxide), culture, and sensitivity test of bronchoalveolar fluid (BAL) aspirate, etc.

MANAGEMENT OF ACUTE RESPIRATORY DISTRESS SYNDROME

Management of ARDS is based on causative agent, severity in terms of PaO_2/FiO_2 ratio, and on associated comorbidities and complications; hence, treating the underlying cause or precipitating factor is the first priority.

Initially, inspired oxygen in moderate-to-high concentrations to obtain PaO_2 >60 mm Hg or SpO_2 >90% is the one required to treat hypoxia. This may result in better oxygenation by clearing alveolar edema clearance in many but some patients may have persistent hypoxemia to put on mechanical ventilator needing different settings such as SIMV (synchronized intermittent mandatory ventilation) and IPPV (intermittent positive pressure ventilation) modes with PEEP (positive end-expiratory pressure) up to 10 cm. High PEEP and low tidal volumes are maintained to prevents ventilator-associated injury.

Though positive fluid balance is avoided, it is very important to maintain euvolemia and mean arterial pressure (MAP) above 60 mm Hg with conservative intravenous (IV) fluid management and inotropic support, not to cause internal dehydration and pulmonary ischemia. Unfortunately patients who manifest resistant respiratory failure may need lung transplantation. In the ventilator management, focus is kept on supportive and lung-protective ventilation to minimize iatrogenic lung injury. The extracorporeal membrane oxygenation (ECMO) is the only option in the patients who continues to deteriorate with adequate ventilator support.

Enteral and parenteral nutritional support should be given during ICU stay along prophylaxis to prevent deep vein thrombosis (DVT).

COMPLICATIONS OF ACUTE RESPIRATORY DISTRESS SYNDROME

There are many complications that develop due to ARDS. They are both pulmonary and extrapulmonary. Important pulmonary complications include barotraumas, pneumothorax, lung collapse, and pulmonary thromboembolism; and extrapulmonary complications include nosocomial infection including ventilator-associated pneumonia (VAP), bleeding dyscrasias, DVT, psychological depression, and neurocognitive impairment.

Specific Fevers with Acute Respiratory Distress Syndrome

Scrub Typhus

Scrub typhus is caused by the organism, *Orientia tsutsugamushi,* transmitted through chiggers (larva of Trombiculid mite). The organism infects vascular endothelium of the skin, liver, kidneys, meninges, and brain. The incubation period is 1-3 weeks. The clinical features include fever with body pains, headache, nausea and vomiting, cough and dyspnea, icterus, delirium, and loss of consciousness. Many organs are affected causing hepatitis, myocarditis, menigoencephalitis, ARDS, and disseminated intravascular coagulopathy (DIC).

Diagnosis of scrubs typhus[4] can be made with Weil–Felix test but more latest, accurate and sensitive tests now available such as ELISA (enzyme-linked immunosorbent assay), immunofluorescence assay to detect IgG and IgM.

Treatment for scrubs typhus[5] includes the first-line antibiotic, doxycycline 100 mg bid, for 7 days. A second-line antibiotic useful in scrub typhus includes azithromycin, rifampicin, chloramphenicol, etc.

Leptospirosis

Leptospirosis is caused by the organism *Leptospira interrogans.* Transmission is through direct contact of skin or mucosa with water contaminated with urine or body fluid of an infected animal.[6,7] The organism infects endothelium of microcirculation causing small-vessel vasculitis. Incubation period is usually 5–14 days.

Clinical features of leptospirosis are characterized by anicteric and icteric phases. During anicteric phase, sudden onset of fever with chills and rigors, body pains, headache, abdominal pain, and skin rash are commonly noted. During icteric phase, which is severe form of leptospirosis, also called as Weil's disease characterized by ictero-hemorrhagica, seen in about 5–15% of leptospirosis patients. The multiorgan damage is most common with hepatitis, nephritis, myocarditis, meningitis, and ARDS.

Diagnosis:[8] Though indirect evidence of abnormal liver function test (LFT), renal function tests (RFTs), and elevated creatine phosphokinase (CPK) levels, spot UACR (urine albumin-to-creatinine ratio), specific tests remains culture of leptospires from body fluids, and positive serology of IgG and IgM by ELISA.

Treatment[9] of leptospirosis includes first-line antibiotic, injection Penicillin G 1.5 MU 6 hourly for 7 days. Second-line drugs include latest-generation cephalosporins with or without oral doxycycline. Intravenous immunoglobulin (IVIG) and plasma exchange can be tried in non-responsive patients.

Malaria

Malaria is a protozoan disease caused by *Plasmodium species* (*P. falciparum, P. vivax*, and *P. malariae*) and transmitted by bite of the vector *Anopheles* mosquito. The parasite infects RBCs and two sequelae are possible: (1) hemolysis of infected RBCs to release schizonts to cause characteristic intermittent fever with chills, duration of fever depends on species, e.g., *Vivax* causing tertian fever and *Malariae* causing quartan fever. The released schizonts reinfect other RBCs and cycle goes on till effective treatment is given. (2) Infected RBCs may be sequestrated by adhering to endothelium causing both obstruction of vessel and vasculitis, which may cause multiple organ damage.

Clinical features include paroxysm of intermittent fever with rigors and chills every 48 or 72 hours. Mild-to-moderate hepatosplenomegaly may be common. Other uncommon, though not rare, features are anemia, acidosis, hypoglycemia, and shock (Algid malaria).

Severe malaria[10] occurs when parasitemia reaches >5%; it may result in cerebral malaria manifesting as seizures and coma, acute kidney injury (AKI) with or without hemoglobinuria (blackwater fever), ARDS, and DIC.

Diagnosis: Though the gold standard tests for the diagnosis of malaria include microscopy with thick and thin smears, rapid diagnostic kits[11] are available with histidine-rich protein (HRP)- and lactate dehydrogenase (LDH)-based immunochromatography with specificity >95%, which helps in rapid initiation of treatment.

Treatment[10] of malaria includes the first-line drug of choice is injection artesunate, intravenously at a dose of 2.4 mg/kg at admission, 12 and 24 hours followed by OD for 7 days with or without oral doxycycline 100 mg bd. Second line of choice is IV injection quinine at the dose of 20 mg/kg loading followed by 10 mg/kg 8th hourly with or without doxycycline.

MANAGEMENT OF UNDIAGNOSED FEVER WITH RESPIRATORY DISTRESS

Sometimes, it is very difficult to differentiate the AFI, probably because of rapidly deteriorating clinical scenario or nonavailability of specific and diagnostic methods. In this situation, it is wise to start with broad-spectrum antibiotics such as injection ceftriaxone 2 g IV twice daily along with azithromycin 500 mg once daily empirically and specific therapy is provided once diagnosis is fully established. Tablet oseltamivir 150 mg is given twice daily, if H1N1 is a possibility and injection remdesivir once daily, if COVID-19 is suspected. Antipyretics for control of fever with IV fluids to maintain adequate hydration are used. Oxygen supplementation with face mask to maintain O_2 saturation >90% by pulse oximetry while critically watching for impending respiratory failure and other organ dysfunctions linked by shock, e.g., prerenal AKI.

■ CONCLUSION

During rainy season, AFI is a very common clinical problem in tropical countries like India which may be complicated further with ARDS. Timely management is extremely important to prevent ARDS-related deaths. Although any severe infection may cause ARDS as secondary complication, any common seasonal infections cannot be ignored. Thus, there is requirement of high index of suspicion for the development of ARDS while treating infections such as malaria, influenza, leptospirosis, and scrubs typhus. Early diagnosis and early intervention for ARDS while treating common fevers could save the life from untimely deaths.

■ REFERENCES

1. Sunit Singhi, Dhruva Chaudhary, George MV, Bhalla A, Karthi N, Kalantri S, et al. Tropical fevers: management guidelines. Indian J Crit Care Med. 2014;18(2):62-8.
2. Patz JA, Graczyk TK, Geller N, Vittor AY. Effects of environmental change on emerging parasitic diseases. Int J Parasitol. 2000;30:1395-405.
3. Marco VR, Gordon DR, Taylo BT, Ferguson ND, Caldwell E, Fan E, et al. The ARDS Definition Task Force. JAMA. 2012;307(23):2526-33.
4. Koh GC, Maude RJ, Paris DH, Newton PN, Blacksell SD. Diagnosis of scrub typhus. Am J Trop Med Hyg. 2010;82:368-70.
5. Rajapakse S, Rodrigo C, Fernando SD. Drug treatment of scrub typhus. Trop Doct. 2011;41:1-4.
6. Sethi S, Sharma N, Kakkar N, Taneja J, Chatterjee SS, Banga SS, et al. Increasing trends of leptospirosis in northern India: A clinico-epidemiological study. PLoS Negl Trop Dis. 2010;4:e579.
7. Kalita JB, Rahman H. Leptospirosis among patients with pyrexia of unknown origin in a hospital in Guwahati, Assam. Indian J Public Health. 2008;52:107-9.
8. Toyokawa T, Ohnishi M, Koizumi N. Diagnosis of acute leptospirosis. Expert Rev Anti Infect Ther. 2011;9:111-21.
9. Charan J, Saxena D, Mulla S, Yadav P. Antibiotics for the treatment of leptospirosis: systematic review and meta-analysis of controlled trials. Int J Prev Med. 2013;4:501-10.
10. World Health Organization. (2010). Guidelines for the Treatment of Malaria, 2nd edition. [online] Available from:https://apps.who.int/iris/bitstream/handle/1 0665/162441/9789241549127_eng.pdf;jsessionid=134154DEB3C8A7AD8E162 D5BF932E06E?sequence=1. [Last accessed on August, 2022].
11. Maltha J, Gillet P, Jacobs J. Malaria rapid diagnostic tests in endemic settings. Clin Microbiol Infect. 2013;19:399-407.

Chapter 21

Fever with Hepatosplenomegaly/ Lymphadenopathy

Alladi Mohan, G Bindhu Madhavi

■ INTRODUCTION

Febrile patients presenting with hepatosplenomegaly/lymphadenopathy is a common clinical problem faced by physicians. Often, hepatosplenomegaly/ lymphadenopathy is evident on clinical examination; sometimes, it may become evident on imaging studies. The diagnostic approach to a patient presenting with fever and hepatosplenomegaly/lymphadenopathy is summarized in this chapter.

■ CLINICAL EXAMINATION: IMAGING CORRELATES

Fever

A temperature of >37.7°C (>99.9°F), which represents the 99th percentile for healthy individuals, defines a fever. The body temperature has a diurnal and seasonal variation, with low levels at 8 AM and during summer and higher levels at 4 PM and during winter season. Fever of >41.5°C (>106.7°F) is termed hyperpyrexia.[1]

Hepatomegaly

The liver is a wedge-shaped organ located in the right hypochondrium of the abdomen. It extends from the right fifth intercostal space to the right costal margin in the midclavicular line, is soft in consistency with a smooth contour. On abdominal ultrasonography, a normal liver span is usually <16 cm in the midclavicular line; however, this may vary with gender and body size. A nonenlarged liver may be palpable on physical examination or may be interpreted as hepatomegaly on imaging due to anatomic variations, such as Riedel's lobe (a downward, tongue-like projection of the right lobe of the liver that extends below the level of the umbilicus) and caudate lobe.

Physical examination of the liver includes abdominal palpation and percussion. While comparing liver size measured by physical examination with the liver size documented on abdominal ultrasonography, it should be remembered that these techniques use two different axes of measurement; physical examination measures liver size in the midclavicular line and abdominal ultrasonography estimates liver size in the transaxial line.

Even though it has been shown that clinical examination by percussion alone may underestimate liver size, if the distance from the upper border of the liver to the percussed liver edge is <13 cm, hepatomegaly is unlikely.[2]

Splenomegaly

The spleen lies within the peritoneal cavity in the posterior portion of the left hypochondrium below the diaphragm and adjacent to the 9th through 11th ribs. Clinically palpable splenomegaly becomes evident when the spleen is enlarged and/or when its texture changes. The spleen must be increased in size by at least 40% to be clinically palpable. While imaging methods of determining spleen size are more accurate than physical examination, especially in individuals with truncal obesity, the clinical or diagnostic significance of a spleen that is enlarged on imaging but is not palpable. Spleen is slightly larger in taller and heavier individuals and in men than women. Hence, height- and sex-corrected values are reported on imaging studies for when reporting spleen size, instead of the commonly used upper limit of normal of 12 cm.

Peripheral Lymphadenopathy

Peripheral lymph nodes are seldom palpable in normal persons. Peripheral lymphadenopathy refers to nodes that are abnormal in size, consistency, or number. Significantly enlarged lymph nodes are generally >1 cm in diameter; palpable supraclavicular, popliteal, and epitrochlear nodes >5 mm, are considered abnormal. In India, in barefoot walkers, clinical significance of inguinal lymphadenopathy should be interpreted with caution. Clinically, lymphadenopathy is classified as localized (when it involves only one region) and generalized when it involves two or more noncontiguous sites.[3]

Fever with Hepatosplenomegaly

Hepatosplenomegaly refers to enlargement of both the liver and spleen. This may be due to infections, vascular congestion, storage disorders, infiltration, autoimmune disorders, obstruction, malignancy, and other miscellaneous causes. Fever associated with hepatosplenomegaly may be seen in case of infection or malignancy arising from the bone marrow or reticuloendothelial system or an autoimmune disorder. Some of the commonly encountered causes of fever with hepatosplenomegaly are summarized in **Table 1**.[4]

Fever with Lymphadenopathy

The combination of fever and lymphadenopathy secondary to infection is more common during childhood, but can also be seen in adults. Fever and lymphadenopathy can be due to various infectious and noninfectious causes (**Table 2**).[5,6]

CHAPTER 21: Fever with Hepatosplenomegaly/Lymphadenopathy

TABLE 1: Some of the commonly seen causes of fever with hepatosplenomegaly.

Infections:	
• Protozoal	• Malaria, kala-azar, and toxoplasmosis
• Bacterial	• Typhoid, sepsis, endocarditis, brucellosis, syphilis, tuberculosis, Rocky Mountain spotted fever, and lymphogranuloma venereum
• Viruses	• Epstein–Barr virus, HIV, and cytomegalovirus
• Mycobacterial	• Disseminated tuberculosis and nontuberculous mycobacterial disease
• Fungi	• Histoplasmosis
Malignancy	Lymphomas, leukemia, and solid tumor metastasis
Autoimmune disorders	Rheumatoid arthritis, (SLE), dermatomyositis, and Sjögren syndrome

(HIV: human immunodeficiency virus; SLE: systemic lupus erythematosus)

TABLE 2: Some of the causes of fever with lymphadenopathy.

Infectious diseases:	
• Viral	• Upper respiratory tract infection, measles, varicella, rubella, hepatitis, HIV, EBV, CMV, adenovirus, hepatitis B, and hepatitis C virus
• Bacterial	• Streptococci, tuberculosis, typhoid fever, septicemia, syphilis, brucellosis, cat-scratch disease (bartonella), endocarditis, plague, and glandular tularemia
• Protozoal	• Toxoplasmosis
• Fungal	• Histoplasmosis and coccidioidomycosis
Noninfectious diseases	Sarcoidosis, SLE, and Kawasaki disease
Malignancy	Metastatic cancer and lymphoma

(CMV: cytomegalovirus; EBV: Epstein–Barr virus; HIV: human immunodeficiency virus; SLE: systemic lupus erythematosus)

EVALUATION OF A PATIENT WITH FEVER WITH HEPATOSPLENOMEGALY/LYMPHADENOPATHY

History and Physical Examination

Several infective and noninfective acute illnesses can present with fever, hepatosplenomegaly, and lymphadenopathy **(Table 1)**. For example, acute clinical presentation with fever, hepatosplenomegaly, and lymphadenopathy can be features of acute presentation of human immunodeficiency virus (HIV) infection, acquired immunodeficiency syndrome (AIDS); disseminated/military tuberculosis (TB); or noninfective conditions such as systemic lupus erythematosus (SLE) and adult-onset Still's disease. A thorough complete history is the first and the most important step in the evaluation of the patient.

History should include the age of the patient, travel, social, and sexual history; family history of malignancy; treatment history (immunosuppressive agents, phenytoin, allopurinol, and antibiotics); possible infectious or toxic exposures through occupation, recent immunizations; and any relevant past medical history of any autoimmune or infectious diseases. Along with this the pattern, character and duration of the fever, associated complaints like pruritus, night sweats, chills and rigor, weight loss, sore throat, arthralgias, and skin rash may contribute important clues to the diagnosis.

After history, a complete physical examination should be done to look at the distribution of lymphadenopathy among all lymph node groups. Lymph node qualities include warmth, overlying erythema, tenderness, mobility, consistency, and fluctuance should be assessed. While evaluating a patient with peripheral lymphadenopathy, a careful search of the draining area must be done to look for clues of origin of lymphadenopathy such as tonsillar, parotid enlargement, and evidence of infection among others. Matting is a characteristic feature of periadenitis in TB lymphadenopathy. A painless, hard, irregular mass or a firm lesion, that is immobile or fixed, may represent a malignancy. Rubbery consistency of the lymph nodes may be evident in Hodgkin's disease. No specific lymph nodal size is indicative of malignancy and the tissue diagnosis should be ascertained by cytopathological/histopathological methods.[7]

Patients presenting with pyrexia of unknown origin (PUO) often present with hepatosplenomegaly/lymphadenopathy; in addition to/in the absence of peripheral lymphadenopathy, intrathoracic, intra-abdominal lymphadenopathy may be evident.

Tender hepatomegaly may be evident in acute hepatitis; in metastatic malignancy, a hard nodular liver may be felt. Patients with pyogenic liver abscess and amoebic liver abscess may present with fever and tender hepatomegaly.

■ LABORATORY EVALUATION

Laboratory studies include routine investigations such as complete hemogram, erythrocyte sedimentation rate, peripheral smear to look for cytopenias, nucleated red cells, red cell abnormalities, abnormal lymphocytes, lymphoblasts, parasites, and Howell-Jolly bodies (seen in case of a hypofunctioning or absent spleen) and serum biochemistry including renal and liver function tests. Serum lactate dehydrogenase levels and uric acid levels are measured to rule out malignancy. Infectious causes can be diagnosed using specific testing based upon the history and physical examination.

Bone marrow aspirate cytopathology and trephine biopsy of the bone marrow with histopathological examination, immunohistochemistry, special stains, flow cytometry analysis, fluorescent *in situ* hybridization (FISH), cytogenetics, and additional molecular testing for particular mutations can be used to detect hematological malignancy.

IMAGING STUDIES

Often hepatosplenomegaly and lymphadenopathies are incidentally picked up on various imaging modalities includes ultrasonography, computed tomography (CT), and ^{18}fluorodeoxyglucose positron emission tomography-computed tomography (^{18}FDG PET-CT).[8] In case of incidentally detected organomegaly or lymphadenopathy, follow-up imaging in short intervals is done to establish a lesion to be unchanged and provide reassurance of its benign nature. Imaging studies are helpful for disease extent documentation and assessing response to treatment.

Fine-needle aspiration cytopathological examination from the most accessible peripheral lymph node is done for investigation of infectious causes. Early biopsy of palpable lymph nodes will lead to early diagnosis; excision biopsy is the gold *standard* and is preferred if malignancy is suspected.

Liver biopsy is indicated for cases of unknown etiology or rapidly progressing diseases. Splenectomy considered in case of persistent symptoms or progressive cytopenias in patients with hematological malignancy or splenic tumors.

TREATMENT

Most of the causes of fever with hepatosplenomegaly/lymphadenopathy are of infectious etiology in children and infectious and malignant etiology in case of adults. Management is based upon the etiology (e.g., short course of antibiotics or anti-TB treatment as appropriate).

> **TAKE HOME MESSAGE**
> - Fever associated with hepatosplenomegaly may be seen in case of infection or malignancy arising from the bone marrow or reticuloendothelial system or an autoimmune disorder.
> - A painless, hard, irregular node or a firm lesion, that is immobile or fixed, may represent a malignancy.
> - In case of incidentally detected organomegaly or lymphadenopathy, follow-up imaging in short intervals is done to determine its nature (benign/malignant).

REFERENCES

1. Surana NK, Dinarello CA, Porat R. Fever. In: Loscalzo J, Kasper DL, Longo DL, Fauci AS, Hauser SL, Jameson JL (Eds). Harrison's principles of internal medicine, 21st edition. New York: McGraw Hill; 2022. pp. 130-3.
2. Castell DO, O'Brien KD, Muench H, Chalmers TC. Estimation of liver size by percussion in normal individuals. Ann Intern Med. 1969;70:1183-9.

3. Ferrer R. Lymphadenopathy: differential diagnosis and evaluation. Am Fam Physician. 1998;58:1313-20.
4. Curovic Rotbain E, Lund Hansen D, Schaffalitzky de Muckadell O, Wibrand F, Meldgaard Lund A, Frederiksen H. Splenomegaly-Diagnostic validity, work-up, and underlying causes. PLoS One. 2017;12:e0186674.
5. Mohan A, Reddy MK, Phaneendra BV, Chandra A. Aetiology of peripheral lymphadenopathy in adults: analysis of 1724 cases seen at a tertiary care teaching hospital in southern India. Natl Med J India. 2007;20:78-80.
6. Gaddey HL, Riegel AM. Unexplained lymphadenopathy: evaluation and differential diagnosis. Am Fam Physician. 2016;94:896-903.
7. Habermann TM, Steensma DP. Lymphadenopathy. Mayo Clin Proc. 2000;75:723-32.
8. Solav SV. FDG PET/CT in evaluation of pyrexia of unknown origin. Clin Nucl Med.2011;36:e81-6.

Fever in Intensive Care Unit

Dhruva Chaudhry, Arpana Chatterjee, Debraj Jash

INTRODUCTION

In our day-to-day clinical practice, temperature is an essential vital sign for bedside assessment of patients in general wards and intensive care units (ICUs). Increased temperature in critical care set up may be due to the new onset of infection or simply may be due to the aggravation of the underlying disease due to any precipitating factors.

DEFINITION

In case of any patient admitted in critical care setting, fever is defined as temperature >101°F or 38.3°C on a single occasion.[1] Temperature exceeding 105.8°F (or 41°C) is known as hyperpyrexia or hyperthermia. For immunosuppressed ICU patient, temperature >101°F (38.3°C) at one episode, or rising above 100.4°F (38.0°C) temperature persisting for >1 hour in any patient with an absolute neutrophil count (ANC) <500 cells/mm.[2,3]

ETIOLOGY

Elevated body temperature enhances immune system and prevents the multiplication of bacteria and virus, which denotes that fever is actually a protective response which helps human body to defend against any infection. Many a cases, infection is present but sometimes absence of infection is not rare. Approximately 60% patients with fever in ICU are caused due to sepsis.[4]

Most important causes of fever in critical care setting are given in **Box 1** and **Table 1**.

In about 50% of the cases, infection is responsible for ICU-acquired fevers.[5,6]

BOX 1: Infectious causes of fever whilst in intensive care unit (ICU).

- Ventilator-associated pneumonia
- Catheter-related blood stream infections
- Urosepsis
- Intra-abdominal infections
- Sinus infections
- Diarrhea

TABLE 1: Noninfectious causes of fever in the intensive care unit (ICU) by organ systems.

Brain	Cerebral infarction/hemorrhage, subarachnoid hemorrhage
Heart	Acute myocardial infarction and pericarditis
Pulmonary	Aspiration, atelectasis, pulmonary embolism, and ARDS
Abdomen	Ischemic bowel gastrointestinal bleeding, pancreatitis, hepatitis, cirrhosis, and adrenal insufficiency
Vascular	Deep vein thrombosis and thrombophlebitis
Cutaneous	Decubitus ulcers
Miscellaneous	Drug fever, reaction to radiological contrast, fat embolism, neoplasms, blood transfusions, transplant rejection, and gout

(ARDS: acute respiratory distress syndrome)

■ HISTORY AND EXAMINATION

For any patient presenting with fever in ICU, detail history taking as well as thorough clinical evaluation is of utmost importance. To differentiate the cause whether infectious or noninfectious is of utmost importance.

- The vulnerable sites of infection as for example, cannulation sites should be thoroughly checked for any foci of impending infection.
- Infective endocarditis, though not so common, but a must be kept in mind etiology, for which proper auscultation of cardiac sounds often helps to detect on bedside.
- Tracheal secretion culture helps in targeting the particular antibiotic choice.
- Dermatological evaluation and soft tissue examination is an important part in any ICU patient with fever, as many a times this can give us a clue for the underlying infection. Among these, abscess.
- Possibility of drug fever should always be kept in mind, while working in ICU.
- Immunocompromised or neutropenic patients hardly present with the typical signs or symptoms. Some typical findings such as erythema multiforme and ecthyma gangrenosum might be the interesting clue to search in this group of patients specifically.

Measurement of Fever

Core body temperature carries most significant role for the measurement of fever in ICU. Pulmonary artery catheter thermistor is not used in ICU, as it is an invasive technique. As urine output is measured in critically ill patients, so bladder thermistor is very important for temperature assessment, Nasopharyngeal, esophageal, rectal, and tympanic membrane measurements are also of special significance.[7] Noninfectious cause carries a significant proportion of fever in ICU, i.e., approximately in 50% cases. The severity of fever does not correlate with the severity of infection.

DIFFERENT CONDITIONS

Systemic Inflammatory Response Syndrome Diagnostic Criteria (Box 2)

> **BOX 2:** SIRS diagnostic criteria
>
> - *Body temperature:* >38°C or <36°C
> - *Heart rate:* >90 beats per minute
> - *Tachypnea:* Manifested by a respiratory rate >20 breaths per minute or a $PaCO_2$ of <32 mm Hg
> - *White blood cell count:* >12,0007 mm^3 or <4,000/mm^3, or the presence of >10% immature neutrophils
>
> (SIRS: systemic inflammatory response syndrome)

Early Postoperative Fever

Increased temperature in postoperative period is of serious concern and common occurrence. In 15–40% of cases of major surgery, fever occurs in the first postoperative day but the actual scenario is, there is not presence of any infection at all in many cases.[8,9] After any major operation, collapse of the basal part of lungs is very common, which is specially associated with general anesthesia.[10] Fevers appearing in the first 24 hours after surgery are the result of the tissue injury sustained during the procedure.

Malignant Hyperthermia

Malignant hyperthermia is generally precipitated by some specific anesthetic drugs which may or may not have the muscle relaxing effect. The classic diagnostic triad consists of skeletal muscle rigidity, elevated body temperature (temperature >40°C or 104°F), and metabolic acidosis.

Blood Transfusions

Blood transfusion is an important cause of chills and rigor. Febrile nonhemolytic transfusion reaction (FNHTR) is the most common type of transfusion reaction occurs specifically in elderly people with more number of units and with red blood cell (RBC) and platelet containing transfusions. FNHTR presents with increased temperature and chills without hemolysis, within the 6 hours' time period since transfusion stops. When donor leukocytes react with the antileukocyte antibodies present inside recipient's body, such type of reaction takes place.

Drug Fever

Drug fever is poorly understood. The clues for drug fever is of typically early onset (7–10 days), unremitting pyrexia, multiple negative blood cultures, relative bradycardia for degree of pyrexia, disproportionately low level of C-reactive protein (CRP), remission on drug withdrawal, and inappropriately well patient. Common drugs are amphotericin, cephalosporin, penicillin, phenytoin, procainamide, and quinidine.

Acalculous Cholecystitis

Acalculous cholecystitis is an acute condition with inflammatory disorder of the gallbladder with multifactorial etiologies, which is seen in few of critically ill patients.[11] Edema of the cystic duct that blocks drainage of the gallbladder, ultimately leads to acalculous cholecystitis.

Endocrine Disorders

Among the endocrine causes, thyrotoxicosis and adrenal crisis play major role for ICU fever. Thyrotoxicosis is not likely to emerge by its own in the ICU, and adrenal crisis occurs as complication of using blood-thinners and disseminated intravascular coagulation (DIC) which lead to adrenal hemorrhage and subsequently crisis.

Iatrogenic Fever

Faulty thermal regulators in water mattresses and aerosol humidifiers can cause fever by transference.

Nosocomial Infections

Pneumonia, urinary tract infection (UTI), sepsis, and postoperative infections make up to 75% of ICU-acquired infections, and three of these infections involve indwelling plastic devices, i.e., 83% of the pneumonias occur in intubated patients, 97% of the urinary tract infections occur in catheterized patients, and 87% of bloodstream infections develop from within the intravascular catheters.

Ventilator-associated Pneumonia

Noninvasive sampling with semiquantitative cultures is the preferred methodology for the diagnosis of ventilator-associated pneumonia (VAP). For patients with suspected VAP, recommendation is using clinical criteria alone, rather than using serum procalcitonin (PCT) and clinical criteria, for making decision regarding initiation of antibiotic therapy **(Flowchart 1 and 2, Box 3).**

CHAPTER 22: Fever in Intensive Care Unit

Flowchart 1: Pathophysiology of ventilator-associated pneumonia.

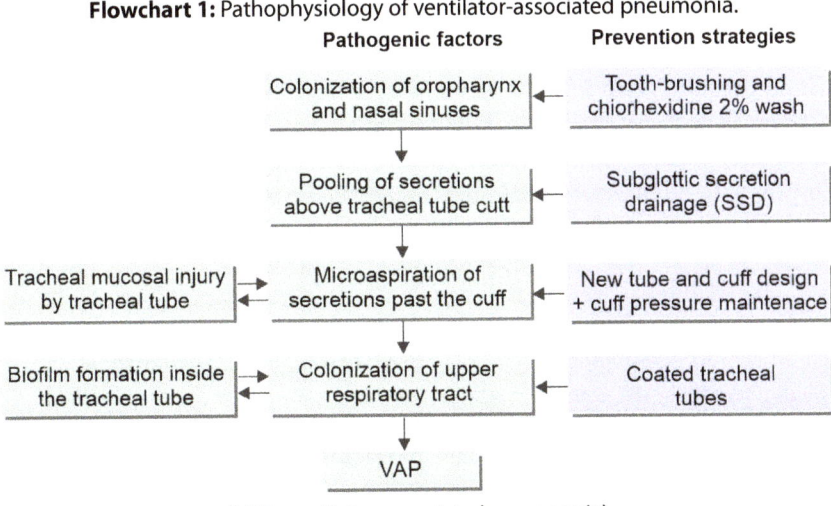

(VAP: ventilator-associated pneumonia)

Flowchart 2: American Thoracic Society (ATS) guideline for the management of hospital-acquired pneumonia (HAP) and ventilator-associated pneumonia (VAP).

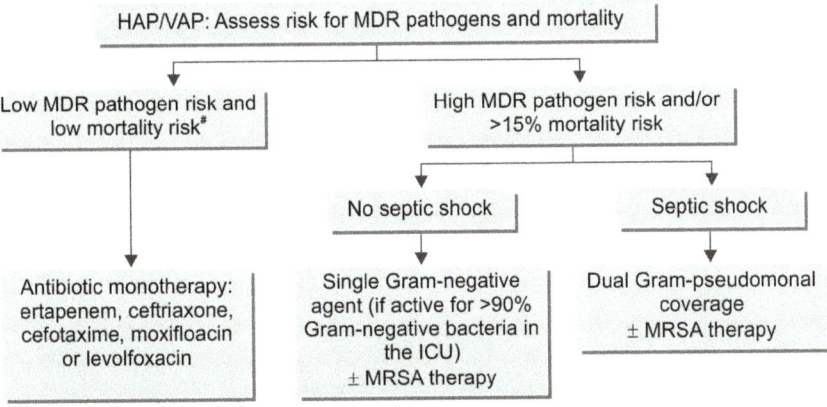

(MDR: multidrug resistant; MRSA: methicillin-resistant *Staphylococcus aureus*)

BOX 3: VAP preventive measures

- Minimize ventilator exposure
- Intensive oral care
- Aspiration of subglottic secretions
- Maintain optimal positioning and encourage mobility
- Prophylactic probiotics

(VAP: ventilator-associated pneumonia)

Clostridium Difficile Infection

Clostridium difficile enterocolitis is a very common entity in critical care, which presents with fever associated with new-onset diarrhea **(Table 2)**. Transmission from patient to patient occurs via the fecal-oral route but patient-to-patient transmission mostly occurs by the hands of hospital personnel.[8] So, proper hand care and use of gloves can reduce this infection.[9] This infection can present in various forms, like with watery diarrhea only, or with fever and

TABLE 2: Management for the *Clostridium difficile* infection according to the severity.

	Description	Primary treatment	Alternative treatment(s)
Mild-moderate disease	WBC count ≤5,000/μL, SrCr <1.5 × baseline	Metronidazole oral 500 mg three times daily for 10–14 days	Vancomycin oral 125 mg 4 times daily for 10–14 days
Severe disease	WBC count ≥15,000/μL, SrCr >1.5 × baseline, albumin <3 g/dL, and abdominal tenderness	Vancomycin oral 125 mg 4 times daily for 10–14 days	
1st recurrence	CDI within 8 weeks of initial episode	Repeat same regimen as initial episode	Consider oral vancomycin if metronidazole use for initial episode
≥2nd recurrence		Taper or pulsed-dose vancomycin oral: 125 mg four times daily for 10–14 days, then 125 mg three times daily for 7 days, then 125 mg twice daily for 7 days, then 125 mg daily for 7 days, then 125 mg every 48 hours for 7 days, then 125 mg every 72 hours for 7 days	• FMT[a] (success rate 83–100%) • Fidaxomicin oral 200 mg twice daily for 10 days • Vancomycin for 10 days, followed by rifaximin[b] or fidaxomicin "chaser"
Severe, complicated disease	Hypotension, shock, ileus, toxic megacolon, high fever, and WBC count ≥35,000/μL	Transfer to hospital for treatment	Offer comfort care for those with "do not hospitalize" goals

(CDI: *Clostridium difficile* infection; FMT: fecal microbiota transplant; SrCr: serum creatinine; WBC: white blood cell)
[a]FMT has not been studied in LTCF populations
[b]Rifaximin is not approved by the US Food and Drug Administration for this indication; it has been studied at doses of 200–400 mg, three times daily

leukocytosis, or in very severe cases, with circulatory shock and multiorgan failure. *Clostridium difficile* cytotoxins in stool by ELISA (enzyme-linked immunosorbent assay) helps in diagnosis, which carries good sensitivity and specificity of this test.[11-13]

Surgical Site Infections

Many a times 5–7 days after surgery, patients present with this scenario. This is very common with deep tissue infections. As for example, sternal infection after open heart surgery may ultimately lead to mediastinitis.[14]

Catheter-related Bloodstream Infection

In critical care units, this is one of the most common infections in daily practices, where microorganisms can make colonization in the intravascular portion of central venous catheters, and subsequent spread in the bloodstream can be grave in up to 25% of cases.[15] With the advancement of medical science, the occurrence of these infections has been lower by almost 60% over the last 10 years.[16]

After the confirmation of the diagnosis of CRBI catheters should be removed and fresh sites to be chosen.[17] Biofilm formation is the major issue which makes decontamination of catheters difficult and in most of the cases infections recur.[18] Antibiotic lock therapy is a unique concept, where mixed solution of different antibiotics are injected inside the catheter lumen for abolishing the micro-organism colonies.

Catheter-associated Urinary Tract Infection

Centers for Disease Control and Prevention (CDC) definition of CAUTI is (1) indwelling urinary catheter for >2 days on the day of the infection, (2) at least one of the following: Fever >38°C, suprapubic tenderness, urinary frequency, dysuria, tenderness or pain in costovertebral angle, and urinary urgency, (3) positive urine culture with two or fewer number microorganisms grown with at least one being bacterium with ≥10^5 CFU (colony-forming unit)/mL **(Flowchart 3 and 4)**.

■ APPROACH TO THE PATIENT

Evaluation

Lactate should be routinely measured as high lactate levels are usually seen in sepsis.

Lactate acts as a marker of decreased tissue perfusion resulting in anaerobic metabolism, as well as reduced clearance from our body due to organ dysfunction. Cut-off level for lactate in our body >2 mmol/L indicates sepsis, also septic shock includes it.[19]

Complete hemogram, urea, creatinine, and liver function tests should be thoroughly evaluated for each patient. To rule out pancreatitis, amylase and lipase level should be sought for **(Flowchart 5)**.

Flowchart 3: Diagnostic approach for the catheter-related bloodstream infection (CRBSI).

```
                            CRBSI
                              │
                              ▼
                        Unspecific
                clinical signs (i.e. isolated fever)
                      │              │
                      ▼              ▼
            Positive blood      Positive blood
            cultures only       cultures and
         (catheter left in      positive catheter tip
              patient)          (catheter removed)
              │    │                 │         │
              ▼    ▼                 ▼         ▼
        Quantitative  DTP         Semi-      Quantitative
        culture      (cultures    quantitative "sonication"-
        (CFU CVC     positive     "roll-plate" method
        blood: CFU   >2 hr        method      (≥1000 CFU)
        peripheral   earlier      (≥15 CFU)
        blood >3.1)  in the
                     catheter
                     blood)
```

(CFU: colony-forming unit; CVC: central venous catheters)

CHAPTER 22: Fever in Intensive Care Unit

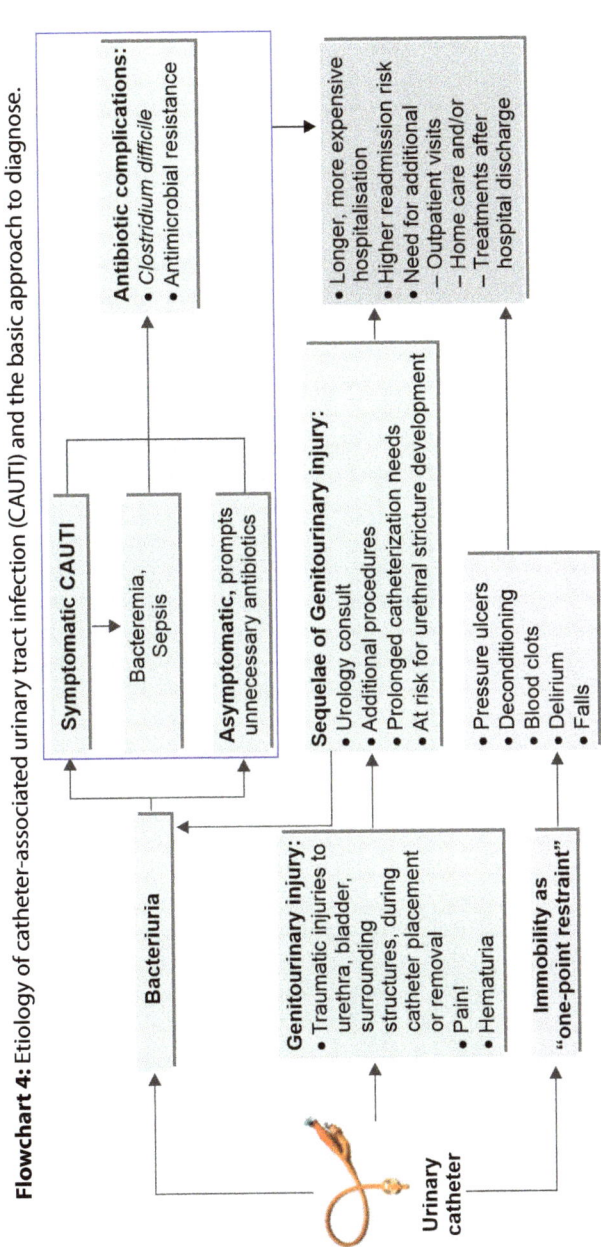

Flowchart 4: Etiology of catheter-associated urinary tract infection (CAUTI) and the basic approach to diagnose.

SECTION 3: Syndromic Approach to Fever

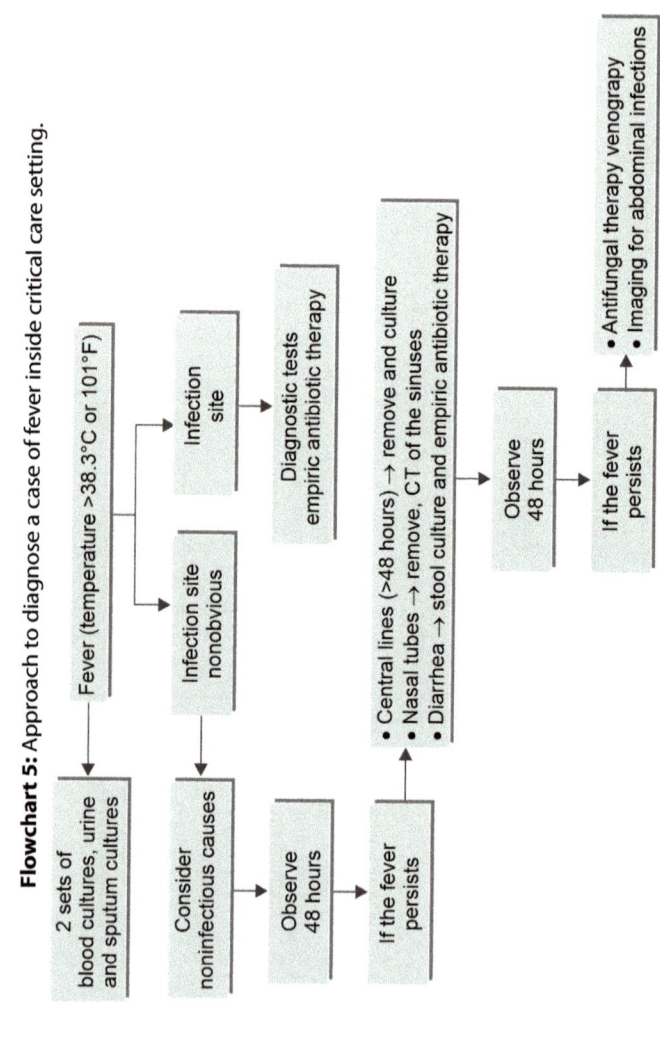

Flowchart 5: Approach to diagnose a case of fever inside critical care setting.

(CT: computed tomography)

Transfusion reactions are very important and commonly occurs. To avoid this troublesome situation, extra precautions such as routine cross matching and exclusion of serological infections should always be done.

For suspected thyroid storm, thyroid hormone levels should be checked. Adrenal insufficiency can be evaluated by free cortisol measurement or adrenocorticotropic hormone (ACTH) test.

Blood culture is gold standard investigation which helps us to proceed and select for the proper antibiotics and thereby early control of the infection, and always should be taken before starting or changing the antibiotics. Different samples are sent in case by case basis, like in ICU, endotracheal secretions, bronchoalveolar lavage are sent in case of lung involvement and suspected pneumonia cases, urine culture, and sensitivity are frequently very much helpful, as significant proportion of patients present with UTI. Raised CRP, which is an acute phase reactant, indicates inflammation, and starts rising in blood as early as 2 hours of infection, reaching in its peak in 48 hours. PCT is superior than CRP in terms of accuracy and assessment of the severity of sepsis. Serum PCT helps as a prognostic marker, helps in the de-escalation of antibiotics in ICU, and also differentiates bacterial from nonbacterial infections.[20]

> **TAKE HOME MESSAGE**
> - Increased temperature is a normal adaptive response that increases the ability for infection eradication.
> - Cooling blankets are notoriously ineffective in febrile response, as it increases cutaneous vasoconstriction and muscle activity.
> - Fever has documented benefits for patients with infection, only early period following cardiac arrest or ischemic stroke are the exception.
> - The logical approach is the ultimate goal. Ordering a barrage of laboratory tests and to culture everything available is the wrong way to proceed.
> - Exact etiology of fever should be searched to evaluate the source as of infectious and noninfectious, as there is always 50–50 chance of getting infection in ICU.
> - Gram-negative aerobic bacilli are of utmost importance, so antibiotic coverage should always be given properly in ICU.
> - Coverage for *Staphylococci* should be included in suspected vascular catheter-related septicemia.
> - An antifungal should be considered when unexplained fever persists for longer than 3 days after the start of empiric antibiotics.
> - Intensive care unit-acquired fever that is associated with new-onset diarrhea should always prompt suspicion of *C. difficile* enterocolitis.

REFERENCES

1. Chamorro C, Romera MA, Balandin B. Fever in critically ill patients. Crit Care Med. 2008;36(11):3129-30; author reply 3130.
2. Freifeld AG, Bow EJ, Sepkowitz KA, Boeckh MJ, Ito JI, Mullen CA, et al. Clinical practice guideline for the use of antimicrobial agents in neutropenic patients with cancer: 2010 Update by the Infectious Diseases Society of America. Clin Infect Dis. 2011;52(4):427-31.
3. Heinz WJ, Buchheidt D, Christopeit M, von Lilienfeld-Toal M, Cornely OA, Einsele H, et al. Diagnosis and empirical treatment of fever of unknown origin

(FUO) in adult neutropenic patients: guidelines of the Infectious Diseases Working Party (AGIHO) of the German Society of Hematology and Medical Oncology (DGHO). Ann Hematol. 2017;96(11):1775-92.
4. Sundén-Cullberg J, Rylance R, Svefors J, Norrby-Teglund A, Björk J, Inghammar M. Fever in the Emergency Department Predicts Survival of Patients With Severe Sepsis and Septic Shock Admitted to the ICU. Crit Care Med. 2017;45(4):591-9.
5. Commichau C, Scarmeas N, Mayer SA. Risk factors for fever in the intensive care unit. Neurology. 2003;60:837-41.
6. Peres Bota D, Lopes Ferriera F, Melot C, Vincent JL. Body temperature alterations in the critically ill. Intensive Care Med. 2004;30(5):811-6.
7. O'Grady NP, Barie PS, Bartlett JG, Bleck T, Carroll K, Kalil AC, et al. Infectious Diseases Society of America. Guidelines for evaluation of new fever in critically ill adult patients: 2008 update from the American College of Critical Care Medicine and the Infectious Diseases Society of America. Crit Care Med. 2008;36(4):1330-49.
8. Samore MH, Venkataraman L, DeGirolami, et al. Clinical and molecular epidemiology of sporadic and clustered cases of nosocomial Clostridium difficile diarrhea. Am J Med 1996; 100:32–40.
9. Johnson S, Gerding DN, Olson MM, Weiler MD, Hughes RA, Clabots CR, et al. Prospective, controlled study of vinyl glove use to interrupt Clostridium difficile nosocomial transmission. Am J Med. 1990;88(2):137-40.
10. Warlitier DC. Pulmonary atelectasis. Anesthesiology. 2005;102:838-54.
11. Mylonakis E, Ryan ET, Calderwood SB. Clostridium difficile associated diarrhea. Arch Intern Med. 2001;161:525-33.
12. Bartlett JG. Antibiotic-associated diarrhea. N Engl J Med. 2002;346:334-39.
13. Yassin SF, Young-Fadok TM, Zein NN, Pardi DS. Clostridium difficile- associated diarrhea and colitis. Mayo Clin Proc. 2001;76:725-30.
14. Loopp FD, Lytle BW, Cosgrove DM, Stewart RW, Golding LAR, Taylor PC, et al. Sternal wound complications after isolated coronary artery bypass grafting: early and late mortality, morbidity, and cost of care. Ann Thorac Surg. 1990;49(2):179-87.
15. Centers for Disease Control and Prevention. Guidelines for the prevention of intravascular catheter-related infections. MMWR. 2002;51:No. RR-10.
16. Centers for Disease Control and Prevention. Vital signs: central line-associated bloodstream infections—United States, 2001, 2008, and 2009. MMWR Morb Mortal Wkly Rep. 2011;60(8):243-8.
17. Mermel LA, Allon M, Bouza E, Craven DE, Flynn P, O'Grady NP, et al. Clinical practice guidelines for the diagnosis and management of intravascular catheter-related infection: 2009 update by the Infectious Diseases Society of America. Clin Infect Dis. 2009;49(1):1-45.
18. Raad I, Davis S, Khan A, Tarrand J, Elting L, Bodey GP. Impact of central venous catheter removal on the recurrence of catheter-related coagulase-negative staphylococcal bacteremia. Infect Control Hosp Epidemiol. 1992;154:808-16.
19. Singer M, Deutschman CS, Seymour CW, Shankar-Hari M, Annane D, Bauer M, et al. The Third International Consensus Definitions for Sepsis and Septic Shock (Sepsis-3). JAMA. 2016;315(8):801-10.
20. Bouadma L, Luyt CE, Tubach F, Cracco C, Alvarez A, Schwebel C, et al. Use of procalcitonin to reduce patients' exposure to antibiotics in intensive care units (PRORATA trial): a multicentre randomised controlled trial. Lancet. 2010;375(9713):463-74.

Approach to an Adult with Pyrexia of Unknown Origin

Chapter 23

Sudhir Mehta, Shaurya Mehta

■ DEFINITION

Clinicians commonly refer to a febrile episode without an initially obvious etiology or without localizing signs as pyrexia of unknown origin (PUO). This usage is not appropriate. PUO refers to a prolonged febrile illness without an established etiology in spite of intensive diagnostic testing as enumerated in the following text.

The definition of PUO defined by Petersdorf and Beeson (1961)[1] has long been the clinical standard, characterized by:
- Fever >38.3°C on several occasions
- Duration of fever for at least 3 weeks
- Uncertain diagnosis after 1 week of evaluation in the hospital.

Nowadays, in-hospital evaluation criterion has been abandoned. The degree and duration of fever are not the only criteria for defining PUO. Prior to concluding that a patient has PUO, the following evaluation should be performed, though not revealing the diagnosis:
- Meticulous history
- Thorough physical examination
- Complete blood count and peripheral smear examination
- Blood cultures
- Routine blood chemistries including liver function tests (LFTs)
- If liver tests are abnormal, hepatitis viral serology
- Urine microscopic examination and culture
- Chest X-ray.

If any signs or symptoms point to a particular organ system, further testing, imaging, and/or biopsy should be performed to pinpoint the diagnosis.

■ CAUSES

Three general categories of illness account for the majority of "classic" PUO cases:
1. Infections
2. Malignancies
3. Systemic rheumatic diseases (e.g., vasculitis and rheumatoid arthritis).

Among infections, tuberculosis and abscesses are the most common etiologies presenting as PUO. Systemic juvenile idiopathic arthritis (formerly called Still's disease) in younger patients and giant cell arteritis in older individuals are the most common rheumatologic disorders presenting as PUO. The most common malignancies to present with PUO are lymphoma, especially non-Hodgkin's, leukemia, renal cell carcinoma, and hepatocellular carcinoma or other tumors metastatic to the liver. Drug fever due to a variety of drugs is also a common cause of PUO.

There are many factors which alter the pattern of PUO. For example, frequent use of empiric antimicrobials can delay the diagnosis of some occult abscesses and infections. Aggressive immunosuppressive regimens, lengthy intensive care unit admissions, and the increase in multiresistant organisms as resident hospital flora have all altered the types of PUOs encountered.

■ EPIDEMIOLOGY

True PUOs are uncommon in western countries. This was illustrated in a report from the Netherlands in which only 73 patients were identified between December 2003 and July 2005 at a 950-bed academic referral hospital and five community hospitals comprising 2,800 hospital beds.[2] However, in healthcare resource-constrained countries, PUO is still a challenging problem for clinicians. Infectious causes of prolonged fever in resource-limited countries include tuberculosis, typhoid, amebic liver abscesses, and acquired immunodeficiency syndrome (AIDS).

■ CLINICAL APPROACH

Assessment of a patient with PUO requires detailed history and meticulous physical examination, which may be repeated at regular intervals, to detect any new sign that may appear later in the course of the disease. It is important to look for uncommon presentations of common diseases rather than looking for rare diseases.

The history and physical examination, such as laboratory tests, have the potential to generate valuable diagnostic clues in patients with PUO. A thorough history should not miss the following information:
- Travel history
- Animal exposure (e.g., pets, occupational, living on a farm)
- Type of immunosuppression
- Drug and toxin history, including antimicrobials
- Localizing symptoms.

Subtle findings, many times, can be uncovered through a careful history-taking. Revisiting the history several times may provide new clues in difficult to diagnose cases. In other words, serial/repeated history-taking and physical examination are important techniques to establish diagnosis of PUO.

The degree and pattern of fever and response to antipyretics have not been found to provide enough specificity to guide the diagnosis of PUO.[3] Fever may be attenuated in older patients and moderated by use of steroids and nonsteroidal anti-inflammatory drugs. However, the fever record may be helpful in determining whether the disease is escalating or not.

INVESTIGATIONS

The list of tests for evaluation of PUO is quite exhaustive, and the extent to which a patient is investigated depends at what point the diagnosis is clinched. A battery of following tests is pursued as part of investigative protocol, in addition to those listed above:
- Erythrocyte sedimentation rate (ESR) or C-reactive protein (CRP)
- Serum lactate dehydrogenase
- HIV immunoassay and HIV viral load for patients at high risk
- Three routine blood cultures drawn from different sites over a period of at least several hours without administering antibiotics
- Immuno-17 profile
- Creatine phosphokinase
- Serum protein electrophoresis
- Computed tomography (CT) scan of abdomen
- High-resolution computed tomography (HRCT) scan of chest
- Markers of malignancies.

Acute Phase Reactants

Almost all clinicians favor obtaining an ESR or CRP, despite their lack of specificity. One study[4] reviewed ESR elevations above 100 mm/h among 263 patients with PUO: 58% had malignancy, most commonly lymphoma, myeloma, or metastatic colon or breast cancer, and 25% had infections such as endocarditis or systemic rheumatic diseases such as rheumatoid arthritis or giant cell arteritis.

In a hospital-based observational cross-sectional study (unpublished data; personal communication), conducted in adults aged 18 years and above, out of 178 patients with extremely elevated ESR (>100 mm/h), infection was the most common cause which included bacterial pneumonia (12.9%), sepsis (11.9%), pulmonary tuberculosis (7.2%), bacterial abscess (4.9%), coronavirus disease 2019 (COVID-19) (4.9%), scrub typhus (2.7%), and HIV (2.2%). Renal insufficiency which included acute kidney injury (10.1%) and chronic kidney disease (3.9%), malignancy (7.8%) and chronic inflammatory conditions such as hypertension (HTN), diabetes mellitus (DM), chronic obstructive pulmonary disease (COPD), and cerebrovascular accident (CVA) were other causes. Extremely elevated ESR was not found in chronic liver disease and malaria.

Drug hypersensitivity reactions, thrombophlebitis, and renal disease may be accompanied by a very high ESR in the absence of infection or malignancy.

A normal ESR or CRP also suggests that a significant inflammatory process is unlikely. However, there are exceptions, e.g., some patients with giant cell arteritis can have a normal ESR.

Procalcitonin, a serum biomarker that is elevated with certain bacterial infections, has no clear role as part of the PUO evaluation; however, it is often used by clinicians to detect occult bacterial infection.

Computed Tomography Scan

Computed tomography scanning of the abdomen is useful in the search for occult abscesses in patients with PUO. The finding of abdominal lymphadenopathy can be a clue to lymphoma or a granulomatous process. The usefulness of CT has resulted in this examination being used in nearly all patients with PUO. While magnetic resonance imaging (MRI) scan can be more sensitive in certain settings (e.g., the diagnosis of spinal epidural abscess), it is rarely required in the initial evaluation of PUO.

For similar reasons, CT scanning of the chest is invaluable in the identification of small nodules (indicative of fungal, mycobacterial, or nocardial infection or malignancy). The identification of hilar or mediastinal adenopathy may prompt biopsy by mediastinoscopy, providing a diagnosis of lymphoma, histoplasmosis, or sarcoidosis.

Nuclear Medicine Testing

Nuclear medicine testing is a more controversial area in the diagnosis of PUO. It is usually ordered when the initial evaluation (including abdominal and chest CT) remains negative and a screening look at the entire body is desired.

Both gallium-67- and indium-111-labeled leukocyte scanning are highly sensitive by virtue of including the whole body. Neither study, however, can pinpoint a diagnosis; they are nonspecific tests to localize a site for more specific evaluation such as with CT. When studied, the overall yield of gallium-67- or indium-111-labeled leukocyte scanning may be higher than with CT or ultrasound.

F-fluorodeoxyglucose positron emission tomography (FDG-PET) appears to be very sensitive in identifying anatomic sites of inflammation and malignancy. This modality may find a valuable place in the evaluation of PUO,[5] but additional data are needed to determine its added value beyond repeated clinical evaluation over time and routine CT.

Specific Tests

When the history, examination, or imaging suggests a possible source, specific testing should be performed. Examples include:
- Subtle central nervous system symptoms or signs should prompt a lumbar puncture and imaging of the head and/or spine.
- A history of trauma, adjacent infection, or intravenous drug use may suggest thrombophlebitis of the legs, arms, or pelvic vessels. Venous duplex imaging can be diagnostic. Fever usually responds to anticoagulation within several days.

Biopsy

Biopsy is a critical modality in the diagnosis of PUO. Examples include:
- Liver biopsy for possible miliary tuberculosis, granulomatous hepatitis, or other granulomatous diseases such as sarcoidosis
- Lymph node biopsy for possible malignancy, especially lymphoma, tuberculosis
- Biopsy of an affected tissue to diagnose a vasculitic process such as polyarteritis nodosa
- Pleural or pericardial biopsy in the evaluation of extrapulmonary tuberculosis
- Bone marrow biopsy is useful in diagnosis of hematological malignancy, disseminated tuberculosis, fungal infections, kala-azar, etc.

Two retrospective reviews of bone marrow biopsies evaluating PUO demonstrated high diagnostic yields and high prevalence of hematologic malignancies.[6,7] Lymphomas constituted >40% of diagnoses, whereas infections were detected in <15% of patients. Other causes of PUO included acute myeloid leukemia, myelodysplastic syndromes, sarcoidosis, systemic mastocytosis, and disseminated granulomatosis. In both studies, hematologic malignancies were strongly predicted by the presence of leukoerythroblastic changes in peripheral blood and a greatly elevated ferritin level (>1,000 ng/mL). The hematologic malignancies were also predicted by the presence of splenomegaly.

CONCEPT OF "THERAPEUTIC TRIAL" IN PYREXIA OF UNKNOWN ORIGIN

Therapeutic trials of antibiotics or steroids, in an attempt to "do something", rarely help in making a diagnosis. In addition, the diagnostic yield of blood cultures and cultures of biopsy material will be affected following empirical antibiotics.

Antibiotics can have effects on other infections than the ones to which therapy is directed. Rifampin, e.g., used in a therapeutic trial for tuberculosis may suppress staphylococcal osteomyelitis or diminish the ability to detect difficult-to-isolate organisms causing endocarditis.

The appropriate duration of a therapeutic trial is also unclear since infections such as endocarditis or pelvic inflammatory disease, may take weeks to normalize fever, even with appropriate therapy. Empiric antibiotics should never be started solely to treat fever; it is irrational and unjustified. Nevertheless, in India, therapeutic trial of antitubercular drugs is often offered to patients in absence of definite diagnosis of PUO.

A therapeutic trial of steroids for an inflammatory disease should not replace relevant biopsies for steroid-responsive diseases such as sarcoidosis, other granulomatous diseases, or vasculitis. A careful evaluation for infection should precede such a trial.

■ OUTCOME OF PYREXIA OF UNKNOWN ORIGIN

The outcome of patients with PUO depends upon the underlying etiology and associated comorbid diseases. Most adults who remain undiagnosed after an extensive evaluation also have a good prognosis. This was illustrated in a study of 199 patients with PUO, 61 of whom (30%) were discharged from the hospital without a diagnosis.[8]

Similar findings were noted in the Netherlands series of 73 patients cited above. Among the 37 patients with no diagnosis who were followed for at least 6 months, 16 spontaneously recovered, 5 recovered with nonsteroidal anti-inflammatory drugs or glucocorticoids, 15 had persistent fever, and 1 died.

TAKE HOME MESSAGE

- Fever of unknown origin (PUO) is defined as fever higher than 38.3°C on several occasions lasting for at least 3 (some use 2) weeks without an established etiology despite intensive evaluation and diagnostic testing.
- Three general categories of illness account for the majority of "classic" PUO cases and have been consistent through the decades. These categories are infections, malignancies, and systemic rheumatic diseases.
- The most important aspects of the evaluation of a patient with PUO are to take a meticulous history, perform a detailed physical examination, and to reassess the patient frequently.
- The diagnostic evaluation may fail to identify an etiology in as many as 30–50% of patients. Most adults who remain undiagnosed have a good prognosis.

■ REFERENCES

1. Petersdorf RG, Beeson PB. Fever of unexplained origin: report on 100 cases. Medicine (Baltimore). 1961;40:1.
2. Bleeker-Rovers CP, Vos FJ, de Kleijn EM, Mudde AH, Dofferhoff TS, Richter C, et al. A prospective multicenter study on fever of unknown origin: the yield of a structured diagnostic protocol. Medicine (Baltimore). 2007;86(1):26.

3. Hirschmann JV. Fever of unknown origin in adults. Clin Infect Dis. 1997;24(3): 291.
4. Zacharski LR, Kyle RA. Significance of extreme elevation of erythrocyte sedimentation rate. JAMA. 1967;202(4):264.
5. Gafter-Gvili A, Raibman S, Grossman A, Avni T, Paul M, Leibovici L, et al. FDG-PET/CT for the diagnosis of patients with fever of unknown origin. QJM. 2015;108(4):289-98.
6. Hot A, Jaisson I, Girard C, French M, Durand DV, Rousset H, et al. Yield of bone marrow examination in diagnosing the source of fever of unknown origin. Arch Intern Med. 2009;169(21):2018.
7. Wang HY, Yang CF, Chiou TJ, Yang SH, Gau JP, Yu YB, et al. A "bone marrow score" for predicting hematological disease in immunocompetent patients with fevers of unknown origin. Medicine (Baltimore). 2014;93(27):e243.
8. Knockaert DC, Dujardin KS, Bobbaers HJ. Long-term follow-up of patients with undiagnosed fever of unknown origin. Arch Intern Med. 1996;156(6):618.

Chapter 24
Emerging Tropical Infections in India

Anupam Prakash

◼ INTRODUCTION

Infectious diseases are a major contributor to morbidity and mortality across the world, especially in the tropical countries. The recent COVID-19 has shown that the world is a global village and infections capable of high transmissibility can spread across several countries with the wink of an eye, and may be unstoppable. Apart from the vulnerability of the world exposed by COVID-19, several diseases already threaten the world, such as yellow fever, poliomyelitis, tuberculosis, for which active surveillance continues round the year in different countries. COVID-19 pandemic exposed our vulnerability and poor preparedness to face the challenges posed by emerging infectious diseases. Apart from COVID-19, several others such as Crimean Congo hemorrhagic fever, Zika virus, and Nipah virus threats are continuously knocking at our doors, and threatening mankind. It is imperative to take cognizance of the emerging infectious diseases and be in a state of preparedness to tackle the threats posed by these diseases.

◼ DEFINITION

Emerging infectious diseases in the simplistic meaning of the term indicate infectious diseases which are newly recognized in a population or in a geographic region. Infectious diseases which are already known but now show a rapid rise in incidence can also be qualified as emerging infectious diseases.[1]

On the contrary, there are diseases which had been controlled or whose incidence was curtailed, but now there is a resurgence in their numbers, such infectious diseases are classified as "Reemerging infectious diseases".

The John Hopkins website indicates that the definition of emerging infectious disease encompasses (1) outbreaks of previously unknown diseases; (2) known diseases which are rapidly increasing in incidence or geographic range in the last two decades; and (3) persistence of infectious diseases that cannot be controlled; as defined by the National Institute of Allergy and Infectious Diseases.[2]

ABOUT EMERGING INFECTIOUS DISEASES

Most of the emerging infectious diseases are zoonotic diseases resulting because of greater human–animal conflicts or interactions, because of reduced forest cover consequent to rapid urbanization and growing human needs. Interestingly, in the last three decades, over 30 new infectious agents have been reported worldwide, most of which are zoonotic diseases and originated in the wildlife. Human immunodeficiency virus (HIV) infections, severe acute respiratory syndrome (SARS), Lyme disease, Hantavirus infection, dengue fever, West Nile virus, and Zika virus are some of the emerging infectious diseases in the USA. India also is a vast country, with so many differing geographic terrains and rich biodiversity. Moreover, the pressure of development, population burden, reducing forest cover, effects of climate change and global warming, the world becoming a global village, and India being a preferred medical tourism destination, are all factors contributing to the changing spectrum of existing diseases, resurgence of diseases and emergence of new diseases. The emerging viral infections in India which pose a threat can be classified into respiratory viral infections, arboviral infections, and bat-borne viral infections.[3,4] The world and India have witnessed the COVID-19 pandemic, and several influenza variants consistently pose a threat, viz. pandemic influenza H1N1pdm09, avian influenza H5N1, and the Middle-east respiratory syndrome (MERS-CoV). Apart from these, Crimean-Congo hemorrhagic fever, dengue fever, chikungunya, Japanese encephalitis, and Kyasanur forest disease (KFD) are arboviral diseases which belong to the category of emerging and re-emerging infectious diseases. Several bat-borne viral diseases also keep threatening, viz. Nipah virus disease outbreaks have been witnessed in Kerala, while Ebola virus disease, Zika virus disease, and severe fever with thrombocytopenia virus also come under the gamut of emerging infectious diseases.

Some of the well-known emerging infectious diseases which have been witnessed in India in the 21st century are shown in **Box 1**. Scrub typhus is another re-emerging infectious disease, which is increasingly being

BOX 1: Emerging infectious diseases seen in India in the 21st century.
- 2001—Nipah virus (Bangladesh and Siliguri, India)
- 2002–2003—SARS coronavirus
- 2003–2004—Avian influenza (H5N1), Thailand
- 2006—Influenza H5N1 (Egypt, Iraq)
- 2007—Nipah virus (Bangladesh and West Bengal, India)
- 2009—Swine flu-influenza H1N1 (Hyderabad, India)
- 2011—Crimean Congo hemorrhagic fever (Rajasthan, India)
- 2018—Nipah virus (Kerala, India)
- 2019–2022—COVID-19 pandemic (SARS-nCoV-2-2019)

> **BOX 2:** Emerging infectious diseases in present day scenario of India.
> - Crimean Congo hemorrhagic fever
> - Ebola and Marburg virus disease
> - Lassa fever
> - MERS and SARS coronavirus fevers
> - Nipah fever
> - Rift valley fever/scrub typhus
> - Chikungunya
> - Severe fever with thrombocytopenia syndrome
> - Zika virus disease
> - Tuberculosis/multidrug-resistant tuberculosis
> - Malaria-ACT resistant
> - Influenza
> - Dengue
> - HIV/AIDS
> - COVID-19
> - Melioidosis
> - Leptospirosis
>
> (ACT: Artemisinin-based combination therapy; AIDS: acquired immunodeficiency syndrome; HIV: human immunodeficiency virus; MERS: Middle East respiratory syndrome; SARS: severe acute respiratory syndrome)

witnessed in the sub-Himalayan areas and the northeastern parts of India.[5,6] Japanese encephalitis is also endemic in Bihar, likewise the acute encephalitis syndrome is also the presentation of Nipah virus outbreaks in Kerala. Further, dengue, chikungunya, malaria, and multidrug-resistant tuberculosis are other emerging infectious diseases which need to be taken care of. Diseases such as leptospirosis and melioidosis are also on the rise. **Box 2** enlists the emerging infectious diseases in the present day's scenario in India.

■ PREVENTION

Early recognition of the disease is important. It is important to be well-versed with the signs and symptoms of these infections. Unusual clinical features, different from the usual clinical features seen with common seasonal diseases, with history of international travel or travel to endemic areas is important for early recognition of the disease. Moreover, employing quarantine and isolation protocols in suspected and confirmed cases respectively is an important step. Adoption of infection prevention and control (IPC) measures are also of utmost importance for the containment of these infectious diseases. Laboratory diagnosis using rapid diagnostic kits and point-of-care tools can be very helpful in having a diagnosis and also help in adoption of containment measures.[7] The discussion of clinical features of each of the emerging infectious diseases is outside the scope of this text.

CHAPTER 24: Emerging Tropical Infections in India

TAKE HOME MESSAGE

- Emerging infectious diseases pose a serious threat to the existence of mankind.
- Most of these diseases are viral infections and zoonotic diseases, arising from the wild.
- Emerging infectious diseases of concern in India can be classified into respiratory viral infections, arboviral infections, and bat-borne viral infections.
- Influenza viruses, corona viruses, Crimean Congo hemorrhagic fever, Japanese encephalitis virus, Nipah virus, and Kyasanur forest disease are the emerging infections of concern in India.
- Dengue, chikungunya, malaria, multidrug-resistant tuberculosis, scrub typhus, leptospirosis, and melioidosis also pose unique challenges to the Indian subcontinent.

REFERENCES

1. McArthur DB. Emerging Infectious Diseases. Nurs Clin North Am. 2019;54: 297-311.
2. John Hopkins Medicine. Emerging Infectious Diseases. [online] Available from www.hopkinsmedicine.org/health/conditions-and-diseases/emerging-infectious-diseases#:~:text=According%20to%20the%20National%20Institute,in%20the%20last%202%20decades. [Last accessed on June, 2022].
3. Mourya DT, Yadav PD, Ullas PT, Bhardwaj SD, Sahay RR, Chadha MS, et al. Indian J Med Res. 2019;149:447-67.
4. Kashyap B, Prakash A. Emerging and re-emerging infectious diseases: a perpetual threat. Indian J Med Spec. 2015;6:79-81.
5. Prakash A. Acharya AS, Jain N, Bhattacharya D, Chhabra M. Scrub typhus- an emerging public health problem in Delhi. Indian J Med Spec. 2014;5:68-72.
6. Prakash A. Emerging and re-emerging infectious diseases: an overview. In: Prakash A (Ed). Emerging Infectious Diseases. Mumbai: Indian College of Physicians; 2019. pp. 1-5.
7. Kashyap B. Laboratory diagnosis of emerging and re-emerging infectious diseases. In: Prakash A (Ed). Emerging Infectious Diseases. Mumbai: Indian College of Physicians; 2019. pp. 6-14.

Neglected Tropical Diseases

Chapter 25

Aritra Kumar Ray

■ INTRODUCTION

Neglected tropical diseases (NTDs) are a varied group of tropical infections which are commonly found in the developing regions of Asia, Africa, and Americas.[1] They are caused by different pathogens, namely bacteria, viruses, parasitic worms, and protozoa and are usually found among the population belonging to the lower socioeconomic conditions.

Reasons for Neglect

- Many of the tropical diseases are asymptomatic.
- Long incubation period.
- Lack of realization of the relation between mortality and NTDs.
- Often high endemicity is found in geographically difficult and isolated regions making prevention and treatment difficult.
- More resources are diverted to the diseases [such as tuberculosis, malaria, human immunodeficiency virus (HIV)/acquired immunodeficiency syndrome (AIDS), etc.] which cause higher morbidity and mortality.
- NTDs are frequently associated with social stigma which leads to decrease in help seeking and treatment adherence.
- Noncommercial and therefore profit has no role in encouraging further research, development, and innovation.
- Lack of effective policy due to lack of awareness.

■ LIST OF DISEASES

According to the World Health Center (WHO) there are some neglected tropical diseases that are enlisted in **Box 1**.

Chagas Disease

Chagas disease, also known as American trypanosomiasis, is caused by *Trypanosoma cruzi* and gets transmitted to people and animals by insect vectors. Infection can also occur through congenital transmission, blood transfusion, organ transplantation, consumption of uncooked food, and

> **BOX 1:** The World Health Organization (WHO) enlisted the following 20 diseases as neglected tropical diseases.
>
> 1. Chagas disease
> 2. Buruli ulcer
> 3. Chikungunya and dengue
> 4. Snakebite envenomation
> 5. Dracunculiasis
> 6. Yaws
> 7. African trypanosomiasis
> 8. Fascioliasis
> 9. Leprosy
> 10. Leishmaniasis
> 11. Onchocerciasis
> 12. Lymphatic filariasis
> 13. Schistosomiasis
> 14. Rabies
> 15. Cysticercosis
> 16. Echinococcosis
> 17. Soil-transmitted helminthiasis
> 18. Trachoma
> 19. Scabies and other ectoparasites
> 20. Mycetoma and deep mycoses

accidental laboratory exposure. Chagas disease is predominantly seen in the rural areas of South America, Central America, and Mexico.

Buruli Ulcer

Buruli ulcer is caused by a bacterium named *Mycobacterium ulcerans* and is predominantly seen in Asia, Africa, and Latin America. Toxin named mycolactone gets produced which leads to destruction of tissues.[2] Mortality associated with Buruli ulcer is usually low but secondary infection, if occurs may lead to dreaded outcomes. Buruli ulcer may lead to disability, deformity, and skin lesions and early interventions with antibiotics and surgery may prevent complications.

Chikungunya and Dengue

Chikungunya is an arboviral infection which gets transmitted by *Aedes aegypti* and *Aedes albopictus*. Chikungunya belongs to the family *Togaviridae* and genus *Alphavirus* and is seen predominantly in Asia and Africa. Symptoms include fever, severe disabling joint pain, headache, joint swelling, muscle pain, or rash. Adequate rest, maintenance of hydration and antipyretics forms the mainstay of treatment.

Dengue fever is caused by *Flavivirus* and gets transmitted through the bite of *A. aegypti* mosquito. Symptoms include fever, rash, nausea, vomiting, retro-orbital pain, joint, and muscle pain. Rest, antipyretics, and maintenance of adequate hydration form the cornerstone of treatment.

Snakebite Envenomation

Snakebite envenomation is caused by the bite of venomous snake and is often seen in Asia, Africa, and Latin America. Elapids (namely cobras, kraits, and mambas), sea snakes, and vipers are mostly responsible for envenomations. Two-puncture wound marks from the animal's fangs is a common sign of a venomous snake bite. Local symptoms include swelling, redness, and severe pain. Sweating, vomiting, bleeding, renal failure, tingling of limbs, and blurred vision may occur. Initial management includes immobilization of the affected limb and cleaning the bite site with soap and water. Antivenom is often very effective in preventing death from snake bites.

Dracunculiasis

Dracunculiasis is caused due to drinking of water contaminated with guinea worm larvae.[3] Symptoms include formation of painful blisters usually on the lower parts of the body. The blisters gradually get bigger and eventually rupture. The worms on getting exposed release thousands of larvae on coming in contact with water. Other symptoms include mild fever, itchy rash, vomiting, nausea, diarrhea, and dizziness. Complications may include abscesses, cellulitis, sepsis, and septic arthritis.

Yaws

Yaws is a chronic debilitating and disfiguring infectious disease which is caused by *Treponema pallidum pertenue*. The disease is predominantly seen among poor communities living in the warm and humid areas of Africa, Asia, Pacific, and Latin America. Yaws mainly affects bone, cartilage, and skin (in the form of ulcers and papilloma). Benzathine penicillin or azithromycin can be used in the treatment of yaws.

African Trypanosomiasis

African trypanosomiasis, also known as African sleeping sickness, is a rare vector-borne protozoal disease which gets transmitted by the bite of tsetse fly.[4] Common symptoms include headache, fever, lymphadenopathy, personality changes, cognitive decline, nocturnal sleeping pattern, and coma. Diagnosis requires demonstration of parasite in any of the body fluids. Pentamidine is the drug of choice for the treatment of early stage of *Trypanosoma brucei gambiense* infection.

Fascioliasis

Fascioliasis is a parasitic infection which is caused by *Fasciola hepatica* (also known as "the sheep liver fluke" or "the common liver fluke"). Infection occurs by eating of raw watercress or other aquatic plants infected with parasite larvae. It primarily affects the liver and the bile ducts though it can affect other body parts as well. In the acute phase, symptoms include gastrointestinal problems in the form of abdominal pain/tenderness, nausea, and vomiting. Fever with rash and respiratory distress may also occur. Diagnosis is done by demonstrating *Fasciola* eggs in fecal specimen under microscopic examination. The first line of treatment is triclabendazole.

Leprosy

Leprosy is an infection caused by *Mycobacterium leprae* and is most prevalent in India, Indonesia, Brazil, Congo, Nigeria, East Africa, and Madagascar. Transmission occurs through droplets from the nose and the mouth of infected individuals.[5] Leprosy mainly affects skin, eyes, nerves, and limbs and it may lead to physical disabilities and disfigurement if not treated early. In very advanced states, loss of sensation leads to multiple injuries and eventually reabsorption of the affected digits occurs over time leading to apparent loss of fingers and toes. Blindness and corneal ulcers may occur if facial nerve gets involved. Saddle nose deformity and loss of eyebrows may also occur. Multidrug therapy (consisting of rifampicin, dapsone, and clofazimine) is the treatment of choice.

Leishmaniasis

Leishmaniasis is a vector-borne protozoal disease which is caused by bite of sandflies. Most of visceral leishmaniasis is found in Brazil, Ethiopia, Bangladesh, India, and South Sudan. Cutaneous leishmaniasis is mainly found in Brazil, Algeria, Afghanistan, Pakistan, Iran, Colombo, Peru, Syria, and Saudi Arabia. Cutaneous leishmaniasis is the most common form in which skin sores are formed within few weeks of sandfly bite. The sores may begin with nodules or papules and may end up with skin ulcers covered with crust or scab. Visceral leishmaniasis can be life-threatening as it affects different internal organs (liver, spleen, and bone marrow). Affected patients may have fever, weight loss, hepatosplenomegaly, and low blood counts. Mucosal leishmaniasis is the least common variant. Diagnosis is done by clinical signs, parasitological, and serologic tests. Liposomal amphotericin B and miltefosine are used in the treatment of leishmaniasis.

Onchocerciasis (also known as "River Blindness")

Onchocerciasis is a vector-borne disease which is caused by infected filarial worms. It is predominantly seen in the rural areas of Sub-Saharan Africa. It may cause skin rashes, skin depigmentation,[6] intense itching, and blindness. Ivermectin is the drug of choice. Prevention can be done only by preventive dosing with ivermectin or by insecticide spraying.

Lymphatic Filariasis (also known as Elephantiasis)

Lymphatic filariasis is a vector-borne disease which is caused by nematodes and gets transmitted by mosquitoes. Though most individuals are asymptomatic, some may develop genital disease (swelling of scrotum and hydrocele), lymphedema of the limbs, and renal damage. It can also lead to tropical pulmonary eosinophilia syndrome. Diagnosis of active infection is done by detection of microfilariae in blood smear. Diethylcarbamazine (DEC) is the drug of choice.

Schistosomiasis

Schistosomiasis is caused by few species of trematodes (flukes) belonging to the genus *Schistosoma* (mainly *Schistosoma haematobium*, *Schistosoma mansoni*, and *Schistosoma japonicum*). Infection occurs when skin comes in direct contact with contaminated freshwater. A person may develop rash or itching within few days of infection. Fever, cough, chills, and muscle aches may develop within 1–2 months of infection. Chronic schistosomiasis may present with abdominal pain, hepatomegaly, blood in the urine or stool, and difficulty in urination. Chronic infection can also lead to enhanced risk of bladder carcinoma or liver fibrosis. Microscopic examination of urine or stool samples for parasitic eggs clinch to the diagnosis. Praziquantel is the drug of choice for both intestinal and urinary schistosomiasis.

Rabies

Rabies is caused by *Lyssavirus* and gets transmitted mainly by direct contact of wounded skin or mucous membranes with saliva from an infected animal. Initial symptoms may include fever, weakness, headache, discomfort, or itchiness over bite site. As the disease progresses, person may develop confusion, anxiety, cerebral dysfunction, delirium, hallucinations, abnormal behavior, insomnia, and hydrophobia. Treatment is mainly supportive.

Cysticercosis

Cysticercosis is a parasitic infection which is caused by the larval cysts of *Taenia solium*. Infection occurs by swallowing of eggs found in the feces of an infected person. Symptoms may include headache, seizures, meningitis, blindness, hydrocephalus, and dementia.[7] Cysts in the muscles can lead to lumps below the skin. Neurocysticercosis is often diagnosed by computed tomography (CT) or magnetic resonance imaging (MRI) of the brain. Blood tests are also often helpful in diagnosing an infection. Prevention is done through livestock confinement, strict meat inspection standards, health education, improved hygiene and sanitation, and treating human and pig carriers.

Echinococcosis

Echinococcosis is a parasitic disease which is caused by infection with tiny tapeworms belonging to the genus *Echinococcus*. Cystic echinococcosis may remain asymptomatic or may cause discomfort, nausea, vomiting, and pain. Alveolar echinococcosis (AE) is a fatal disease with high mortality rates and it may affect brain, lungs, and liver. Symptoms of AE include pain, discomfort, malaise, and weight loss but it can also lead to hepatic failure and death. Ultrasonography, CT scans and MRIs are often used to detect cysts. Once cysts are detected, confirmation of diagnosis is done by serologic tests. Modalities of treatment include PAIR (percutaneous aspiration, injection of chemicals, and reaspiration), chemotherapy, cyst puncture, and surgery.

Soil-transmitted Helminthiasis

Soil-transmitted helminthiasis refers to the intestinal worms which get transmitted to humans through contaminated soil. These include *Trichuris* (whipworm), *Ascaris* (roundworms), *Ancylostoma duodenale*, and *Necator americanus* (hookworms). Infection occurs on putting contaminated fingers or hands inside mouth or by consuming fruits and vegetables which are not properly washed, peeled, or cooked. Affected individuals may remain asymptomatic or may present with diarrhea, abdominal pain, rectal prolapse, blood loss, and cognitive and physical growth retardation. Albendazole or mebendazole is the treatment of choice. Prevention can be done through improved sanitation, hygienically prepared food, clean water, health education,[8] and periodic deworming.

Trachoma

Trachoma is an infectious disease which is caused by the bacterium *Chlamydia trachomatis*. Transmission occurs either by direct or indirect contact with an infected person's eyes or nose. Symptoms include internally scarred eyelids, conjunctivitis, swollen eyelids, pain, eye discharge, trichiasis, corneal ulceration, and eventually blindness. Azithromycin or topical tetracycline are commonly used in the management of trachoma. Surgery is often helpful in cases of trichiasis and lid contour abnormalities.

Scabies

Scabies is a skin infestation caused by the itch mite, *Sarcoptes scabiei*.[9] Severe pruritus, especially at night, is the most common and earliest symptom of scabies. A papular itchy rash and tiny burrows can be found over penis, armpit, between the fingers, elbow, wrist, waist, nipple, and buttocks. Intense itching leads to scratching which further leads to skin sores and additional secondary bacterial infection. Diagnosis is made based on the clinical appearance, distribution of rashes, presence of burrows, and identification of the mite or mite eggs. Drug of choice is permethrin.

Mycetoma and Deep Mycoses

Mycetoma is a chronic infection caused by either fungi (eumycetoma) or bacteria (actinomycetoma) found in water and soil. Symptoms consist of triad of painless, firm lump under the skin, grainy discharge, and multiple weeping sinuses. Biopsy of the infected area and culture (growing the fungi or bacteria in the laboratory) are helpful in the diagnosis of mycetoma. X-ray, ultrasonography, and MRI are often essential to see the extent of damage to the bones and muscles. Actinomycetoma is generally treated with antibiotics and eumycetoma with long-term antifungal medicine. Surgery or amputation may be needed in some cases.

■ EFFECTS FOR PATIENTS

The severe deformities caused by different NTDs (e.g., leprosy, filariasis, etc.) result in social stigma which leads to inability to work, denial of marriage, and disturbance of family life. Economic prospects may also get affected. Infected individuals are predisposed to poor mental health conditions. Such individuals are found to be cut off from different aspects of society via educational opportunities, civic rights, and employment. Prevalence of depression and post-traumatic stress disorder (PTSD) is found to be high among the snakebite survivors. The cost of treatment of some of the NTDs is very high which leads to financial ruins and deferral of treatment. Government also suffers in terms of lost worker productivity through shortened lifespan and increased morbidity.

■ SOCIAL AND ECONOMIC IMPACT OF NEGLECTED TROPICAL DISEASES

- The inability to perform traditional farming practices necessary for survival in rural areas.
- Inability to play any social and economic role within family and community.
- Cost of inappropriate management (e.g., traditional healers) which enhances cycle of poverty and poor health.
- Loss of opportunities of education leading to the creation of a generation of individuals with minimal education.

■ PREVENTION, TREATMENT, AND ERADICATION

Eradication and prevention are essential because of the stigma, blindness, disabilities, and disfigurement caused by NTDs.

Policy Initiatives

With the aim of eradication and prevention, campaigns are funded by WHO and other nongovernmental organizations (NGOs). Incentives are granted to companies to invest in new vaccines and drugs for tropical diseases.

Deworming Treatment

Deworming treatment improves nutrition as worm infestation causes malnutrition[10] in infected children. Sanitation and hygiene behaviors need to be improved as well to achieve health gains in the long term.

Integration of Treatment

Many prevalent diseases and NTDs share common vectors (e.g., mosquitos, black flies, sandflies, etc.) and hence medicinal as well as vector control efforts can be combined.

Integration with Wash Programs

Water, sanitation, and hygiene (WASH) interventions are important in preventing several NTDs (e.g., soil-transmitted helminthiasis). WASH and other public health programs must be integrated to accelerate eradication of NTDs. This plan aims to eliminate and control certain NTDs in specific geographical regions.

■ CONTROL OF NEGLECTED TROPICAL DISEASES

World Health Organization recommends five interventions to control and combat NTDs:
1. Innovative and intensified disease management (IDM)
2. Preventive chemotherapy and transmission control (PCT)
3. Vector ecology and management
4. Veterinary public health services
5. Safe WASH.

■ CONCLUSION

A high level of commitment is required from endemic countries, charities, and NGOs. To enhance compliance and to improve geographic and therapeutic coverage, strengthening of capacity from center to the communities needs to be prioritized.

> **TAKE HOME MESSAGE**
> - Government should adopt new policies and launch awareness programs among the population.
> - Cross-border collaboration is very essential in achieving control and eradication of NTDs.
> - Control of NTDs is very essential as it is considered an economic burden for a country and causes social and mental agony to an individual.
> - NTDs should be diagnosed and treated early as several NTDs cause deformities and disabilities.

REFERENCES

1. Hotez PJ, Aksoy S, Brindley PJ, Kamhawi S. What constitutes a neglected tropical disease? PLOS Negl Trop Dis. 2020;14(1):e0008001.
2. World Health Organization. "Buruli Ulcer". [online] Available from https://www.who.int/news-room/fact-sheets/detail/buruli-ulcer-(mycobacterium-ulcerans-infection). [Last accessed July 2022].
3. World Health Organization. "Dracunculiasis". [online] Available from https://www.who.int/news-room/fact-sheets/detail/dracunculiasis-(guinea-worm-disease). [Last accessed July 2022].
4. World Health Organization. "World Health Day 2014: small bite, big threat". [online] Available from https://www.who.int/westernpacific/news/item/04-04-2014-world-health-day-2014-small-bite-big-threat-. [Last accessed July 2022].
5. World Health Organization. "Leprosy". [online] Available from https://www.who.int/news-room/fact-sheets/detail/leprosy#:~:text=Key%20facts,20%20years%20or%20even%20more. [Last accessed July 2022].
6. World Health Organization. "Onchocerciasis". [online] Available from https://www.who.int/news-room/fact-sheets/detail/onchocerciasis#:~:text=Onchocerciasis%2C%20commonly%20known%20as%20%E2%80%9Criver,the%20parasitic%20worm%20Onchocerca%20volvulus.&text=Symptoms%20include%20severe%20itching%2C%20disfiguring,live%20in%2031%20African%20countries. [Last accessed July 2022].
7. World Health Organization. "Signs, symptoms and treatment of taeniasis/cysticercosis". [online] Available from https://www.who.int/news-room/fact-sheets/detail/taeniasis-cysticercosis#:~:text=Abdominal%20pain%2C%20nausea%2C%20diarrhoea%20or,may%20live%20for%20several%20years. [Last accessed July 2022].
8. World Health Organization. "Soil-transmitted helminth infections". [online] Available from https://www.who.int/news-room/fact-sheets/detail/soil-transmitted-helminth-infections. [Last accessed July 2022].
9. Centers for Disease Control and Prevention. "Epidemiology & Risk Factors".
10. Taylor-Robinson DC, Maayan N, Donegan S, Chaplin M, Garner P. Public health deworming programmes for soil-transmitted helminths in children living in endemic areas. Cochrane Database Syst Rev. 2019;9(11):CD000371.

Chapter 26

Health Policies and Economic Impact of Fever on Indian Society

Saswati Chaudhuri, Biswajit Mandal, Swati Pal

■ INTRODUCTION

Epidemiology is a branch of study that traditionally comprises of technical study of incidence, distribution, and both short and long run health effects of a disease. It also has something to do with economics as a subject. The main intersection between economics and epidemiology is the changing behavior of people, whose optimization techniques and reactions are primarily dealt with in economics, in response to the possibility of various illness or diseases. When the diseases are highly contagious such as common cold, human immunodeficiency virus (HIV), and influenza, these create a bunch of economic externalities which one must take into account while framing sustainable economic and health policy. So, calculating excess burden of disease is an important task to be accomplished by the policy makers. In this context, most researchers use the popular and easily tractable SIR (Susceptible, Infected, and Recovered) model to trace how an infectious disease evolves over time. It also predicts the time when the population is most vulnerable, and shows the reciprocal relationship between prevalence of the disease and self-protection through vaccination, etc. The set of transition equations and the steady-state solution to this SIR model shows that the size of the susceptible population is inversely related with infectivity parameter and directly related with recovery rate. Eventually it explains why a policy of vaccine subsidy is effective in reducing the number of infected people in the steady state.

Recent global outbreak of COVID-19-related illness is a classic example of how an infectious disease, causing fever, and other illness can jeopardize the system in its entirety. It started in 2019 in China, and the whole world is still struggling to cope with the massive devastating effects of such virus. India is no exception. Our country is still under the Omicron-fueled fourth wave of COVID-19.

Unlike the coronavirus (COVID-19), which originated at Wuhan city of China in early December 2019, the Omicron variant was first reported in South Africa's Gauteng province on November 24, 2021. This variant boasts of a high transmissibility rate and within 2 weeks, the COVID-19 case counts in

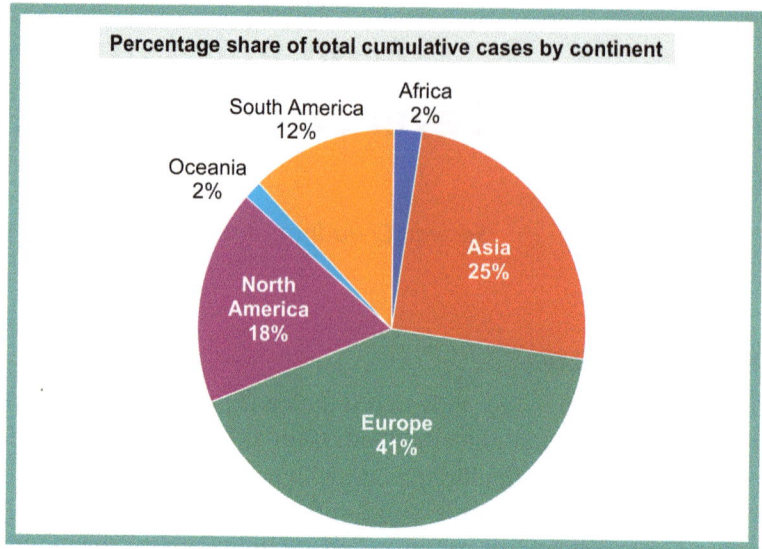

Fig. 1: Spread and incidence of coronavirus across the globe.
Source: WHO database and authors' own calculation.

the country had surpassed all previous records, with the variant spreading to 60 countries. This characteristic of a much higher transmissibility is ominous it could mean a much higher caseload in a much shorter time than the second wave. There already exists inter-regional disparity in healthcare facilities and the fiery spread of the omicron variant would prove to be detrimental to the already dilapidated healthcare facilities in the districts.

The spread and incidence of coronavirus across the globe and across various countries in Asian subcontinent are shown in **Figures 1 and 2**.

■ ECONOMIC REPERCUSSIONS

Bloom et al.[1] reiterates that new and resurgent infectious diseases can have far-reaching economic repercussions. The relentless efforts of the medical fraternity throughout the world have gone a long way in abating the infectious diseases and its associated mortality, but nevertheless, they still pose a significant threat throughout the world. Old diseases such as plague have not yet been entirely eliminated from the face of the earth and here we are still resisting the newer ones like the HIV, and the onslaught of COVID with its ever-increasing mutant varieties such as Delta and Omicron. When we try to map out the risks entailed by these diseases on the economy, we tend to take into account not only the health risks but also the fear and panic that accompany them.

First, there is no doubt that the health system of the economy, both public and private, is severely compromised. A large outbreak can jeopardize the

CHAPTER 26: Health Policies and Economic Impact of Fever on Indian Society

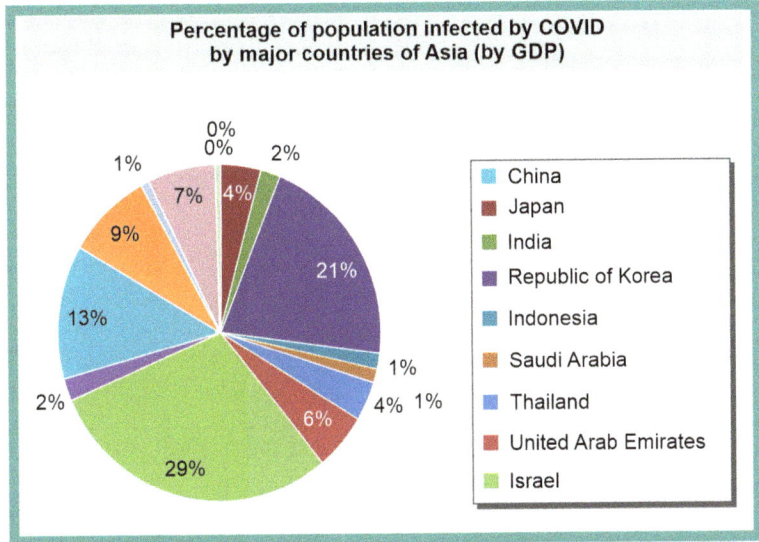

Fig. 2: Spread and incidence of coronavirus among the Asian countries.
Source: WHO database and authors' own calculation.

health system, routine health issues systematically suffers, and magnify the problem in the process. Epidemics also coerce both the one who has been infected and their caretakers to take leave from work or be less effective at their jobs, leading to lowering of productivity and even disrupting it at various times. The fear of infections like the one witnessed during the COVID pandemic had led to worldwide lockdowns, closure of schools, enterprises, commercial establishments, transportation, and public services—all of which disrupt economic and other socially valuable activity. Thus, the economic risks of epidemics cannot be trivialized on any account. Even when the health impact of an epidemic is not very large, its economic consequence can be a huge one as was seen with the recent Ebola outbreak in Liberia, which witnessed a decline of 8% points in gross domestic product (GDP) growth from 2013 to 2014. The world has witnessed a gradual decline in GDP as well during this period. This trend is shown in **Figure 3**.

Epidemics and outbreaks also result in disproportionate impacts on various sectors of the economy and cohorts of the population group.

The pharmaceutical companies as producers of vaccines, antibiotics, or other products crucial to combat the outbreak are potential beneficiaries. On the flip side, the life insurance companies are likely to be hit with enormous costs, at least in the short term. The livestock producers would also be on the losing side in the event of an outbreak linked to animals. The poor are likely to have less access to health care and lower savings to protect against financial catastrophe and hence suffer disproportionately. Such income inequality

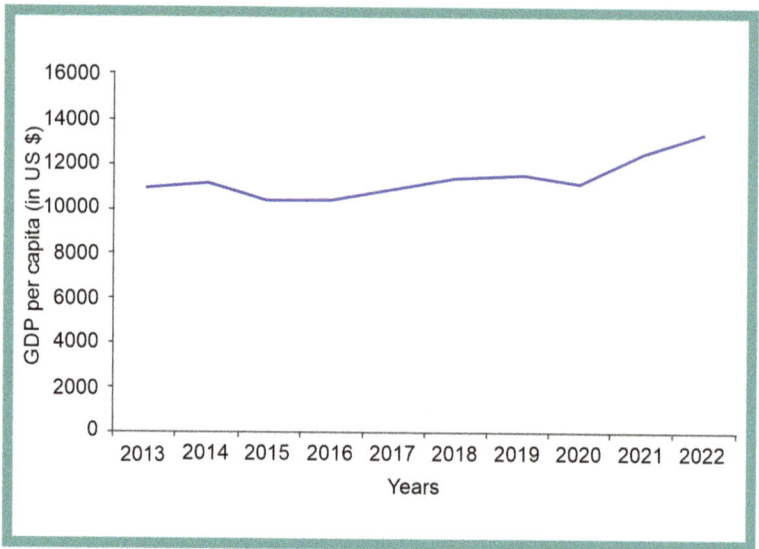

Fig. 3: Trend line of world gross domestic product (GDP) per capita (in US $).
Source: IMF.

and health inequality nexus become more distended during the outbreak of any infectious disease like what we have been experiencing for 3 years now.

■ COVID AND THE INDIAN ECONOMY

COVID-19 had been successful in magnifying the cracks in the socioeconomic fabric and the healthcare infrastructure of the Indian economy. An estimated 10 million migrant workers lost their livelihoods as the first wave of COVID hit the country in 2020. They had to return to their native places mainly the rural hinterlands of the country after the imposition of the lockdown. The existing vulnerabilities in the Indian economy were further brutally exposed in the second wave of COVID-19. As shops, eateries, factories, transport services, business establishments had to shut down, the lockdown had a disastrous impact on slowing down India's $2.9 trillion economy. The informal sectors of the economy have been worst hit by the global epidemic. Furthermore, rising inequality and a pull back by the household's strained budget have constrained the recovery phase. From growing only 4% in 2019–2020 to contracting 7–8% in 2020–2021 to staring at another low economic growth recovery in 2021 to staring at the face of stagflation, the Indian policymakers have their task cut out. Therefore, a judicious mix of fiscal and monetary policy must lend a generous helping hand to lead vulnerable businesses and households toward economic recovery.

As per the official data released by the ministry of statistics and program implementation, the Indian economy clocked an 8.4% uptick between July and September, 2021 compared with the same period last year. Besides, in

Indian context, the government went for *Atmanirbhar Bharat* in 2020 as an economic recovery mechanism to come out of the sluggish performance due to countrywide spread of coronavirus. The economic rationale and effectiveness of this program have been explained in great detail by Mandal and Chaudhuri.[2]

■ MOVEMENT OF PEOPLE AND THE SPREAD OF INFECTION

Migration is nothing but the survival instinct that goads human beings in search of better prospects or "greener pastures".[3] Global migration is thus a part of ongoing historical process. Since the middle of the 20th century, there has been unparalleled increase in the volume, speed, and geographical extent of travel and has been instrumental in characterizing migration.[4] The causes of migration generally owe their roots to certain economic, sociocultural, and environmental factors. Economic justifications largely concentrate on the search for better income and employment opportunities, the sociocultural explanations center on the migrants' desire to break the shackles of traditional constraints and inequalities, and also the lure of the cities while the environmental considerations border on shoving the migrants receive in their land of origin due to disaster and calamities.[5] Thus, undeniably people often move in search of a better life and job and sometimes to escape life full of uncertainty. Therefore, income inequality and lack of employment opportunities, along with political instability and conflict, can be reasons for people's movements away from their homes.[6]

Geographic movement of people produces varied kinds of health shock which can affect both the migrant and the host population. To put things in a proper perspective, it would not sound totally unconvincing if we say that population mobility has been the cause of epidemics throughout history.[7] We can justify this by saying that first, the condition which lead people to migrate is very similar to those conducive to the surfacing of new infections. Not only that, a collapse of systems to control infections that were previously researched well has also been noted. Economic failure resulting in poverty not only encourage the people to migrate but also leads to a caving in of public health infrastructure and hinders proper provisioning of adequate housing, sanitation, drinking water, etc. Second, the process of migration can also throw up not only socioeconomic challenges but also psychological and physical one.

If the displaced people are malnourished and live in over-crowded set-ups, they are more prone to fall sick. Third, migration brings people in contact with new microbes and vectors, as well as new gene pools and immunological make-ups all of which influence the risk of infections.

The low-income countries have given shelters to most of the world's displaced people (around 6.9 million), though most of them are temporary in nature.

In the overcrowded environment of theirs, person-to-person contact is generally amplified leading to devastating epidemic infections. A case to illustrate the above point is the death of 50,000 people in the refugee camps, who had fled to Zaire from Rwanda and died due to epidemics of cholera and dysentery.[8] Malaria epidemics in the refugee camps are well-documented for instance in the case of Afghanistan and Pakistan.[9]

■ EFFECT ON EMPLOYMENT

The Indian economy witnessed a downward spiral effect as the lockdown due to COVID increased inequality dramatically. People at the low end of income distribution experienced a near wipe-out of their income. The workers in the informal sector saw its *income* fall by a sizeable 40 to over 80%, not only during the lockdown but even in the later months as reported by Centre for Monitoring the Indian Economy (CMIE). Households responded to this precarious situation by disposing off their assets in lieu of cash or by borrowing. The latter resulted in debts ranging from two to six times of the earnings of the households. In fact, the COVID-19 Livelihoods Survey of vulnerable households, conducted by Azim Premji University,[10] found that the bottom 25% of the households had debt burdens nearly four times their monthly household income.

The vulnerable households need to be compensated for the loss of their earnings. This can be accomplished only by designing a comprehensive policy. The wage subsidies routed through the EPF (Employees Provident Fund) announced under Atmanirbhar Bharat Rozgar Yojana can presumably promote hiring of salaried workers and an appreciated move. A guarantee of alternative employment sources can provide the much needed support to the daily wage workers and self-employed. The program budget of MGNREGA or programs like this need to be expanded on a priority basis. This would help to meet the demand for employment as well as to extend the number of guaranteed days that people can expect to be employed. In urban areas as well, an employment guarantee scheme needs to be urgently devised and implemented. The urban employment regeneration program can play an important role in providing a bare minimum level of earning while also developing public infrastructure. Such initiatives would invariably have multiplier impacts by increasing demand at a local level.

■ HUMAN CAPITAL AND PRODUCTIVITY IN DAYS TO COME

Another undeniable economic setback would follow through the channel of quality of human capital. In this context, health becomes the most predominant factor. Following Becker,[11] Grossman[12] was among the very few to formally establish the connectedness among health and improvement in health as investment in human capital. Improvement in health not only enhances productivity immediately, it also adds to the stock of human capital and increases the rate of human capital formation for augmenting productivity in future. Productivity rises in both manual and psychological fronts. Hence the link between health, human capital, and economic growth is apparent. Acemoglu et al.,[13] Kalemi-Ozcan et al.,[14] Summers et al.,[15] Well,[16] etc., are some notable works to explore further the adage—healthier is wealthier.

But, unfortunately, accessible health infrastructure in various countries is showing signs of waning in their incessant warfare against the pandemic. In what follows, we observe a gradual deteriorating health condition of the society. This obviously calls for a significant amount of government money being justifiably siphoned off for treating corona patients and for protecting the others. Thus, the governments would be left with no choice but to cutback spending to finance other programs including health and human capital for future. So, it goes without saying that the niggling question coming to the fore is who is going to substitute human capital? What would happen to mental health, happiness, social capital, etc.? These are some worrying difficulties one has to get to grip with even if we pull through the current quandary.[2]

■ CONCLUSION

Policymakers have a whole range of tools at their disposal which can be deployed to minimize the likelihood of these epidemical outbreaks or at least to limit their spread or proliferation, minimizing the health impact such outbreak or the economic impact. Thus, improved sanitation, provisioning of clean drinking water, and better infrastructural facilities can reduce the interaction of the humans and the pathogens to a great degree. The need of the hour is a focus on building a strong health system with proper nutrition so that the body becomes equipped enough to fight infections.

Economic growth and development strengthens the basic systems and upgrades the economic infrastructure. However, policies to expand government expenditure in these areas even when budgets are constrained can help safeguard developing economies from major health crises. In turn, it would prevent these shocks to deliberately impede economic growth through the channel of adverse impact on human capital.

Trust among people and on the government also plays a very engaging role to ensure higher effectiveness of any socioeconomic policies. However, this very issue has not received much attention in the mainstream literature hitherto, whereas the role of social capital has been accepted as a major catalyst for development. Very recently Chaudhuri and Mandal[17] focused on such dimension of valuation of trust with the efficacy of social capital as a harbinger of desired pattern of economic development even during pandemic such as COVID-19.

It is impossible for us to predict which pathogen will prompt the subsequent epidemic, the place of origin of the epidemic, or how ominous the result will be. But as long as humans and infectious pathogens coexist, outbreaks and epidemics are certain to occur. Not only would they occur, they would also impose considerable costs. The positive aspect is that we can take hands-on measures to manage the risk of epidemics and moderate their impacts. Intensive and rigorous action at the local, national, and multinational levels can go a long way toward protecting our collective well-being in the future.

> **TAKE HOME MESSAGE**
> - Contagious disease usually creates economic externalities which policy makers must take into account while framing sustainable economic and health policy.
> - SIR (Susceptible, Infected, and Recovered) model helps predicting the time when the population is most vulnerable.
> - Epidemics coerce both the infected and their caretakers to be less effective at their jobs, leading to lowering of aggregate productivity.
> - Another undeniable economic setback would follow through the channel of formation of bad quality human capital for future.
> - We need to take proactive steps to minimize the risk of epidemics and alleviate their possible long run economics upshots.

REFERENCES

1. Bloom DE, Cadarette D, Sevilla J. Epidemics and economics. *Finan Dev.* 2018;55(2):64.
2. Mandal B, Chaudhuri S. Trade, protectionism, and self-reliance: a sense of déjà vu. AIC Commentary, No. 11. 2020.
3. Chaudhuri, S. In the midst of dire hopelessness: An analysis of poverty, social capital and migration behaviour of Kolkata's rural in-migrants. In: Internal Migration within South Asia. Singapore: Springer; 2022. pp. 183-204.
4. Colin J, Lee K. Globalisation and transborder health risk in the UK. Case studies in tobacco control and population mobility. London: The Nuffield Trust; 2003.
5. Sundari S. Migration as a livelihood strategy: a gender perspective. Economic and Political Weekly; 2005. pp. 2295-303. [online] Available from https://www.epw.in/journal/2005/22-23/review-labour-review-issues-specials/migration-livelihood-strategy.html. [Last accessed May 2022].
6. UNFPA. (2003). China–United Nations Population Fund Fifth Country Programme (2003–2005), Project document between the government of the People's Republic of China and the United Nations Population Fund on the project of reproductive health/family planning, CPR/03/P01, May. [online] Available from https://www.gov.uk/research-for-development-outputs/unfpa-china-reproductive-health-family-planning-project-cpr-03-p01-baseline-survey-key-findings. [Last accessed May 2022].
7. Wilson ME. Travel and the emergence of infectious diseases. Emerg Infect Dis. 1995;1(2):39.

8. Centers for Disease Control and Prevention (CDC). Cholera Outbreak among Rwandan Refugees—Democratic Republic of Congo. MMWR. 1998;47(19); 389-91.
9. Molyneux DH. Control of human parasitic diseases: context and overview. Adv Parasitol. 2006;61:1-45.
10. Azim Premji University. COVID-19 livelihoods survey: early findings from phone surveys. Bangalore: Azim Premji University; 2020.
11. Becker GS. Investment in human capital: A theoretical analysis. J Polit Econ. 1962;70(5 Part 2):9-49.
12. Grossman M. On the concept of health capital and the demand for health. J Polit Econ. 1972;80(2):223-55.
13. Acemoglu D, Johnson S. Disease and development: the effect of life expectancy on economic growth. J Polit Econ. 2007;115(6):925-85.
14. Kalemli-Ozcan S, Ryder HE, Weil DN. Mortality decline, human capital investment, and economic growth. J Dev Econ. 2000;62(1):1-23.
15. Summers LH, Pritchett L. Wealthier is healthier. J Human Resources. 1996;31(4): 841-68.
16. Well DN. Accounting for the effect of health on economic growth. Q J Econ. 2007;122(3):1265-306.
17. Chaudhuri S, Mandal B. A note on valuation of trust, social capital and development. Trade Dev Rev. 2020;13(1).

Index

Page numbers followed by *b* refer to box, *f* refer to figure, *fc* refer to flowchart, and *t* refer to table

A

Abscess
   bacterial 227
   epidural 25
   intracerebral 25
   spinal epidural 228
Acetaminophen 68, 183
Acidosis 56
Acinetobacter baumannii 9
Acquired immunodeficiency syndrome 133, 209, 226, 234, 236
Acrophobia 189
Actinomycetoma 241
Acute febrile encephalopathy 21
   causes of 188
Acute respiratory distress syndrome 21, 27, 31, 41, 55, 86, 87, 88*f*, 199-202, 204, 214
   Berlin criteria for diagnosis of 200*b*
   causes of 200
   complications of 203
   course of 201
   diagnosis of 203
   management of 203
Acute undifferentiated febrile illness 84, 149, 150*b*, 153*fc*
   pathogenesis of 148
Acute undifferentiated fever 20, 147
   classification of 148*f*
Acyclovir 195
Adenosine
   monophosphate 15
   triphosphate 14
Adenovirus 97, 98, 100
Adrenocorticotropic hormone test 223
Aedes
   aegypti 11, 35, 91, 94, 164, 188
   africanus 90
   albopictus 36, 91, 94, 237
African trypanosomiasis 238
Alanine aminotransferase 149, 186
Albendazole 126, 195

Albuminuria 85
Alkylphosphocholine 69
Allopurinol 210
Alpha coronaviruses 100
Alveolar echinococcosis 240
American Thoracic Society 217*fc*
American trypanosomiasis 10
Amikacin 9
Amodiaquine 60
Amoxicillin 9, 111
   plus clavulanic acid 9
Amphotericin 68, 140, 216
Ancylostoma
   braziliense 165
   duodenale 241
Anemia 66
   mild 109
   severe malarial 55, 56
Anicteric syndrome 83
Ansuvimab 178
Antibiotic 210
   lock therapy 219
   short course of 211
   therapy 110, 111*t*
Antibody dependent enhancement 36
Antifungal therapy 140
Antigen detection 86
Antileishmanial drugs 68
Antimicrobial 8, 226
   treatment 88
Antineutrophil cytoplasmic antibody 184
Antinuclear antibody 184
Antipyretics 18, 183
Antiretroviral therapy 143
Antirheumatic drug, disease-modifying 96
Antiviral drugs 47
Arboviral infection 21, 75
Arena virus 173
Arrhythmias 87
Artemether 60
Artemisinin-based combination therapy 234
Arterial blood gas 203

Arteritis 190
Artesunate 59
Arthralgia 38, 91
Ascaris 241
Aspartate
　aminotransferase 186
　transaminase 26
Aspergillus galactomannan 139
Assist control volume control mode 87
Athlete's foot 135
Atmanirbhar bharat 249
Atoltivimab 178
Autoimmune disorders 209
Ayurvedic drugs 156
Azithromycin 77, 80, 88, 110, 111, 185, 192, 204, 241
Aztreonam 10, 110, 111

B

Bacillus thuringiensis israelensis 48
Backache 38
Bacteremia
　primary 106
　secondary 106
Bacteria 19, 236
　anaerobic 167
Barotraumas 203
Bartonella 19
Basidiobolomycosis, gastrointestinal 135
Basidiobolus ranarum zygospore 140*f*
Biopsy 229
Blastomyces dermatitidis 137
Blood 56
　culture 29, 110, 184
　feeding insects 125
　pressure 56
　sucking arthropod 126
　transfusion 22, 44, 60, 215
Bloodstream infection, catheter-related 219, 220*fc*
Bone
　marrow cultures 29
　pain 38
Brain
　abscess 191
　computed tomography of 120, 121*f*
　magnetic resonance imaging of 29, 121*f*
Brainstem 189
　encephalitis 25
　evoked response audiometry 120
Bronchoalveolar lavage 102
Brown adipose tissue 14
Brucella 19
　melitensis 191
Brucellosis 4, 21-23, 191
Brugia
　malayi 125
　timori 125
Bruise, pulmonary 200
Burkholderia pseudomallei 190
Buruli ulcer 237

C

Cardiovascular system 83
Carrico index 199
Cefixime 111
Cefotaxime 88, 111
Cefpodoxime proxetil 111
Ceftriaxone 88, 111
Cell culture 75
Central motor conduction time 120
Central nervous system 16, 117, 188, 190
　dysfunction 188, 190, 193, 195
Central venous pressure 31
Cephalosporin 195, 216
　fourth-generation 10
　third-generation 10, 192
Cerebellar ataxia 25, 189
Cerebral
　hemorrhage 16
　malaria 53, 193
　　pathogenesis of 54*f*
Cerebrospinal fluid 29, 75, 84, 91, 117, 119, 153, 189
　study 119
Cerebrovascular accident 227
Chagas disease 10, 236
Chaka's disease 188
Chandipura virus 190
Chemoprophylaxis 179
Chest X-ray 88*f*
Chikungunya 19, 21, 23, 25, 75, 90, 94, 96, 171, 189, 233, 234, 235, 237
　fever 24, 91*t*, 94, 159
Chills 210
Chlamydia trachomatis 241
Chloramphenicol 77, 204
Cholecystitis, acalculous 41, 83, 216
Cholestasis 84
Chromoblastomycosis 131, 135, 136, 138, 142
Ciprofloxacin 111

Clindamycin 9
Clofazimine 239
Clostridium
    difficile 218, 219
        infection 218, 218t
    tetani 192
Coccidioidomycosis 171
Coma 25
Common cold 245
Complete blood count 109, 186
Computed tomography 120, 121f, 191f, 222, 228
Conduction 15
    abnormalities 41
Confusion 25
Conidiobolus coronatus 140f
Conjunctiva 173
Conjunctival suffusion 85
Conjunctivitis 91
Contagious disease 252
Convulsions 55, 56
Coronavirus 97, 98, 100
    incidence of 246f, 247f
    spread of 246f, 247f
Corticosteroid therapy, intravenous 89
Cough 201
COVID-19 84, 103, 180, 227, 245, 248, 250, 251
    pandemic 4, 232, 247
Coxsackie 164
Cranial nerve palsy 25, 191
Cranial neuropathy 23
C-reactive protein 17, 86, 216, 227
Crimean-congo hemorrhagic fever 173, 233
Cryotherapy 143
Cryptococcosis 171
Cryptosporidiosis 21
Culex
    pseudovishnui 115
    vishnui 115
Cyclic adenosine monophosphate 16
Cyclooxygenase inhibitors 18
Cystic fibrosis transmembrane conductance regulator 106
Cysticercosis 240
Cytokine 16
    storm 201
Cytomegalovirus 19, 170, 181, 184, 196, 209
Cytopenias 41, 199

D

Dapsone 239
Delirium 25
Dengue 19, 21, 23-25, 28, 35, 75, 84, 180, 182, 184, 185, 187, 188, 234, 235, 237
    diagnosis of 149
    fever 23, 35, 38, 39, 91t, 158, 164, 177, 185t, 233
        pathogenesis of 182fc
    hemorrhagic fever 84, 182
    infection 35, 41t
        pathophysiology of 37f
    severe 36
    shock syndrome 35
    syndrome, expanded 40, 41
    virus 35, 36, 149, 165, 182
        infection 37
Dermatophytic infections 135t
Dermatophytosis 138, 141
Dialysis, different forms of 87f
Diaphoresis 201
Diarrhea 238
Dihydroartemisinin 59, 60
Direct fluorescent antibody 102
Disability-adjusted life years 7
Disse space 181
Disseminated intravascular coagulation 60, 84, 182
Dizziness 238
Doxycycline 9, 74, 77, 80, 88, 129, 179, 191, 195
Dracunculiasis 21, 238
Drug
    fever 216
    hypersensitivity reactions 228
    induced hypersensitivity syndrome 161
Dyspnea 201

E

Ebola 19
    prevention of 179
    viral disease 177
Echinococcosis 240
Echovirus 164
Ecthyma gangrenosum 162
Edema, pulmonary 56
Electroencephalogram 120
Elephantiasis 239
Elevated creatine phosphokinase 204
Emerging infectious diseases 233, 233b, 234b, 235

Emergomyces africanus infection 134*f*
Emergomycosis 136, 139, 142
Empiric antimicrobials 226
Encephalitic syndrome, acute 21
Encephalitis 23, 25, 41, 95, 191, 192
Encephalomyelitis 192
    acute disseminated 118, 188
Encephalopathy 25, 31, 41
    syndrome 195
Endocarditis 227
Endocrine disorders 216
Enteric fever 21-25, 29, 84, 105, 106, 109*f*, 110, 111*t*, 192
Enterica serovar typhi 105
Entomophthoromycosis 135, 138
Enzyme-linked immunoassay 75, 76, 79, 85, 93
    tests 78
Eosinopenia 109
Eosinophilia 128
Epidermophyton 134
Epstein-Barr virus 171, 181, 184, 209
Eruption 24
Erythema 183*f*
    infectiosum 157
    nodosum 83, 163
Erythrocyte sedimentation rate 86, 119, 227
Ethambutol 190
Eumycetoma 131, 142, 241
Exanthem subitum 157
Extended spectrum beta-lactamase enzymes 9
Extracorporeal membrane oxygenation 203

F

Facial plaques 134
Faine's criteria, modified 85*t*
Falciparum malaria 21, 185
Fasciola hepatica 238
Fascioliasis 238
Fat embolism 200
Febrile
    encephalopathy, acute 21
    illness 119
        acute 84, 199
    nonhemolytic transfusion reaction 215
    syndromes 23*t*
Fecal microbiota transplant 218
Fever 14, 17, 20-22, 24-26, 26*fc*, 27, 30, 31, 85, 91, 107, 156,165*t*, 166*t*-168*t*, 180, 88, 195, 199, 207, 208, 209, 209*t*, 213, 240
    bacterial hemorrhagic 177, 178
    causes of 157*t*, 164, 180, 209*t*
    clinical features of 183*f*
    consequences of 17
    differential diagnosis of 166*t*, 171
    early postoperative 215
    etiology of 181*t*
    hemorrhagic 173, 174*t*, 177
    iatrogenic 216
    infectious causes of 213*b*
    malarial 148*fc*
    measurement of 214
    mild 238
    noninfectious causes of 214*t*
    nonmalarial 148*fc*
    parasitic hemorrhagic 177
    paratyphoid 105
    pathogenesis of 15*fc*
    pathophysiology of 14
    relapsing 23
    rheumatic 23
    rickettsial spotted 23
    scarlet 24
    spotted 75, 79
    trench 79
    tropical 1, 3, 19, 33, 195*t*
    viral hemorrhagic 163, 176
Fight infections 251
Filarial infection 129
Filariasis 21, 125, 188, 242
Filarioidea 125
Flagellar H antigen 105
Flavivirus 90, 182, 188, 237
Fosfomycin 10
Fulminant hepatic failure 41
Fungal infection 22, 131, 132*t*, 135, 138, 138*t*
    disseminated 24
    tropical 136
Fungus 19

G

Gamma-glutamyl transpeptidase 186
Gastrointestinal system 83
Gentamycin 9
German measles 23
Giant cell
    arteritis 226
    multinucleated 171
Glasgow coma score 56

Glomerulonephritis 41
Glycophosphatidylinositol 55
Gomori methenamine silver 137
Gonococcal infection 22
Granulomatous diseases 229
Guanosine triphosphatase 106
Guillain-Barré syndrome 25, 41, 83, 95, 118, 188, 189

H

Haemophilus influenza 168
Hand-foot-and-mouth disease 159
Hantavirus 84, 173, 177, 182, 184, 185
  infection 21, 233
Headache 25, 85, 107, 194, 240
Helminthiasis 125
Helminthic disease 25
Hemagglutination inhibition 119
Hematocrit, implication of 185t
Hematuria 183
Hemodialysis, intermittent 87
Hemoglobin 56, 109, 186
Hemoglobinuria 205
Hemolysis, elevated liver enzymes and low platelets syndrome 46, 83
Hemolytic uremic syndrome 41
Hemoptysis 201
Hemorrhage 84, 91
  conjunctival 40f
  intracerebral 25
  intracranial 41
  pulmonary 41, 176
Henoch-Schönlein purpura 25, 165
Hepatitis 41
  A 21, 84
  acute viral 149
  B 22, 171
    surface antigen 184
    virus 165, 170
  C 22, 171
    virus 165, 170
  granulomatous 229
  viral 21, 184
Hepatomegaly 41, 207
Hepatorenal syndrome 84, 180, 181t, 184
Hepatosplenomegaly 20, 107
High positive-end expiratory pressure 87
Histidine-based rapid test 29
Histoplasmosis 228
Hookworms 241
Horowitz index 199
Howell-Jolly bodies 210

Human immunodeficiency virus 3, 19, 57, 65, 66, 69, 75, 133, 136, 143, 153, 156, 163, 165, 166, 170, 196, 209, 234, 236, 245
  infection 66, 233
Human metapneumovirus 97-99
Hydrocele 239
Hydrocephalus 191f
Hydrophobia 189
Hypercarbia 199
Hyperintense fluid-attenuated inversion recovery 121f
Hyperparasitemia 56
Hyperthermia 17
  malignant 215
Hypoalbuminemia 65
Hypoglycemia 56, 59
Hypoxia 199

I

Icteric leptospirosis 83
Idiopathic thrombocytopenic purpura 41, 165
Immune fluorescence assay 80
Immunization 112
Immunochromatographic test 75, 76, 78
Immunofluorescent assay 75, 76, 79
Immunoglobulin
  A nephropathy 41
  E 184
  G 75, 78, 84, 110
  intravenous 122
  M 75, 78, 79, 91, 110, 119, 184
Indian tick typhus 79
Indirect fluorescent antibody 29, 75
Indirect immunoperoxidase test 75, 76
Infections 208
  bacterial 190
  phases of 39
  tropical 186t, 187t
Infectious diseases 209, 232
Influenza 19, 84, 98, 206, 245
  A 97
  B 97
  viruses 97
Ingestion 21
Intensive care unit 199, 213, 213b, 214t
Interferon-gamma 55, 65
Interleukin 15, 118f
Intracranial pressure 31, 119, 195
  raised 119
Intrauterine growth restriction 57

Intravenous fluids 183
   judicious use of 87
Invasive ventilation 87
Iridocyclitis 191
Isavuconazole 140
Isoniazid 190
Itchy rash 238
Ivermectin 126

J

Japanese encephalitis 21, 23, 25, 29, 115, 123, 190, 233
   pathogenesis of 118*f*
   transmission of 116*f*
   vectors of 116*f*
   virion, structure of 116*f*
   virus 23, 115
Jaundice 26, 30, 56, 85, 183*f*
Jock itch 135

K

Kala-azar 21, 64
Kawasaki disease 160
Keloid blastomycosis 136
Keloidal skin lesion 134
Kidney
   injury, acute 55, 86, 182, 205, 227
   replacement treatment 86
      continuous 87
      prolonged intermittent 87
Kyasanur forest disease 233

L

Lactate dehydrogenase-based rapid test 29
Larva migrans, cutaneous 22
Lassa fever 176
Legionella pneumophilia 153
Leishmania 19, 195
   chagasi 64
   donovani complex 64
   infantum 64
Leishmaniasis 64, 193, 239
   cutaneous 64
Leprosy 239, 242
Leptospira 19, 82, 83
   interrogans 204
Leptospirosis 21, 23, 25, 29, 75, 82, 83, 86, 88*f*, 149, 158, 171, 173, 181, 183, 184, 187, 204, 206, 235
   clinical features of 204

   pathogenesis of 84*f*c
   treatment 185*t*
Leukemia 25, 226
Leukocytosis 86
   polymorphonuclear 119
Leukopenia 66, 91
Linezolid 10
Lipopolysaccharide 15, 84
Liposaccharide O antigen 105
Liver
   biopsy 211
   failure, acute 26
   function test 86, 186
      abnormal 204
Lobomycosis 131, 136, 138, 142
Lockdowns 247
Loop-mediated isothermal amplification 67, 102
Lumbosacral plexopathy 188
Lumefantrine 60
Lung
   collapse 203
   injury 200
   protective ventilation 87, 203
Lyme disease 21, 23, 25, 171, 191
Lymphadenopathy 20, 27, 41, 207-209, 209*t*
   peripheral 208
Lymphatic filariasis 125, 239
   elimination of 126
Lymphatic vessels 127
Lymphoblasts 210
Lymphocytes, abnormal 210
Lymphoedema 129
Lymphohistiocytosis, hemophagocytic 41
Lyssavirus 240

M

Macular rash 24
Maculopapular rash 22, 24
Maftivimab 178
Magnetic resonance imaging 29, 57, 120, 121*f*, 194*f*
Major histocompatibility complex 38
Malaria 3, 21-23, 25, 26, 28, 28*f*, 52, 56*t*, 61, 75, 84, 183-185, 187, 205, 206, 234, 235
   diagnosis of 149
   drug treatment of 59*b*
   severe 53, 59, 61, 205
   treatment of 185*t*, 205
   uncomplicated 59, 185

Malarial parasite, life cycle of 53*f*
Mansonella
  ozzardi 125
  perstance 125
  streptocerca 125
Mean arterial pressure 203
Measles 19, 22, 24, 157
Mechanical ventilation 87
Mefloquine 60
Melioidosis 21-23, 25, 180, 190
Meningism 85, 189
Meningitis 25, 95, 190, 191, 195
  lymphocytic 191
Meningococcal diseases 75
Meningococcemia 84
Meningoencephalitis 23, 25
Mental status, altered 23
Meropenem 111
Metapneumovirus 97
Methicillin-resistant Staphylococcus aureus infection 3
Methotrexate 96
Metronidazole 9
Microglia hypertrophy 117
Microscopic agglutination test 85, 175
Middle east respiratory syndrome 100, 233, 234
Miliary neurocysticercosis 194*f*
Miltefosine 69
Monkeypox 21
Monocytosis 109
Mononeuritis multiplex 25
Mononeuropathy 41, 188
Mononuclear pleocytosis 192
Mononucleosis, infectious 157
Motor evoked potentials 120
Mucormycosis 22
Mucosal leishmaniasis 64
Mucous membrane 173
Multidrug-resistant tuberculosis 234, 235
Multiorgan dysfunction 21, 73, 180, 193
  syndrome 181, 202
Myalgia 38
Mycetoma 135, 136, 241
  diagnosis of 242
Mycobacterium
  fortuitum 22
  leprae 239
  marinum 22
  tuberculosis 8, 184
Mycoplasma pneumoniae 153
Mycosis 141
  tropical 140

Myelitis 25, 191
  transverse 25, 41, 118
Myelopathy 25
Myocarditis 41, 68, 83
Myoclonus 25

N

Nakayama vaccine 122
Nausea 68, 238
Necator americanus 241
Neck rigidity 25
Neglected tropical diseases 10, 10*b*, 236, 237*b*, 242
  control of 243
Neisseria meningitides 168
Nephritis 181
Nerve injury, immune-mediated 188
Neurocysticercosis 25, 188, 194
Neuropathy 25
  peripheral 23
Neutrophils 201
  count, absolute 213
  polymorphonuclear 202
Night sweats 210
Nipah virus 19, 23, 25
  encephalitis 189
Nitrofurantoin 9
Nitrogen retention 85
N-methyl-D-aspartate 118
Nodular lesion 24
Nonsteroidal anti-inflammatory drugs 43, 93
Nosocomial infections 216
Nuclear medicine testing 228
Nucleic acid
  amplification tests 57, 102
  sequence-based amplification 102

O

Odesivimab 178
Onchocerca volvulus 7, 125, 165
Onchocerciasis 239
Onychomycosis 135
Opsoclonus myoclonus 25
Optical immunoassay 102
Organ systems 214*t*
Orientia tsutsugamushi 71, 177, 182, 192, 204
  isolation 75
  transmission of 72*f*
Orthomyxoviridae 97

P

Pain
  bone 38
  chest 201
  muscle 85
Pancreatitis 41, 83
Pancytopenia 66
Paracoccidioides brasiliensis 140
Paracoccidioidomycosis 131, 138, 143
Parainfluenza 97, 98, 99
  virus 97, 99
Paramyxoviridae 97, 189
Parasite 210
  detection 67
  specific lactate dehydrogenase 29
Parasitic disease 24
Parechoviruses 97
Paromomycin 69
Parotitis, acute 41
Penicillin 88, 216
Penicilliosis 136
Pericarditis 41
Peripheral blood 229
  smear 42, 75
Phaeohyphomycosis 131
Phenytoin 210, 216
Photodynamic therapy 143
Picornaviruses 97
Piperaquine 60
Pityriasis versicolor 134, 141
  superficial infection of 131
Plague 21
Plasma glucose 56
Plasmapheresis 89
Plasmodium
  falciparum 7, 28, 52, 57, 149, 177, 193
    malaria 59
      parasitemia 56
  knowlesi 52
  malariae 22, 52
  ovale 8, 52
  vivax 8, 22, 52, 62, 177
    infection, diagnosis of 150
    malaria, chloroquine sensitive 59
Plateau pressure 87
Platelet 109
  transfusion 44t
Pneumonia
  bacterial 227
  hospital-acquired 217fc
Pneumonitis 41
Pneumothorax 203

Poecilia reticulata 48
Poliomyelitis 21
Polyarthralgia, post-chikungunya 96
Polyenes 140
Polymerase chain reaction 42, 67, 75, 76, 79, 102, 110, 119, 175, 184
Polymyxin B 10
Polyneuropathies 41
Polysaccharide capsule 105
Post-kala-azar dermal leishmaniasis 64, 66, 70
Praziquantel 195
Pregnancy 45
  acute fatty liver of 83
Procainamide 216
Prostaglandin E 15
Prostration 56
Protein, histidine-rich 205
Proteinuria 41
Protozoa 19
Protozoal disease 25
Pruritus 166t, 210
Pseudallescheria boydii 136
Pseudomonas aeruginosa 167
Psychiatric illness 23
Purpura 25
Pustular rash 24
Pyrazinamide 190
Pyrexia of unknown origin 210, 225, 229
  diagnosis of 226
  outcome of 230
Pyrogens 15

Q

Q fever 4, 21, 22, 79
Quinidine 216
Quinine 59

R

Rabies 189, 240
Radiation 15
Radiculopathy 25
Rapid
  antigen test 28
  detection tests 29
  diagnostic test 57, 67
Rash 20, 22, 24, 39f, 91, 156, 157t, 166t, 168t
  distribution of 22
  morphology of 165t, 169t
Rat bite fever 158
Red blood cell 52-54, 215

Renal cell carcinoma 226
Renal failure 27, 30
   acute 27, 41
Renal function tests 204
Renal replacement therapy
   continuous 31, 87
   prolonged intermittent 87
Renal tubular necrosis 84
Respiratory distress 31, 199
Respiratory syncytial virus 97, 98
Respiratory tract infections 97
   lower 97
Reticuloendothelial system 106
Reverse transcription polymerase chain reaction 50, 86, 91, 102
Rhabdomyolysis 83
Rheumatoid arthritis 225, 227
Rhinovirus 97, 98, 101
Ribonucleic acid 90
Rickettsia 19, 173, 192
Rickettsial
   diseases 71, 78, 79, 79*t*, 80
   organism 71
   pox 24, 79
Riedel's lobe 207
Rifampicin 77, 190, 191, 204, 239
Rigor 210
River blindness 126, 239
Rocky mountain spotted fever 23, 79
Rotavirus 19
Roundworms 241
Rubeola 22, 157

S

Saint Louise virus 173
Salmonella 19
   enterica 105
      serovar typhi 192
   hirschfeldii 105
   paratyphi 105
   schottmuelleri 105
   typhi 105
   virulence of 105
Sarcoidosis 228, 229
Sarcoptes scabiei 241
Scabies 241
Schistosoma 19, 240
   haematobium 108, 240
   japonicum 193, 240
   mansoni 165, 240
Schistosomiasis 22, 193, 240
Scrotum, swelling of 239

Scrub typhus 21, 23, 24, 29, 71, 74, 75*t*, 77, 77*t*, 79, 79*t*, 84, 158, 182–184, 187, 204, 206, 227, 235
   differential diagnosis of 75*t*
   diagnosis of 204
Seizure 25, 194
Sensorium, altered 25
Sepsis, bacterial 21
Serological tests 67, 102
Serum agglutination test 85
Severe acute respiratory syndrome 100, 233, 234
Sexually transmitted
   diseases 167
   infection 163
Shock 56, 91, 199
   compensated 56
   decompensated 56
Skin rash 183
Smallpox 24
Snakebite envenomation 237
Sodium stibogluconate 68
Soil-transmitted helminthiasis 241, 243
Splenic tumors 211
Sporotrichosis 131, 134, 138, 141
Squamous cell carcinoma 135
Staphylococcal scalded skin syndrome 161, 167
Staphylococcal toxic shock syndrome 160
Staphylococcus aureus 15
   infection 3
Stenotrophomonas maltophilia 167
Stevens-Johnson syndrome 166, 167
Still's disease 159
Streptococci viridians 167
Streptococcus pneumoniae 167
Stress disorder, post-traumatic 242
Stroke 25
   hemorrhagic 188
Strongyloidiasis 22
Sulfamethoxazole plus trimethoprim 9
Sulfasalazine 96
Surgical site infections 219
Syphilis 22, 159, 171
Systemic inflammatory response syndrome 202, 215
Systemic lupus erythematosus 166, 209
Systemic rheumatic diseases 225, 227

T

Tachycardia 201
Tachypnea 201

Taenia solium 194, 240
Talaromyces marneffei 137
Talaromycosis 136, 139, 142
Tetanus 192
Tetracycline 77
Thermotherapy 143
Thrombocytopenia 30, 86, 91, 173
    immune-mediated 93
Thromboembolism, pulmonary 203
Thrombophlebitis 68
Thrombotic thrombocytopenic purpura 25, 83
Tigecycline 10
Tinea
    capitis 134*f*, 135
    cruris 135
    incognito 135
    pedis 135
    unguium 135
Togaviridae 90, 237
Total leukocytic count 109
Toxemia, pre-eclamptic 46
Toxic epidermal necrolysis 165-167, 170
Toxic shock syndrome 167
Toxoplasmosis 21, 22, 171
Trachoma 241
Treponema pallidum pertenue 238
Trichuris 241
Tropical fever 1, 3, 19, 33, 195*t*
    drug discovery for 7
    etiology of 4, 19*t*
Tropical infection 186*t*, 187*t*
    treatment of 30
Tropical pulmonary eosinophilia syndrome 239
Trypanosoma 19
    brucei gambiense infection 238
    cruzi 8, 165, 236
Tsutsugamushi triangle 71, 72
Tubercular meningitis 190
Tuberculosis 19, 22, 23, 181, 190, 191*f*, 229
    drug-resistant 3
    pulmonary 227
Tularemia 21
Tumor necrosis factor 15, 16, 65, 118*f*, 148
Typhidot 29, 110
Typhoid 75
    fever 23, 158
        complications of 107
        vaccines 112, 113*t*
    toxin 105
Typhus 23, 71
    endemic 23, 79
    epidemic 79
    fever 79

U

Urinary tract infection 216
    catheter-associated 219, 221*fc*
Urticaria eruption 24
Uveitis, chronic 83

V

Vaccines 47, 61
Varicella 24, 161, 164
    zoster 19
Vascular cell adhesion molecule 53
Vasculitis 225
    systemic 25
    urticarial 162
Venovenous
    hemodialysis, continuous 87
    hemofiltration, accelerated 87
Ventilation, noninvasive 87
Ventilator-associated pneumonia 204, 216, 217, 217*fc*
    pathophysiology of 217*fc*
Vesiculobullous lesion 24
Viral capsid antigen 184
Virchow Robin spaces 117
Virus 19, 35, 188, 236
Visceral leishmaniasis 64, 69
    coinfection 66, 69
Vomiting 68, 238

W

Weakness 240
Weight loss 210
Weil's disease 204
Weil-Felix test 29
West Nile
    fever 23
    virus 23, 233
Whipworm 241
White blood cell 54, 175, 186, 218
Widal test 29, 110
Wolbachia bacteria 127, 129
Worms, parasitic 236
Wuchereria bancrofti 125

Y

Yaws 238
Yellow fever 21, 27, 177, 179
    virus 173

Z

Zika 90, 96, 180, 189
    fever 91*t*
    virus 23, 25, 90-93, 96, 233
        infection 90
        outbreaks of 92*f*

EU GSPR Authorised Reprsentative
Logos Europe, 9 rue Nicolas Poussin
1700, La Rochelle, France
Phone: +33 (0) 6 67 93 73 78
E-mail: contact@logoseurope.eu

www.ingramcontent.com/pod-product-compliance
Ingram Content Group UK Ltd.
Pitfield, Milton Keynes, MK11 3LW, UK
UKHW050428150426
5217IPUK00019B/1287